Creative CBT with Youth

Robert D. Friedberg • Erica V. Rozmid
Editors

Creative CBT with Youth

Clinical Applications Using Humor, Play,
Superheroes, and Improvisation

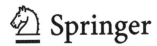 Springer

Editors
Robert D. Friedberg
Palo Alto University
Palo Alto, CA, USA

Erica V. Rozmid
Clarity CBT & DBT Center
Los Angeles, CA, USA

ISBN 978-3-030-99668-0   ISBN 978-3-030-99669-7   (eBook)
https://doi.org/10.1007/978-3-030-99669-7

This Springer imprint is published by the registered company Springer Nature Switzerland AG
The registered company address is: Gewerbestrasse 11, 6330 Cham, Switzerland

To my mom whose writing, perspicacity, and creativity never received the attention it deserved but who nurtured my efforts. You are the true superhero. (R. D. F.)
To all the children, adolescents, and families for whom I have treated and to those who I will work with in the future. (E. V. R.)

Acknowledgments

First and always, to my brilliant wife Barbara whose own writing career is a model and catalyst to my creativity. I really don't deserve you, but I treasure you anyway!! Second, huge kudos and gratitude to my fantastic co-author, Dr. Erica Rozmid, whose intelligence, clinical skillfulness, and creativity are unparalleled. Everyone should have a colleague like her! Loud shoutouts to the individual chapter authors whose outstanding work filled the pages of this volume. Thank you to the many patients who entrusted their care to me over the years. Finally, to the late Aaron T. Beck, M.D. who sadly passed away shortly before the publication of this book, I am forever indebted to you for your inspiration, wisdom, friendship, pioneering leadership, and encouragement to find my own CBT voice. (R. D. F.).

Dr. Robert D. Friedberg started out as my mentor and became a colleague; I am so incredibly honored to co-author this book with him! It is because of him that I am an evidence-based clinician, and I am eternally grateful for his clinical and academic expertise. To my husband, Ramsey, thank you for always being my number one fan and cheerleader. I especially appreciate how you committed to watching the *entire* Star Wars series with me after I realized I couldn't skillfully edit a chapter with my little Star Wars knowledge. I'd also like to acknowledge my parents, who live and breathe the concept of "one to many." I truly hope that this one book has the impact on many children around the world. 100 years on this Earth, but lifetimes of impact. Dr. Aaron T. Beck, this book would not have existed without you. Thank you for paving the way, tirelessly and effortfully creating and studying CBT throughout your life. Lastly, huge shoutouts to the wonderful expert authors of this book. Their creativity and expertise in CBT have inspired me to incorporate more fun and humor into my own clinical work. (E. V. R.).

Contents

Contributors

William M. Buerger Cognitive and Behavioral Consultants, LLP, White Plains, NY, USA

David Castro-Blanco Department of Counseling and Clinical Psychology, Medaille College, Buffalo, NY, USA

Mamatha Challa Department of Psychiatry, Harvard Medical School, Cambridge Health Alliance, New York, MA, USA

Rishi Chelminski Pace University, Dyson College of Arts and Sciences, New York, NY, USA

Debora J. Dartnell West Chester University, Morgantown, PA, USA

Ryan C. T. DeLapp Department of Psychiatry and Behavioral Sciences, Montefiore Medical Center/Albert Einstein College of Medicine, New York, NY, USA

Anxiety and Mood Program Child Outpatient Psychiatry Division, Bronx, NY, USA

Christy Duan Private Psychiatric Practice, New York, NY, USA

Mind Body Seven, Brooklyn, NY, USA

Eva L. Feindler Clinical Psychology Doctoral Program, Brookville, NY, USA

Robert D. Friedberg Palo Alto University, Palo Alto, CA, USA

Jennifer Herren Pediatric Anxiety Research Center, Bradley Hospital and Department of Psychiatry and Human Behavior, Warren Alpert Medical School of Brown University, East Providence, RI, USA

Anna Charlton Kidd Department of Psychology and Neuroscience, Baylor University, Waco, TX, USA

Rachel E. Kim Judge Baker Children's Center, Boston, MA, USA

Susan M. Knell Private Practice, Highland Heights, OH, USA

Kelsey Largen Stephen D. Hassenfeld Children's Center for Cancer and Blood Disorders, Department of Child and Adolescent Psychiatry, New York, NY, USA

Drea Letamendi Counseling and Psychological Services, Student and Campus Resilience, UCLA, Los Angeles, CA, USA

Becky H. Lois Department of Child and Adolescent Psychiatry, Hassenfeld Children's Hospital at NYU Langone, New York, NY, USA

Alec L. Miller Cognitive and Behavioral Consultants, LLP, White Plains, NY, USA

Gian Ramos Monserrate Universidad Central del Caribe School of Medicine, Bayamon, Puerto Rico

Diana Mujialli Worcester, MA, USA

Laura Nabors Health Promotion and Education Program, School of Human Services, University of Cincinnati, Cincinnati, OH, USA

Alayna L. Park Department of Psychology, University of Oregon, Eugene, OR, USA

Briana A. Paulo Department of Applied Psychology, Bouvé College of Health Sciences, Northeastern University, Boston, MA, USA

Sandra S. Pimentel Department of Psychiatry and Behavioral Sciences, Montefiore Medical Center/Albert Einstein College of Medicine, Bronx, NY, USA
Anxiety and Mood Program Child Outpatient Psychiatry Division, Bronx, NY, USA

Erica V. Rozmid Clarity CBT and DBT Center, Los Angeles, CA, USA

Christina G. Salley Department of Child and Adolescent Psychiatry, Hassenfeld Children's Hospital at NYU Langone, New York, NY, USA

Olutosin Sanyaolu Health Promotion and Education Program, School of Human Services, University of Cincinnati, Cincinnati, OH, USA

Elena Schiavone Florida International University, Miami, FL, USA

Alexandra Mercurio Schira Ridgewood, NY, USA

Elaine Shen Department of Psychiatry and Behavioral Sciences, Northwestern University Feinberg School of Medicine, Chicago, IL, USA

Hara Stephanou St. John's University, Jamaica, NY, USA

Thomas W. Treadwell Center for Cognitive Therapy, University of Pennsylvania and West Chester University, Philadelphia, PA, USA

Chapter 1
Incorporating Humor, Superheroes, and Improvisational Theatre Exercises into CBT with Youth: *"Just Because Something Works, It Doesn't Mean It Can't Be Improved"*

Erica V. Rozmid and Robert D. Friedberg

Keywords Cognitive behavioral therapy · Youth therapy · Play therapy · Superhero therapy · Cinemedicine · Evidence-based treatment

1.1 A CBT Origin Story

> How many times do I have to teach you: just because something works doesn't mean it can't be improved.
> **Shuri, Black Panther (2018)**

Once upon a time a long, long time ago in a place familiar to some, psychotherapy was ruled by two giants. Let's call them Psychoanalysis and Behavior Therapy. These two heavyweights dominated the scientific and clinical landscapes. But a new contender came along to join these kingpins. Hmm…Let's call this outsized dark horse candidate Cognitive Behavioral Therapy (CBT). CBT offered a new direction and therapeutic promise. However, this contender was dwarfed by the big shots. Now, CBT is the gold standard. Indeed, CBT's origin story is a compelling one.

Dozois et al. (2019) reported that CBT first popped onto the psychotherapy scene in the 1970s. Beck, Ellis, Kendall, Kazdin, and Meichenbaum among others were

E. V. Rozmid (✉)
Clarity CBT and DBT Center, Los Angeles, CA, USA
e-mail: erozmid@claritycbt.com

R. D. Friedberg
Palo Alto University, Palo Alto, CA, USA
e-mail: rfriedberg@paloaltou.edu

the first pioneers. However, scholars and clinicians trace CBT's roots back much farther (Benjamin et al., 2011; Pies, 1997). Pies (1997) noted that ancient philosophers such as Epictetus, Aurelius, Spinoza, and Maimonides form the historical foundations for the phenomenological approach which characterizes modern CBT. Benjamin et al. (2011) emphasized that operant and classical conditioning models shaped the development of the paradigm. Further, the emergence of information processing models and social learning theory with its focus on self-efficacy expectations were powerful influences. Thus, while CBT was somewhat of an upstart, the approach is deep-seated in philosophical, theoretical, and empirical traditions.

In order to earn its place in the psychotherapy universe, CBT needed to empirically demonstrate its effectiveness. Fortunately, over the years, CBT's outcome research portfolio is robust and far-reaching. CBT is effective for childhood anxiety obsessive-compulsive, trauma, and disruptive disorders as well as depression (Chorpita & Weisz, 2009; Davis et al., 2019). The approach appears widely acceptable to diverse problems, settings, and populations (Friedberg & Paternostro, 2019; Norris & Kendall, 2020).

However, despite the far-reaching appropriateness and robust clinical potential, not all youth respond to a traditional approach (Kendall & Peterman, 2015). When deciding to write a book for clinicians, we asked ourselves where the current gaps exist in typical treatments for youth. While cognitive and behavioral therapies are the gold standard treatment for many youth with psychiatric disorders, there are still children and adolescents who receive treatment and do not get better. Early dropout rates, missed sessions, and lack of individualized and engaging treatment account for the lack of symptom improvement. Unfortunately, dropout rates are extremely high, with approximately 33% of patients dropping out after one session and 28–75% of patients prematurely terminating psychotherapy (Olfson et al., 2009; Barrett et al., 2008) with ethnically minority youth having the highest dropout rates (de Haan et al., 2018).

While CBT is the most effective treatment for youth psychopathology, no treatment is perfect. In fact, nothing in life is perfect and we can always do better. Knowing which patient groups respond best to therapy allows the field to accurately assess the gaps and implement changes. Multiple studies found that initial symptom severity determined the strength of treatment gains (Kennedy et al. 2021; Wergeland et al., 2021; Kunas et al., 2021). Further, early to mid-treatment success predicted post-treatment gains (Kennedy et al. 2021). While these studies and meta-analyses revealed mixed findings (e.g., higher symptom severity either led to more or less improvements), it is clear that patient characteristics impact treatment trajectory. While those who enter treatment at higher levels of psychopathology have greater room to improve, Kennedy et al. (2021) suggested that moving to behavioral experiments and exposures more quickly may lead to higher therapeutic gains. Additionally, Kunas et al., 2021 found that parental symptomology significantly impacted anxious youth's treatment gains. Therefore, when parental psychopathology is present, parents should be referred for their own therapy as a means to improve their quality of life and their child's. Last, older youth improved the most over the course of treatment (Wergeland et al., 2021). One possible interpretation is that older youth have a higher cognitive load and can engage in treatment more similarly to adults; younger children are pre-operational and require more tangible and concrete teaching methods, such as metaphors and play. Overall, CBT is extremely effective in both laboratory studies and routine clinical care. Nevertheless, we have set out to improve the clinical care of youth.

We agree with Shuri, the Princess of Wakanda, that just because something works does not mean, it cannot be improved. Indeed, this is the precise reason we curated this book. CBT's robust theoretical foundations and strong empirical support create launching pads for innovations that augment its muscular procedures. Integrating humor, play, superheroes, and improvisational theatre techniques with CBT represents promising creative applications. In this introductory chapter, we highlight the chapters to follow and emphasize their compelling nature.

1.2   What you Will Discover in this Book?

Chapter 2 provides a humbling reminder that most of the youth who enter treatment only attend a couple of sessions—not nearly enough for adequate change. Castro-Blanco identifies barriers that clinicians face when attempting to engage youth in therapy and demonstrates methods to utilize humor as a vehicle for increasing therapeutic participation. As providers, we all know the trials and tribulations of attempting to captivate a child or adolescent in therapy. Showing our patients that therapy will help improve their quality of life is no easy task. This fundamental chapter reviews the basics of utilizing humor to increase engagement in the therapeutic process. Readers will greatly benefit from the proposed guidelines on using humor with their youth patients.

In dialectical behavior therapy, irreverence is the stylistic tool that most therapists struggle to achieve and strive to perfect. Well-intentioned therapists who use a confrontational tone or express ideas in an unconventional manner fear damaging the therapeutic relationship. Using humor with dysregulated teenagers proves risky at times. In Chap. 3, Buerger and Miller provide a crash course on DBT, case conceptualization of maladaptive behaviors, and recommendations on how to apply humor as a means of strengthening patient-therapist rapport and treatment effectiveness. The numerous clinical examples illustrate the dos and don'ts of irreverence and the specifics on when and why to implement a particular stylistic tool. Working clinicians will greatly benefit from the clearly outlined recommendations on utilizing humor with dysregulated teenagers.

Humor with Pediatric Patients (Chap. 4) illustrates how humor is an effective cognitive behavioral tool to ease the challenging therapeutic nature of pediatric care. In a hospital setting, humor acts as a normalizing mechanism for children seeking medical treatment, enabling laughter as a common bond for the clinician and patient relationship. Stephanou and colleagues claimed that clowns and art therapy are common vehicles of humor to assist youth confronting difficult medical procedures, such as blood draws and preparation for surgery. From relationship and rapport building, to coping and exposure to medical procedures, humor decreases negative emotions and unites the clinician and patient to a common message. Throughout this chapter, clinicians learn how to leverage humor at the individual level with a cultural lens to improve pediatric-focused patient care.

Cognitive Behavioral Play Therapy (CBPT; Chap. 5*)* instructs readers on the tenets of integrating puppets, stuffed animals, and toys with evidence-based practice. Clinical vignettes augment the expertise of Knell's novel treatment. For example, Knell recruited a stuffed animal bear to assist a five-year-old in mastering toilet training, a usually daunting experience for parents. CBPT is applicable for youth in developmental stages from different cultures and families. This chapter reviews the empirical evidence for CBPT and empowers all clinicians to benefit from Knell's expert guidance with a step-by-step plan on implementing CBPT.

Park and Kim (Chap. 6) propose cogent guidelines as clinicians consider how to prioritize evidence-based treatment with the integration of play and fun. This chapter reviews the appropriateness of when to use play, like in the beginning of treatment to assess youth's symptoms, or during parent coaching to improve the parent–child relationship. Clinicians learn how to adapt play based-CBT treatment in different settings, cultures, and delivery modes. They propose interventions that can be flexibly implemented and incorporate sample treatment plans, examples of play activities based on developmental level, and comics used to demonstrate psychoeducation. Park and Kim's comprehensive chapter leaves most clinicians yearning to be a child therapist!

Young children who unremittingly exhibit aggressive behaviors are at a higher risk for subsequent psychological sequela (Evans et al., 2019). Fortunately, play is an effective medium to teach youth about the roles of emotions and emotion regulation. Turtle Magic Intervention (TMI) developed by Feindler and Schira integrates the use of cognitive behavioral and play therapy within an individual or group setting for aggressive pre-school aged youth. Children learn about the engaging story of Timmy Turtle as they acquire skills about emotional identification, relaxation, positive self-talk, and problem-solving. In Chap. 7, Feindler and Schira provide a detailed account of TMI, a list of materials required to carry out the intervention, as well as the intervention manual. This chapter is an excellent resource for any clinician working with young children who desire a ready-to-use and accessible treatment manual.

Herren et al. describe a family-oriented approach to cognitive behavioral therapy for treating pediatric obsessive-compulsive disorder (Chap. 8). Herren and colleagues promote the use of play to enhance engagement and willingness which paves the way to exposure treatment. This chapter describes typical cognitive behavioral techniques such as psychoeducation, hierarchy building, and relapse prevention while simultaneously highlighting the unique use of art and play to enhance OCD treatment. Interventions such as the Fear Thermometer, Climbing the Fear Ladder, Creating a Sticky Note Ladder, and Video Game Levels are illustrated to equip clinicians with tangible treatment mechanisms. Tangible strategies and games assist clinicians as they collaboratively work with their youth patients and families to combat pediatric obsessive-compulsive disorder.

While traditional cognitive behavioral therapy approaches are not always relatable to children, Chap. 9 describes how to leverage superhero narratives and characters to improve clinical outcomes. The use of superheroes for youth allows for an accessible, creative, and playful approach to therapy. Clinicians grasp how the intersection of case conceptualization and superheroes drives a more engaged treatment plan. While children have their own personal stories that brought them to therapy, superheroes also have their own tales of highs, lows, and lessons learned. Youth learn their own form of superpowers, which we clinicians call skills, such as coping, problem-solving, and emotional recognition and expression. The work by Pimentel and DeLapp is suited for clinicians looking to put on their CBT cape, and harness new superpowers (or skills) to improve patient outcomes for youth.

In their riveting chapter on using superheroes as the medium to teach youth about conquering their fears with medical procedures, Nabors and Sanyaolu (Chap. 10) present an in-depth discussion on superhero play with a boy who experiences migraine headaches and stress. The authors depict the metaphoric nature of superheroes as youth with chronic illness tackle common medical challenges, overcome obstacles, and achieve success. Readers will discover that a child's struggles parallel the stories that superheroes encounter; superheroes embody the lessons and tools that children can leverage in their real lives. For example, children re-imagine themselves as superheroes- and their skills as superpowers. Alongside superheroes, play via puppets, stuffed animals, and LEGOs create a fun environment where children are amenable and excited about therapy. This chapter offers a broad approach that is easily adaptable for working with children who suffer from fatigue, chronic pain, and medical issues.

Letamendi (Chap. 11) ties together two seemingly disparate topics of Star Wars and Mindfulness in a cognitive behavioral approach to youth anxiety, stress, and mood disorders. The concept of The Force unifies Star Wars fans and practicing clinicians alike in a fun and relatable analogy tackling specific problem areas among children and adolescents. Mindfulness and CBT-based skills are designed to increase resilience and are powerful tools for recognizing and regulating emotions. Mindfulness training, like Jedi training, leads to improvements in self-awareness, expands outward awareness, and acts as a grounding mechanism. After re-watching a few Star Wars movies, readers will be well on their way to incorporate the gems of Star Wars in their therapy sessions.

Steven Universe, a Cartoon Network animated series, tells the story of a boy coming-of-age alongside diverse characters, relationship dynamics, LGBTQ+ representation, and mental health challenges. Steven Universe is an acclaimed series that connects children of all demographics by depicting life lessons, adversity, and success stories. In Chap. 12, clinicians learn to leverage the cartoon's use of gems, weapons, and objects to create illustrative examples of the challenges that young patients face daily. The cognitive behavioral triangle and various worksheets are adapted to the cartoon world of Steven Universe. The inclusive television series offers an approachable medium for clinicians to utilize in their therapy sessions.

In Chap. 13 by Treadwell and Dartnell, you are invited to experience a moment of surplus reality through Cognitive Behavioral Experiential Group Therapy (CBEGT). Through experiential therapy (also known as psychodrama), youth display their inner feelings, desires, struggles, and fantasies through dramatic re-enactments. In this group therapy context, youth learn how to express emotions and effectively problem-solve with the assistance of other group members as they act out of scenes from their lives. Psychodrama is an appealing and fun way for youth to participate in therapy. The group instructor, or clinician, guides the youth through traditional CBT skills with the integration of acting and experiencing activities. In addition to the clear outline of how to run a group therapy session from beginning to end and the detailed CBT worksheets, this chapter demonstrates the application of CBEGT through an intriguing clinical vignette.

Chapter 14 integrates popular culture and improv theatre into the CBT supervisory relationship. The most efficient way to teach the upcoming generation of clinicians is through supervision. How else can we expect providers to seamlessly integrate improvisational theatre, humor, and superheroes into CBT? Not to mention, the beginning stages of becoming a therapist are quite scary and daunting. Friedberg and Rozmid offer compelling vignettes, real-life examples, and exciting improv activities to propel a fun and low-risk learning environment. Recommendations and debriefing questions are provided to assist CBT supervisors as they reflect on the effectiveness of interventions. This chapter is designed for both aspiring and established supervisors.

1.3 Conclusion

As I look back over the past 65 years, my professional life has been filled with what I can best describe as a continual series of adventures. For the most part, the challenges that I've confronted were of my own making: Like Theseus in the labyrinth, whenever I seemed to find a solution to a problem, I was confronted with another problem (Beck, 2019, p. 16).

As you are probably aware, this is not your typical CBT textbook. Aaron T. Beck, MD, the superhero of CBT, epitomizes the notion of trying to continually improve without seeking perfection. In this way, he and Shuri are alike. Further, the current CBT maxim, balancing theoretical fidelity with flexibility, espoused by yet another CBT hero Phil Kendall and his colleagues (2008), is entirely consistent with the idea of extending a successful paradigm through innovations. Flexibility involves the creative application of empirically supported principles and practices to personalize treatment. However, according to Kendall and associates, flexibility is not a blank check to modify CBT in a haphazard manner. The creative applications must remain faithful to a cognitive behavioral case formulation, adhere to treatment goals, and maintain an action-oriented approach to treatment. Throughout this text, the individual chapters meet all these criteria.

We are humbled and honored to introduce the chapters that follow to you. They are filled with creative application of CBT augmented by real world clinical experiences. Readers will find worksheets, exercises, techniques, and resources that ideally will apply to your diverse settings. Enjoy the journey that lies ahead.

References

Barrett, M. S., Chua, W. J., Crits-Christoph, P., Gibbons, M. B., & Thompson, D. (2008). Early withdrawal from mental health treatment: Implications for psychotherapy practice. *Psychotherapy: Theory, Research, Practice, Training, 45*(2), 247.

Beck, A. T. (2019). A 60 year evolution of cognitive theory and therapy. *Perspectives on Psychological Science, 14*, 16–20.

Benjamin, C. L., Puleo, C. M., Settipani, C. A., Brodman, D. M., Edmunds, J. M., Cummings, C. M., & Kendall, P. C. (2011). History of cognitive-behavioral therapy in youth. *Child and Psychiatric Clinics of North America, 20*, 179–190.

Chorpita, B. F., & Weisz, J. R. (2009). *Modular approach to therapy for children with anxiety, depression, trauma or conduct problems (MATCH-ADTC).* Practicewise.

Davis, J. P., Palitz, S. A., Knepley, M. J., & Kendall, P. C. (2019). Cognitive-behavioral therapy in youth. In K. S. Dobson & D. J. A. Dozois (Eds.), *Handbook of cognitive behavioral therapies* (4th ed., pp. 349–382).

de Haan, A. M., Boon, A. E., de Jong, J. T., & Vermeiren, R. R. (2018). A review of mental health treatment dropout by ethnic minority youth. *Transcultural Psychiatry, 55*(1), 3–30.

Dozois, D. J. A., Dobson, K. S., & Rnic, K. (2019). Historical and philosophical bases of the cognitive behavioral therapies. In K. S. Dobson & D. J. A. Dozois (Eds.), *Handbook of cognitive-behavioral therapies* (4th ed., pp. 1–31).

Evans, S. C., Frazer, A. L., Blossom, J. B., & Fite, P. J. (2019). Forms and functions of aggression in early childhood. *Journal of Clinical Child & Adolescent Psychology, 48*(5), 790–798.

Friedberg, R. D., & Paternostro, J. P. (Eds.). (2019). *Handbook of cognitive behavioral therapy for pediatric medical conditions.* Springer.

Kendall, P. C., & Peterman, J. S. (2015). CBT for adolescents with anxiety: Mature yet still developing. *American Journal of Psychiatry, 172*(6), 519–530.

Kennedy, S. M., Halliday, E., & Ehrenreich-May, J. (2021). Trajectories of change and intermediate indicators of non-response to transdiagnostic treatment for children and adolescents. *Journal of Clinical Child & Adolescent Psychology, 50*, 904–918.

Kunas, S. L., Lautenbacher, L., Lueken, U., & Hilbert, K. (2021). Psychological predictors of cognitive-behavioral therapy outcomes for anxiety and depressive disorders in children and adolescents: A systematic review and meta-analysis. *Journal of Affective Disorders, 278*(1), 614–626.

Norris, L. A., & Kendall, P. C. (2020). A close look into coping cat: Strategies within an empirically supported treatment. *Journal of Cognitive Psychotherapy, 34*, 4–20.

Olfson, M., Mojtabai, R., Sampson, N. A., Hwang, I., Druss, B., Wang, P. S., … Kessler, R. C. (2009). Dropout from outpatient mental health care in the United States. *Psychiatric Services, 60*(7), 898–907.

Pies, R. W. (1997). Maimonides and the origins of cognitive behavioral therapy. *Journal of Cognitive Psychotherapy, 1*, 21–36.

Wergeland, G. J. H., Riise, E. N., & Öst, L. G. (2021). Cognitive behavior therapy for internalizing disorders in children and adolescents in routine clinical care: A systematic review and meta-analysis. *Clinical Psychology Review, 83*, 101918.

Chapter 2
Humor and Engagement with Children and Adolescents

David Castro-Blanco

Keywords Engagement Humor Working Alliance Breach Dropout · Attrition

2.1 Introduction

UFO's/The Loch Ness Monster. Yeti. Elvis sightings. Easily engaged children and adolescents in psychotherapy. What do these five things have in common? They're reported by hundreds and believed by thousands. The available evidence for each of them has been the subject of deep and extensive study. So far, the evidence (or lack of it) raises serious questions about how real they are.

While space aliens and cryptids have been a wellspring of "speculative reality" television, spurred countless books and articles and provided entertainment for many, the effective engagement of children and teens in mental health treatment is serious business. Globally, it is estimated that nearly 20% of adolescents are likely to experience at least one episode of serious mental illness with self-harm, constituting a serious risk for death in people ages 15–24 (UNICEF, 2020). Similar estimates of psychopathology prevalence are found in the United States (Weller et al., 2018).

At the time of this writing, the SARS-CoV2 (COVID) pandemic effected major changes in the everyday life of people worldwide. Not least of these changes are a general shift to telehealth delivery for many healthcare disciplines. Though years-old, the delivery of psychotherapy via telehealth gained prominence in the face of demands for safe, socially distant mental health services and moving traditional psychotherapy from face-to-face to remote delivery. Challenges to providers and therapy clients abounded as these alterations to the traditional service delivery model were adopted, and successfully engaging both new and existing clients in remotely delivered formats emerged as a vital aspect of treatment (Bachireddy et al., 2020; Dixon et al., 2016).

D. Castro-Blanco (✉)
Department of Counseling and Clinical Psychology, Medaille College, Buffalo, NY, USA
e-mail: David.R.Castro-Blanco@medaille.edu

R. D. Friedberg, E. V. Rozmid (eds.), *Creative CBT with Youth*,
https://doi.org/10.1007/978-3-030-99669-7_2

The imposition of restrictions on in vivo mental health treatment for children and adolescents has only served to exacerbate the challenges of successfully engaging this vulnerable population in therapy (van Dyk et al., 2020). This only heightens concerns about successfully engaging young people in mental health treatment.

2.1.1 With All Due Respect to Fritz Perls

Though the Empty Chair Technique enjoys classic status in psychotherapy, since being pioneered by Gestalt Therapy founder Fritz Perls, when children and teens present for treatment disguised as empty chairs, psychotherapy is a daunting task. No matter how creative, sophisticated, or potentially impactful an intervention might be, if the intended target is nowhere to be found, it is bound to fail.

2.1.2 Why this Matters

Young people with mental health problems face many challenges. Accurate identification of their psychopathology, availability of and access to adequate treatment resources, and recognition of factors and stressors contributing to risk and resilience all pose demands on the families of young people with mental health issues and their would-be providers. Many children and adolescents in need of mental health treatment are not able to access needed resources (UNICEF, 2020) or are at-risk for premature treatment dropout (Castro-Blanco et al., 2010), de Haan et al., 2013).

Psychopathology first emerging in youth has a major impact on adult interpersonal and emotional functioning. The antecedents of adult pathology are often found in earlier life experiences and challenges. This only heightens the importance of delivering effective, timely treatment to young clients. The child literally is the parent of the adult.

2.1.3 It's Not Vaccines, It's Vaccinations

A truism in pediatric medicine holds that immunizations for common childhood diseases are only effective when they are administered and received. Put more bluntly, no treatment is effective unless it is taken. Despite the apparent need for timely and efficacious treatment of psychological and behavioral problems in young people, and, despite their apparent availability, connecting these treatments with those in need has proven a major challenge.

While intervention for many children and teens might clearly be indicated, benefitting from such treatment is far from a certainty. Young people face a number of potential barriers to receiving adequate treatment. Some of these are circumstantial and reflect economic and insurance impediments, logistical challenges indicative of lack of physical proximity, available transport, and sufficiency of treatment resources. Other limitations, reflective of familial commitment to treatment, concerns about stigmatization, and incorporation of family members into therapy can also impede the availability and delivery of effective intervention.

As the rest of this book will demonstrate, there is no shortage of innovative interventions available for young people at-risk for mental health problems. The challenge is making sure these treatments reach their intended targets. It is not about vaccines, it's about vaccinations.

Engaging clients in treatment is a challenge for even the most talented clinicians. The professional literature is replete with studies and recommendations about engaging individuals in therapy. One of the key variables associated with successfully engaging clients in treatment is the Working Alliance (or Therapeutic Alliance). Introduced as a transtheoretical concept by Bordin in 1979, the alliance describes the mutually goal-directed and respectful relationship between the client and therapist in treatment. Put simply, three dimensions define the alliance relationship:

- Collaborative agreement between therapist and client about the _**Goals**_ of treatment.
- Collaborative agreement between therapist and client about the _**Tasks**_ of treatment.
- Respectful, interpersonal bond between therapist and client, emphasizing the best interests of the client.

Bordin's conceptualization of the alliance was intended to demonstrate that the important constant relationship between the client and therapist is in psychotherapy, transcending specific theoretical approaches and models. Research has supported the importance of the alliance, suggesting it to be the single greatest predictor of a positive treatment outcome (Norcross & Lambert, 2018).

2.2 The More Things Change

Most of the research looking into the nature and effects of the working alliance has taken place with adult patients. While a degree of coercion may mark the entry of some adults into treatment (e.g., relational stress, difficulties at the workplace, etc.), the decision to enter treatment is usually made by the client him or herself. This is far less often the case with young people. Faced with little choice, it ought to come as no surprise, that many young clients are reluctant to enter in treatment or engage in the therapy process. How much of a challenge is it to engage young people in treatment.

2.3   How Few Is Few?

Nearly three decades ago, DiGiuseppe et al. (1993) suggested that the modal number of sessions attended by children in psychotherapy was four. While estimates of the modal number (most often repeated) of sessions have varied in the intervening years, the overall picture is not an encouraging one.

Kazdin et al. (1997) suggested that the number of sessions attended by young patients tended to vary between four and nine, depending on parental commitment to treatment and the influence of potential financial and environmental barriers to engaging services. Spirito et al. (2011) reported that adolescents referred for outpatient psychotherapy subsequent to hospitalization for a suicide attempt attend an average of eight sessions.

A 40-year review of psychotherapy engagement research with child and adolescent clients reported that nearly 50% of young people referred for treatment received no psychotherapy at all (Becker et al., 2018). Hoyt et al. (2018) suggest that providers working with adolescent clients may have an average of a single session and point to the importance of effective engagement with young people.

2.4   What Do Birds of Paradise, Sea Horses, and Therapists Have In Common?

Given the scant number of sessions typically attended by young patients, what's a therapist to do? Many seem to take a page out of popular nature programs on television. Exotic species such as Birds of Paradise and sea horses are renowned for their elaborate courtship rituals. Displays of plumage, ritualized dances, and extensive efforts to attract and retain companions are common. Similarly, many therapists engage in actions every bit as exotic and elaborate, attempting to win over reluctant clients. They may become familiar with popular music, and gaming trends utilize social media and appear conversant in the latest popular slang in order to demonstrate their trustworthiness and appeal as someone to whom the young people can relate.

These efforts often demonstrate a misguided attempt to appear likeable and compatible with their young clients. While therapist likeability may, in fact, increase following such efforts, the result may well be a more likeable therapist confronting an empty chair when their hard sought client no longer attends treatment sessions.

2.5 Engagement

While establishing an effective working alliance between therapist and adult clients might seem a fairly straightforward endeavor, it is a complex and difficult process. Among the first priorities facing the therapist is framing issues to foster collaboration. Forging agreement about goal-setting and defining the tasks of therapy occurs in the context of a professional, client-focused relationship. This can result in significant challenges to both, the therapist and client. These challenges are further complicated when the clients do not choose to be in treatment. Effecting engagement with reluctant young people poses many concerns to therapists. Doing so takes considerable patience and clinical awareness. It also requires a sense of humor. Humor?

2.6 One Doesn't Have a Sense of Humor: It Has You (*Larry Gelbart*)

Humor is not necessarily thought of as a major component of psychotherapy training or practice. Many people succeed in becoming psychotherapists without being particularly funny or using humor directly in their work. Why would it be important in the engagement of child and adolescent clients? Demonstrating humor does not necessarily equate with being funny. It entails appreciating the unusual and sometimes even the absurdity of situations and responding to those situations in a way that is gentle and emphasizes appreciating their unusual aspects.

2.7 Like Beauty

Humor is often in the eye (or ear) of the beholder. What might seem funny isn't necessarily humorous, particularly where psychotherapy is concerned. Typical examples of funny situations include watching episodes of a favorite situation comedy, a stand-up comedy special or cartoons in which the characters mutually antagonize each other. All of these may appeal to some of us and seem funny. Not all of the themes would be appropriate to bring into therapy with adult clients. This is even more the case when our clients are children or teens. Why?

2.8   Humor Is the Affectionate Communication of Insight (*Leo Rosten*)

Using humor during the course of therapy can prove highly productive while also posing a considerable risk. Through humor, many clients experience a greater degree of engagement, which may be strengthened by the therapist's strategic use of humor, and the client's receptivity to it.

Humor often softens the edges of potentially uncomfortable situations and interactions. It also provides a supportive entrée to discussing unpleasant truths and emotions, allowing otherwise easily rejected or disputable points to be raised and discussed.

On the other hand, while humor can prove a helpful and useful tool in treatment, like so many tools, if misapplied, it can prove destructive and damaging. Using humor as an engagement tool requires sound judgment and delicate timing. It also requires something far more important and far less tangible.

2.9   It's the Ability to *Take* a Joke, Not Make a Joke, that Proves You Have a Sense of Humor (*Max Eastman*)

Using humor in treatment is based on a few, important assumptions on the therapist's part. The first is that the therapist frames events, situations, and concerns in a humorous manner. The second is that the intended recipient of the humor receives and recognizes the content as humorous. Finally, and perhaps most importantly, the therapist understands whether the timing and situation permit a humorous approach.

One way of gauging the appropriateness of humor and the readiness of the client to accept such an approach involves the use of self-deprecating humor by the therapist. Gently poking fun at oneself is a way of lightening the mood in session; however, this has to be done judiciously. This is especially the case when working with young people, as the therapist often represents an imposing adult figure and authority. Making a humorous observation about some aspect of the therapist is far different from positioning oneself to appear a buffoon and threaten the loss of credibility.

While mild self-deprecation sometimes lends a more humanizing tone to the therapist–client interaction, the working alliance is based on an ability to cooperatively develop goals and tasks of treatment in the context of the client-centered relationship. The therapist's motives for engaging in self-deprecating humor should be congruent with those of other interactions: To further treatment and advance the interests of the client. How can this play out when dealing with younger clients, though?

2.10   If this Is the Stuff Adults Have to Think About, I Never Want to Grow Up (*Stephen King*)

The principles of the alliance are the same for both adult and younger clients. An effective alliance is based on agreed-upon goals and tasks as well as a strong, respectful interpersonal bond. On paper, that sounds fine, but how do therapists working with (typically) reluctant clients engage them in treatment? This is where a more sophisticated view of both, humor and treatment engagement can be helpful/.

2.11   Everything Is Funny, As Long As It's Happening to Someone Else (*Will Rogers*)

Therapists seeking to enlist the participation of younger clients are liable to overdo their efforts to be humorous and engaging. This frequently results from overestimating one's own sense of humor, as well as disregarding the client's sense of humor.

If handled properly, mild self-deprecation is an effective tactic for use with younger people. With adolescent clients, pointing out confusion with the workings of social media, lack of familiarity with some aspects of popular culture or technical advances may allow the therapist to appear more approachable. More importantly, doing so may aid the therapist in appearing more authentic.

2.12   There's Something Very Authentic About a Sense of Humor. Anybody Can Pretend to Be Serious, But You Can't Pretend to Be Funny (*Billy Collins*)

Authenticity is, in many ways, a therapist's "secret weapon." Knowledge of psychopathology, therapy approaches, and diagnostic experience working with a variety of clients and complaints and technical prowess are all important. More important still is the therapist's conveyance of authenticity and genuineness. Adolescents are particularly sensitive to slights and what they perceive as inauthentic interactions and messages. Some of this sensitivity seems rooted in developmental limits, coupled with a heightened sense of idealism. Whatever the origins of their intolerance of disingenuous interactions, many teens are quick to dismiss as inauthentic, efforts to enlist their cooperation with reference to issues they perceive to be their exclusive province.

2.13   If It Bends, It's Funny. If It Breaks, It Isn't Funny
(*Lester, in Crimes and Misdemeanors*)

Engaging young patients with humor is challenging, but often worthwhile. The cautionary note here is ensuring, <u>both</u> therapist and client recognize and appreciate the humor involved. Similar to the sentiment expressed above is the following idea: If <u>everyone</u> laughs, it's a joke. If <u>not everyone</u> laughs, it's an insult.

Authentic humor involves finding areas of commonality and those of potential conflict. Humor is a means to addressing potentially uncomfortable, and therefore, often avoided topics. Taking risks and pushing limits are common in therapy. Ruptures to the working alliance are a frequent risk in every session, but there is a substantial body of research suggesting that repairs of these ruptures are not only possible but also can strengthen the overall therapeutic relationship and outcome.

Translating this point into more accessible terms, if the therapist can raise potentially uncomfortable or challenging topics and issues in a gentle, humorous manner, repairs to any alliance rupture may be swifter and more complete. Threading the needle between posing challenges and avoiding a tome or words that suggest mocking or ridicule can be a very delicate task. What are some practical ways of addressing these challenges?

2.14   Wish I Wasn't Here

One of the first keys to utilizing humor in the effort to engage young clients is recognizing that most children and adolescents do not self-refer for treatment. In plain words, most do not want to be there, and do not want to have anything to do with the therapist.

Treatment reluctance may be daunting and prove challenging to clinicians, but this very fact may make the use of humor even more appealing. Recognizing and acknowledging the likelihood that the young client would prefer not to be participating in treatment is both a demonstration of authentic and a possible entryway to a stronger alliance. The therapist using humor may face this challenge head-on and take advantage of the young person's reluctance.

2.15   The Problem with Having a Sense of Humor Is that Often, the People You Use It on Aren't in a Very Good Mood (*Lou Holtz*)

Many younger clients who are made to attend treatment (and often are described as being the problem) present with resentment and anger. They approach therapy with a mix of defiance and a determination not to cooperate or aid the therapist, who they may see as working with or for their parents. It might seem these angry and resentful children and teens are anything but open to humor, yet, this is not necessarily the case.

It is important to keep in mind that the therapist's primary task in working with young clients is their engagement in the treatment process. The most thoughtful and sophisticated interventions and treatment tactics will fall flat if the intended target is not receptive or engaged. The beginning of treatment is a critical point for the therapist to establish a sincere commitment to the young client, which can be facilitated through humor. The principal goal is not to cheer up the client, or make the young person laugh. Rather, establishing the therapist as a genuine ally, sincere in the promise of collaboration and cooperation is essential.

2.16 Sometimes a Smile Is Better than a Laugh

Using humor as an engagement tool does not mean "performing" during sessions. At least no more so than for any other clinical interaction. Appreciating and acknowledging the probable reluctance of the client often position the therapist in a more positive light as far as the adolescent client is concerned. The belief that therapy is a punishment for some perceived wrongs, or that the referral for treatment is designed to have the adolescent "shape up and get in line" predisposes the young person to be resistant to engaging with a process seen as coercive and unpleasant. How can humor help soften some of the edges associated with these views?

It is imperative that the therapist makes treatment participation minimally coercive. Recognizing the young client's power to frustrate parents or others in authority by being uncooperative provides the therapist with a potential advantage. Leveraging this ability serves to empower the young person and strengthen the alliance between therapist and the child/adolescent client.

Humor can be especially helpful here, as it permits the therapist to communicate the client's ability to exercise agency while not inadvertently guiding the client to become even more overtly resistant or adversarial.

2.17 How to Get that Smile

Therapists seeking to engage a reluctant or resistant youth in treatment need to tread carefully. Appearing to agree with the client that therapy is unjustified or is an unfair imposition can lead to a seemingly strong alliance between the therapist and client, but to what end? If the alliance is between the individuals rather than between both parties and the treatment process, not only will that alliance be short-lived, but it will also be counterproductive. The client can actually feel positively disposed toward the therapist and still be resistant to therapy and refuse to attend or participate in treatment sessions. Once again, therapy with an empty chair proves unsatisfying to all involved.

Can the therapist acknowledge the coercive nature of treatment referral and still refute the assertion that therapy is not indicated or warranted? Yes. Acknowledging the young client's reluctance to participate and resentment at being forced to attend sessions is not an endorsement of that reluctance. Rather, seizing the opportunity to point out that parental demands are unpleasant and frequently pejorative. Treatment offers the young person the prospect of easing parental disapproval, even if it is not the young person's idea to be there in the first place. Introducing as a goal of treatment, effecting changes in the interaction patterns between parents and clients is a powerful intervention. In other words, getting one's parents off their back is introduced as a central focus of treatment.

While this approach does not ensure cooperation, it can go a long way toward doing so. One of the major complaints made by young people referred to treatment is the belief that s/he is to blame for problems that either do not exist (at least in the estimation of the client) or are not the young person's fault. Recognizing that the primary goal of treatment does not have to be "fixing," the broken young person offers the alternative of therapy accomplishing worthwhile change. Once the therapist is established as a collaborator and ally, the young person is able to gauge the authenticity of the therapist, rather than pre-emptively rejecting treatment and dismissing the efforts of the clinician.

2.18   I Think the Next Best Thing to Solving a Problem Is Finding some Humor in It (*Frank Clark*)

It has frequently been said that children and adolescents are not motivated for change. Nothing could be further from the truth. Not only are they able to recognize the need for change, they are often highly motivated for change to occur. Unfortunately, this often involves the desire to have others change their behaviors rather than directly changing their own. This is both a boon and a source of difficulty to therapists seeking to secure the engagement of the young person in treatment.

Engagement in therapy is predicated on the belief that problems have solutions, and treatment is an avenue to problem-solving. The process of converting complaints into problems is sometimes a complex one. This is especially so for younger clients. Their ability to articulate perceived problems and provide a clear sense of their feelings make the therapist's job all the more challenging.

In order to convert complaints into problems, therapists effectively translate personal, subjective, and often vague statements (e.g., "I hate my parents," "I don't like school") into actionable targets for change. This might sound simple but coming up with the right problems is challenging. Humor offers a helpful adjunct to this important task, enhancing the young client's understanding when this translation is handled in a gentle, humorous way.

Seeing the potential humor in converting complaints into problems requires the therapist to avoid making statements suggesting the client's concerns are not being taken seriously. Qualifying statements, such as "It sounds as if…" "If I am hearing you correctly…" and "I think what you are telling me is…" can permit gentle probing about the nature of the complaint. Where is the humor in that?

Taking a somewhat playful approach allows the client to expand upon the complaint in their own words, while the therapist frames the issue more constructively. For instance, the complaint "I hate my parents" could be responded to with the observation that many young people believe this to be true and request the specific reasons why these parents are worthy of being hated. The greater the client's specificity in framing the nature of the complaint, the more effectively the therapist can convert the complaint and its circumstances into a treatable problem.

2.19 Converting Problems into Goals

After converting complaints into problems, the next step involves generating specific goals to address the problem. Problem-framing greatly influences the goals formulated and how these are articulated. For the reluctant adolescent client complaining about parental demands, are respect and compliance the appropriate goals to get the parents to change their demands, or to get them off the teen's back? While the client might prefer that her/his parents change, and that change to be absolute, it is far more likely and realizable to form a goal for the child to feel less criticized. Crafting such a goal requires the therapist to realistically point out the lower probability of the parents spontaneously desisting and focus on what can actually be attained.

2.20 Part of Something Usually Beats All of Nothing

One of the methods for engaging the young client in realistic goal-setting is pointing out the likely outcomes of differing scenarios. While absolute change on the part of the other may seem desirable, and a firmly stated preferred outcome, the probability that this will actually occur is extremely low. Borrowing from negotiation techniques, therapists can seek to enhance engagement by expanding on the potential range of outcomes. In other words, therapists can try to shape expectations less absolute and more pragmatic.

While adult clients might more readily grasp revising expectations and making goals more realizable, humor may aid achieving this task with younger clients. Pointing out the absurdity of extreme goal-setting can be accomplished by probing the young person to identify the perceived demands and expectations of their parent.

Identifying the unrealistic aspects of absolute thinking can then be brought to the discussion of the teen's own goals. Approaching this process with humor, rather than rancor can help advance both, the engagement of the young person in the process of treatment, and the specific definition and attainment of goals for the treatment.

Much like the candidate for class president in third grade, promising no homework and ice-cream for lunch every day in exchange for election, many young clients enter treatment with ideal desires as their expected outcomes. Asking the young person about how those promises of homework-free life, filled with ice-cream worked out can open the door to more realistic discussion of the potential for treatment to help decrease distress and effectively address problems.

2.21   Humor Is Laughing at What You Haven't Got when You Ought to Have It (*Langston Hughes*)

While part of something might be better than all or nothing, noting that fact may not be enough to convince a young client of the value of therapy. Pointing out the absurdity of external demands and desired outcomes may not mitigate beliefs about wanting change and dissatisfaction with the status-quo. Being able to discuss the challenges and potential difficulties posed by change can prove daunting to the therapist seeking to engage young, ambivalent clients. Acknowledging possible inequities and unsatisfied desires can help the client become more engaged in the treatment process. Pointing out some of the inconsistencies involved in the young person's life and how it is perceived can aid in gently offering a supportive, but goal-centered environment in which the client can better engage with the therapist.

Framing goals in terms of what the young person could gain, in ways that reinforce the contrast between the current and desired situation can also emphasize the ability to view these contrasts in humorous ways. This is not to suggest that what are perceived to be losses or deficits are funny or amusing, but that if, in fact, humor is the ability to laugh at what is not possessed, when it is felt it should be, the therapist can indeed facilitate this process.

Listing ways in which the young client is fortunate not to have what is desired is an example of pointing out the humor of a perceived deficit. This can lead to constructing a list of benefits provided by not having the desired outcome, increasing in absurdity and reinforcing not only the desirability of achieving a solution but discussing practical methods for doing so.

2.22   The Absolute Truth Is the Thing that Makes Most People Laugh (*Carl Reiner*)

Engaging young people in treatment requires the therapist to be clear-eyed about the potential goals and outcomes of therapy, and to be as authentic and transparent as possible in communicating these. Attempting to somehow soften or lessen the reality of the effort required and likely outcomes proves a disservice to the client and to the treatment process. An important reminder for therapists is the distinction between what constitutes humor and what is disrespectful or ridicule. Authenticity is predicated on truth and genuine efforts to communicate. This goal, in many ways, frames virtually all communication between therapists and clients as potentially humorous.

2.23   When Humor Works, It Works Because It's Clarifying What People Already Feel (*Tina Fey*)

Humor bridges difficult breaches in treatment and the alliance between therapists and clients. This does not suggest that therapists attempt to be funny, nor that the very serious situations and concerns expressed by clients are trivial or not concerning. The essence of humor is the ability to regard the truth and permit an opportunity for compassionate self-observation. Due to limits in development, experience or both, many young people are not optimally positioned to observe their circumstances with the distance and compassion necessary to recognize the disarming aspects of humor.

Therapists can play a pivotal role in the effort to engage child and adolescent clients in treatment. Given their tendency to resent being referred for therapy and typical reluctance to engage, young people are often at-risk for premature treatment dropout or receiving inadequate treatment dosage. Efforts to engage young clients can prove frustrating and misdirected, leading to a variety of tactics, designed to enlist the young person as an active treatment participant, but instead backfiring and contributing to high rates of attrition and the low number of treatment sessions attended by this vulnerable group.

Humor engages young people in treatment. It is essential that when employed, humor is not defined unilaterally by the therapist. Some simple do's and don'ts regarding humor may be helpful to remember.

2.24   Humor Do's and Don'ts

Humor can be a powerful tool in the effort to increase treatment engagement with young clients. It can also be a hazardous and damaging tactic that can increase the breaches in therapeutic alliance and make even more difficult efforts to engage young clients. Some core issues to consider in employing humor in treatment include:

- Remember humor and being funny are not necessarily the same.
- Children and adolescents tend to regard humor differently than do adults.
- If everyone laughs, it's a joke. If _not_ everyone laughs, it's an insult.
- Humor is based on truth and authenticity, not ridicule or disrespect.
- Humor is a gentler way to convey painful truths and challenging the status-quo.
- Humor helps engagement by aiding a unified way of looking at reality.
- Humor in treatment should _always_ emphasize the client's best interests.
- When used properly, self-deprecating humor by the therapist can aid treatment engagement.
- Humor can _assist in_ clarifying, destigmatizing, and legitimizing the goals and desires of young people in treatment.

2.25   Conclusion

Young people referred for treatment face many challenges. Literature accumulated over decades suggests that many children and adolescents referred for therapy, even consequent to major, high-risk events, such as suicidal behavior, are likely to attend only a handful of therapy sessions (Yan et al., 2014).

Barriers to treatment attendance have long been noted to further future difficulties for young people in therapy. Limited engagement in treatment adds to these already existing difficulties. While many approaches to enlist young clients in treatment have been developed and applied, the majority appear not to have significantly improved the engagement of this vulnerable population.

The use of humor as a vehicle for increasing engagement proves a useful and exciting tool in clinical work with young clients. Before leaping into efforts to employ humor in the engagement of young people, it is imperative that clinicians observe some basic truths regarding how children and teens attend to and appreciate humor and adhere to fundamental principles of authenticity, gentleness, and honesty in doing so.

References

Bachireddy, C., Chen, C., & Dar, M. (2020). Securing the safety net and protecting public health during a pandemic: Medicaid's response to COVID-19. *Journal of the American Medical Association, 323*, 2009–2010. https://doi.org/10.1001/jama.2020.4272

Becker, K. D., Boustani, M., Gellatly, R., & Chorpita, B. F. (2018). Forty years of engagement research in children's mental health services: Multidimensional measurement and practice elements. *Journal of Clinical Child and Adolescent Psychology, 47*, 1–23. https://doi.org/10.108 0/15374416.2017.1326121

Bordin, E. (1979). The generalizability of the psychoanalytic concept of the working alliance. *Psychotherapy: Theory, Research and Practice, 16*, 252–260. https://doi.org/10.1037/h0085885

Castro-Blanco, D., North, K., & Karver, M. (2010). Introduction: The problem of engaging high-risk adolescents in treatment. In D. Castro-Blanco & M. Karver (Eds.), *Elusive alliance: Treatment engagement strategies with high risk adolescents*. American Psychological Association. isbn: 13-978-1-4338-0811-1.

de Haan, A. M., Boon, A. E., DeJong, J. T. V. M., Hoeve, M., & Vermieren, R. R. J. M. (2013). A meta-health care. *Clinical Psychology Review, 33*, 698–711. https://doi.org/10.1016/jcpr.2013.04.005

DiGiuseppe, R., Leaf, R., & Linscott, J. (1993). The therapeutic relationship in rational-emotive therapy: Some preliminary data. *Journal of Rational-Emotive and Cognitive Therapy, 11*, 223–233. https://doi.org/10.1007/BF01089777

Dixon, L. B., Holoshitz, Y., & Nossell, I. (2016). Treatment engagement of individuals experiencing mental illness: Review and update. *World Psychiatry, 15*, 13–20. https://doi.org/10.1002/wps20306

Hoyt, M. F., Bobele, M., Silva, A., Young, J., & Talman, M. (2018). *Single-session therapy by walk-in or appointment: Administrative, clinical and supervisory aspects of one-at-a-time services*. Routledge. https://doi.org/10.4324/9781351112437

Kazdin, A. E., Holland, L., & Crowley, M. (1997). Family experience of barriers to treatment and premature termination from child therapy. *Journal of Consulting and Clinical Psychology, 65*, 453–463. https://doi.org/10.1037/0022-006X.65.3.453

Norcross, J. C., & Lambert, M. J. (2018). Psychotherapy relationships that work III. *Psychotherapy, 55*, 300–315. https://doi.org/10.1037/pst0000193

Spirito, A., Esposito-Smythers, C., Wolff, J., & Uhl, K. (2011). Cognitive-behavioral therapy for adolescent depression and suicidality. *Child and Adolescent Psychiatric Clinics of North America, 20*, 191–204. https://doi.org/10.1016/j.chc.2011.01.012

UNICEF. (2020). *Adolescent mental health matters: A landscape analysis of UNICEF's response and agenda for action*. Author.

van Dyk, I. S., Kroll, J. L., Martinez, R. G., & Emerson, N. D. (2020). COVID-19 tips: Building rapport with youth via telehealth. https://doi.org/10.13140/RG2.223293.10727.

Weller, B., Blanford, K. L., & Butler, A. M. (2018). Estimated prevalence of psychiatric co-morbidities in U.S. adolescents with depression by race/ethnicity 2011–2012. *Journal of Adolescent Health, 62*, 716–721. https://doi.org/10.1016/j.jadohealth2017.12.020

Yan, S., Fuller, A. K., Solomon, J., & Spirito, A. (2014). Follow-up treatment utilization by hospitalized suicidal adolescents. *Psychiatric Practice, 20*, 353–362. https://doi.org/10.1097/01.pra.0000454780.59859.9e

Chapter 3
Humor, Irreverent Communication, and DBT

William M. Buerger and Alec L. Miller

Keywords Irreverent communication · Humor in psychotherapy · DBT with suicidal · Multi-problem adolescents

3.1 Introduction to DBT, and the Strategy of Irreverent Communication

Dialectical Behavior Therapy (DBT) was created in 1993 by Marsha Linehan, who sought to address a gap in care for individuals living with chronic suicidality (Linehan, 1993). A trained behaviorist, Dr. Linehan had attempted to provide interventions focusing on behavioral change, only to find her clients protest that she was demanding too much and failing to acknowledge the severity of their difficulties. When Dr. Linehan changed her clinical approach to be more supportive in nature, she again received negative feedback from her clients, who wondered why she was not putting greater effort into helping them change the circumstances that were causing such pronounced suffering. Dr. Linehan sought to resolve this impasse by addressing both needs concurrently, prescribing behavioral interventions that would reduce her clients' suffering while also validating the difficulty of implementing these changes. This dialectical approach of allowing two ostensibly contradictory ideas to coexist permeates throughout DBT and provides the theoretical foundation upon which all DBT treatment plans are built. To help clients move more seamlessly through the treatment, making it an "easier pill to swallow," Linehan developed a balanced set of communication strategies: irreverent and reciprocal communication.

W. M. Buerger (✉) · A. L. Miller
Cognitive and Behavioral Consultants, LLP, White Plains, NY, USA
e-mail: wbuerger@cbc-psychology.com; amiller@cbc-psychology.com

R. D. Friedberg, E. V. Rozmid (eds.), *Creative CBT with Youth*,
https://doi.org/10.1007/978-3-030-99669-7_3

As will be described throughout this chapter, irreverence and humor are integral to the work we do with DBT clients and especially with teens.

3.1.1 What Is DBT?

DBT treatment focuses on using behavior chain analyses to clarify how the client's emotions, thoughts, urges, and behaviors interact to generate and maintain their difficulties. The clinician incorporates a range of change-oriented strategies, including DBT skills, to help clients more effectively navigate these difficulties and work towards their self-identified "life worth living goals." DBT skills are taught to the adolescent client and their caregivers in a multi-family group format, and fall into five modules:

1. Mindfulness Skills (increasing attentional control as well as non-judgmental awareness of internal experiences, thereby improving the client's ability to recognize maladaptive thoughts, feelings, urges, and implement more adaptive solutions).
2. Distress Tolerance Skills (skills for moments of pronounced distress, in order to allow the client to "survive the crisis without making it worse through impulsive action" (Rathus & Miller, 2015, p. 126)).
3. Emotion Regulation Skills (skills that allow the client to change one's emotional experience, e.g., increase positive emotions, reduce vulnerability to negative emotions).
4. Interpersonal Effectiveness Skills (helping the client establish and maintain healthy relationships, while also communicating their needs and maintaining their self-respect).
5. Walking the Middle Path Skills (using dialectical thought and communication to help clients and their parents/guardians understand and shape each other's perspectives, using validation of self and others to convey greater acceptance and understanding, and applying behavioral principles to effect change in self and others).

DBT is a principle-based treatment, meaning that while some components are necessary to the treatment (e.g., the client completing a weekly diary card monitoring their experiences and use of skills; a session agenda that addresses life-threatening and treatment-interfering behaviors before all other treatment targets), the clinician is encouraged to select interventions based on what is indicated by the guiding principles of dialectics and behaviorism. Clinicians strive to consistently adopt and convey the central dialectic of acceptance of the client's difficulties and efforts while at the same time encouraging positive changes to the client's behaviors, emotions, urges, and cognitions. This is achieved by deliberately striking a dialectical balance between empathically taking the client's agenda seriously (i.e., "reciprocal communication"), and interjecting comments that are intended to knock the client "off balance" and shift thoughts, emotions, or behaviors (i.e., "irreverent communication").

Both forms of communication can be achieved verbally and nonverbally. In reciprocal communication (e.g., nodding along with the client's story, making statements that affirm their thoughts and feelings), the clinician aims to validate the client's understanding of their experiences. The response is in-line with what the client expects and hopes to hear. On the other hand, irreverent communication (e.g., an exaggerated eye roll, expressing dissent in a way that is satirical and noncombative) challenges the client's understanding of their experiences. This intervention is often unexpected by the client, knocking them off a track that the clinician believes to be problematic.

While the use of humors falls within the category of irreverent communication, irreverent communication need not be humorous. This chapter will provide a set of guiding principles for how this broader category of irreverence can be used effectively, so that the reader will understand ways of making use of humor within this framework. In-line with DBT being a principle-based treatment, emphasis will be placed on "function over form" by describing the rationale for selecting certain irreverent strategies, rather than listing specific statements that qualify as "irreverent." Implementing a list of humorous or irreverent phrases whenever an opening presents itself is not enough. Clinicians must have a firm understanding of the function of each irreverent statement, and whether irreverence will act in service of their therapeutic goal in that moment. The authors' intention here is to provide guidance on how this might be achieved using theory and clinical anecdotes.

3.1.2 Humor as a Reciprocal Communication Strategy

Within this chapter's focus on irreverence, it is important to consider the utility of humor as a reciprocal strategy. While humor can be used to "grease the wheels" of change, it also serves an important affiliative function, strengthening the relationship between the clinician and the client. Empirical support for this function can be found across the lifespan, including in children and adolescents, for whom the use of humor has been shown to result in improved interpersonal relationships (Cameron et al., 2010; Erickson & Feldstein, 2007; Führ, 2002; Geiger et al., 2019). There has been much debate about the primacy of this relationship in the therapeutic process, and there is broad consensus that a strong therapeutic alliance is a predictor of positive treatment outcomes (Horvath et al., 2011; Martin et al., 2000). Although empirical evidence that humor contributes directly to this relationship is hard to come by, anecdotal support might be found by reflecting on the people in your life whom you feel connected to and go to for advice and support. How many of those people do you feel comfortable laughing with, and how many do you feel incapable of connecting with through humor? For the majority of individuals, the former category is more well populated than the latter.

Humor also offers a dialectical balance to the seriousness of the topics discussed in psychotherapy. Clients do not seek out psychotherapy to discuss their favorite TV shows or most recent successes, but instead their fears, doubts, regrets, and difficulties finding a "life worth living." (Linehan, 1993, p. 99). These conversations can feel austere, somber, or frantic, and benefit from being balanced by interactions that introduce a certain amount of levity and play. This emphasis on levity may be why research suggests that not all forms of humor are created equal. Specifically, humor whose focus is "benign" or "benevolent," meaning that it reflects positively on self or others, has been shown to improve mental health, while that which is critical of self or others often has the opposite effect (Kuiper et al., 2004; Martin et al., 2003). More specifically, "affiliative humor," which involves laughing with others in an effort to improve relationships, and "self-enhancing humor," which uses perspective-taking to improve emotion regulation and ability to cope with stressful events, are both associated with cheerfulness, high self-esteem, and psychological well-being, and negatively associated with anxiety and depression.

Although using humor to increase positive interactions and feelings of connectedness may come naturally to many, a more difficult maneuver is to use humor as a dialectical strategy to encourage change. Within DBT, this takes the form of irreverent communication, which are intended to cause the client to "jump the track," or "(1) to get the patient's attention, (2) to shift the patient's affective response, and (3) to get the patient to see a completely different point of view" (Linehan, 1993, p. 393).

This definition succinctly describes the purpose of irreverent communication but offers little instruction on how and when the technique should be implemented. Irreverent statements are not inherently effective and cannot be used in all clinical scenarios. This difficulty is further complicated by the fact that interactions that naturally pull for irreverence can often be characterized by feelings of frustration or irritation within the clinician. This potential pitfall was highlighted by Miller et al. (2007) who stated that "It is essential, however, never to use it in a mean-spirited way; the therapist must be mindful of his or her intentions and attitudes while using irreverence." (Miller et al., 2007, p. 68) For this reason, DBT emphasizes "function over form," focusing on the use of specific forms of irreverence in specific clinical scenarios, rather than on what words or phrases qualify as being "irreverent." As an example, a clinician could collect a list of irreverent statements (e.g., "Sounds like we're both going to need more therapy after this session."; "Well, that would be wildly ineffective."; "What a dreadful plan! Please don't."), but these phrases would be useless if they are not used at the right time, with the right client, for the right purpose. The pertinent question is not "what is irreverence?" but instead "when and how can irreverence be used effectively?" In order to answer this question, one must first understand how DBT conceptualizes mental health difficulties.

3.1.3   DBT Case Conceptualization

When looking to understand clinical complaints and how they can be addressed, DBT clinicians deemphasize diagnostic criteria in favor of problem areas, which correlate with the five aforementioned adolescent DBT skills modules. Specifically, clients are assessed for difficulties in the areas of:

1. Self-Dysregulation (e.g., confusion about self, sense of emptiness, lack of focus, low awareness, or other deficits in mindfulness skills)
2. Behavioral Dysregulation (e.g., impulsive behaviors, including non-suicidal self-injury and substance use, as well as extreme avoidance behaviors, or other deficits in distress tolerance skills)
3. Emotional Dysregulation (e.g., difficulty modulating distress, exacerbated by increased sensitivity to environmental cues, or other deficits in emotion regulation skills)
4. Interpersonal Dysregulation (e.g., interpersonal problems, chaotic relationships, ineffective help-seeking, loneliness, or other deficits in interpersonal effectiveness skills)
5. Cognitive and Familial Dysregulation (e.g., ineffective judgments of self or others, rigid or black-and-white thinking, or other deficits in walking the middle path skills)

Once these areas of dysregulation are identified, the ways that they interact with one another and with the environment are clarified and used to identify alternative, more effective approaches. As an example, when people have difficulty managing their anger (emotion dysregulation), they sometimes say things that they wish they could take back (interpersonal dysregulation), thereby creating discord within their family (familial dysregulation).

However, one of the primary barriers to this process is that the client often lacks awareness of these patterns of dysregulation, which have become the status quo and often serve a reinforcing (e.g., negative reinforcement) function (e.g., self-harm may be an effective way of reducing distressing emotions, albeit in the short term). Irreverent communication provides one means through which the clinician can highlight these problematic patterns for the client and redirect the conversation towards more effective ways of being. This is particularly useful when discussing self-harm behaviors with adolescents, who sometimes describe self-injury in a flippant or frivolous manner. Irreverence allows the clinician to block this problematic pattern, diverting the narrative by treating self-harm as a serious treatment target.

3.1.4   Use of Humor as an Effective Therapeutic
Change Strategy

In order to understand how to most effectively use irreverent communication and the related concept of humor, let us briefly review what differentiates humor from sarcasm or insult. While attempts to explain the nature of humor date back to Aristotle, the most modern and widely accepted guiding framework is known as "benign violation theory" (McGraw & Warren, 2010). Building off the work of linguist Tom Veatch, benign violation theory suggests that humor requires three conditions be met for a situation to be perceived as humorous; (1) the situation is appraised to be a "violation," or one in which norms and expectations are violated, (2) this violation is not experienced as threatening and hence is interpreted as "benign,", and (3) these two perceptions occur simultaneously.

This framework provides an explanation for why failed attempts at humor are often either too unprovocative (not appraised as a "violation") or too risqué (not interpreted as "benign"). Clearly, "teasing" is more likely to be received positively if it is not targeting traits that are relevant to an individual's self-concept, and if the teasing is exaggerated and able to be interpreted multiple ways (Keltner et al., 2001; McGraw & Warren, 2010). This finding highlights how benign violation theory may offer guidance on how to use irreverent communication effectively, because irreverence, while not "teasing," does consist of statements directed towards the client that also "violate" their expectations. Clinicians should therefore consider whether this violation will be interpreted as "benign" by the client or will instead be perceived as a threat or attack.

The proposed guidelines for effectively using irreverence are as follows:

Implementing Humor Within DBT

Identify whether the client is (or the client and clinician are) stuck in a maladaptive pattern that has gone unrecognized or been accepted as the status quo.

Select a form of irreverent communication that can be used to highlight and break this problematic pattern. The form of irreverence that will most likely be effective will depend on the nature of the problematic pattern. In other words, what strategy is most likely to make the client "jump the track" depends on which "track" the client is stuck on.

Implement this strategy (verbally or nonverbally) in a manner that will be perceived by the client as "benign."

3.2 Clinical Applications

The remainder of this chapter will focus on how to effectively implement this process with six unique strategies of irreverent communication. While these strategies do not constitute all of the ways that irreverence can be used within DBT, they are among the most commonly implemented techniques. Particular focus will be placed on clarifying the conceptual rationale for discerning which irreverent strategy is most likely to be effective, given a particular maladaptive action urge, thought, or emotional response. Focus on this conceptual rationale will provide more specific clinical instruction on how to use irreverent communication effectively and encourage the reader to adopt a clinical approach that emphasizes "function over form."

3.2.1 Reframing in an Unorthodox Manner

Reframing in an unorthodox manner involves restating the client's words such that attention is redirected away from their intended message and towards a new area of focus. In some scenarios, the primary intention is to pull away from a particularly ineffective idea or communication by treating it with little regard or seriousness. Such was my (WB) intention in responding to a client who expressed frustration with her family members and peers, who she suggested held unrealistic expectations about her academic performance. I had good reason to believe that this interpretation was inaccurate, and that her interpersonal difficulties had more to do with her impulsive behaviors, such as when she locked her sister outside in the snow following an argument. I therefore said, "People aren't disappointed because you get bad grades or are unlikely to become president, they're disappointed because you make them act out The Revenant." Here, my intention was to respond in a manner that the client likely did not anticipate, thereby blocking the problematic interpretation held within the initial statement.

This intervention can take the form of not only redirecting an ineffective statement, but also highlighting unintended aspects of what is being communicated. An opportunity later arose with the same client, who stated that only taking two AP courses made her "worthless," and that she might as well kill herself if she could not get into AP Calculus. Not wanting to allow this problematic conclusion to pass by unnoticed, I (WB) responded by saying, "You're ready to accept death, but not Algebra II?" Here, my intention was to place increased emphasis on those aspects of the thought process that were difficult for the client to defend. Although I felt an urge to validate the reasons that academic performance held such weight in the client's mind, I decided to instead highlight how her concerns about her mathematical prowess had grown so immense that they eclipsed even death. The irreverent communication served the purpose of blocking a maladaptive thought process, and also highlighting the specific aspect that made it problematic. Fortunately, the client responded as I had hoped; a wry grin, followed by a somber glance, and a description of the client's fear and shame. "Fine, Will. We both know I'm not going to kill myself over some numbers…I just can't have more proof that I'm not as smart as everyone else."

This emphasis on "maladaptive functions" also indicates which clinical scenarios are most likely to benefit from reframing in an unorthodox manner: *situations in which a maladaptive pattern is explicitly (verbally) being presented as the status quo*. This might take the form of statements suggesting that the maladaptive decision is actually effective (e.g., "You can say I shouldn't have left her out in the cold, but my sister got the message not to talk to me like that.") or the client's explanation that presents some maladaptive behavior as an acceptable status quo (e.g., "So naturally, I locked her outside in the snow.") Reframing these statements in an unorthodox manner (e.g., "Who told you that banishing your siblings into the wilderness was an effective way of resolving familial disputes? Do you live in some sort of Medieval Fiefdom?") helps to challenge and ultimately change this maladaptive cognition by treating these statements as anomalies that should not pass by unquestioned. This sudden shift in focus draws attention to these patterns and allows the clinician to highlight those aspects that make them ineffective. If the clinician approached this clinical situation with a more traditional therapist response, i.e., validating (reciprocal) communication (e.g., "Wow, sounds like your sister must have been really annoying you for you to decide to leave her out there in the cold."), this client would likely have felt empowered to make such a decision (e.g., "Exactly. That's what you get for being so ridiculous and annoying.")

The clinician must have a clear conceptualization of what makes the behavior, urge, or thought maladaptive, and an ability to describe this rationale if questioned by the client. This is because reframing in an unorthodox manner can be detrimental rather than benign if the strategy is used to target a pattern that is not actually maladaptive. For instance, imagine that the same client shared passive suicidal ideation that she noticed after not getting into AP Calculus, stating "I wish those thoughts weren't there, but they are. I just get so angry at myself, and I guess I start feeling hopeless that I'll never be good enough. I know the bar I set for myself is too high, but it still hurts when I jump and don't catch it." Here, the client's description of their emotions, thoughts, and behaviors is not maladaptive, only painful. The client is noticing suicidal thoughts following a performance that she has historically deemed to be unacceptable, thoughts that she is not engaging with nor suggesting are wise to act on, but instead sharing as indicators of underlying emotions. For this reason, the aforementioned irreverent phrase of "You're ready to accept death, but not Algebra II?" would be clinically contraindicated.

Additionally, we believe it is generally most effective to direct the unorthodox reframe towards the maladaptive urge, thought, or behavior, rather than the individual presenting the maladaptive urge, thought, or behavior as the status quo. For instance, there is a difference between saying, "well, that sounds ridiculous" and "you're ridiculous." While therapists naturally become frustrated with clients from time to time, making the clinician's irritation the primary focus of conversation is seldom helpful. Exceptions might be made when implementing the DBT practice of "radical genuineness" or "self-involving self-disclosure," but even here the disclosure of the clinician's irritation would be used to highlight the interpersonal impact of the client's behaviors rather than condemn their character. The goal is to allow the client and clinician to direct their attention towards the maladaptive behavior or thought pattern, not elicit shame within the client, who is assumed to be "doing the best he or she can." As such, we recommend the clinician will be more effective focusing on the words rather than on the speaker.

3.2.2   Plunging in Where Angels Fear to Tread

Psychotherapy inherently involves discussions of difficult topics. While the stigmatization of mental illness has decreased in recent years, it is still common for people to feel shame related to their difficulties establishing and maintaining a sense of internal stability and comfort. The difficulty of having these conversations is further complicated by the fact that people unintentionally contribute to their own suffering by responding in ways that serve some protective function but ultimately exacerbate their suffering (e.g., avoiding social scenarios that invoke anxiety, thereby decreasing distress in the short term but exacerbating their functional impairment in the long term). The client and clinician therefore have the difficult task of discussing topics and identifying patterns that the client may prefer to ignore.

Plunging in where angels fear to tread involves pushing past this discomfort and engaging in direct conversation in spite of the anxiety, shame, or anger that may follow. One such opportunity emerged during a conversation with one of my clients who was expressing feeling "rage" towards his coach and boyfriend and was considering quitting his team and ending his relationship. I (WB) had seen this pattern of anger emerge time after time and was concerned about the loneliness and regret that often followed acting on these urges. Pushing aside the anxiety that accompanied what I was about to say, I offered, "Yeah, but you hate everyone, sometimes. You hate me, sometimes. You've fired me a bunch of times." Here, I made the decision to ignore social niceties, and dive directly into the discomforting topic. "Dive" is the operational word, as I was not dipping my toes into the water (e.g., "I wonder if you've ever had these feelings before? If there have been other times where perhaps been this angry at other people? Maybe even me?") but rather I dove in head-first.

My client appeared taken aback, and the intervention served its purpose. He redirected away from arguing that he ought to leave his job and boyfriend and went on to describe how he "hates [me] and hates the Uber driver that brought [him] here," and concluded with his conviction that "he will probably hate three people on [his] way home." Acknowledging the fluctuations in his feelings towards other people allowed my client to see that his urges to end his relationships would likely also change with time. He agreed that it was therefore in his best interest to acknowledge and address his frustrations within his relationship with his coach and boyfriend, but not dissolve these relationships outright.

This technique differs from reframing in an unorthodox manner, which requires that a maladaptive pattern be explicitly (verbally) presented as the status quo. Instead, plunging in where angels fear to tread is best when this *maladaptive pattern is being implicitly (nonverbally) presented as the status quo*. In other words, a maladaptive pattern is presenting itself within the therapy room, and neither the clinician nor the client is highlighting it as problematic. The problem is therefore not so much the words being spoken as what is remaining unsaid.

This framing highlights the interrelated nature of therapy, and the way in which maladaptive patterns of emotions, thoughts, and behavior occur not only within clients, but also within clinicians. While the subject of this intervention may be the client's problematic patterns, the primary barrier to using this intervention is generally the clinician's hesitation to engage in a difficult discussion. With teens, this could include frank discussions about sexual activity, drugs, cheating, etc. This hesitation can be due to any number of factors, including anticipated consequences (e.g., expressed anger from the client, who may leave the room or treatment entirely), and the therapist's vulnerability factors (e.g., a well-intentioned desire to invoke feelings of comfort rather than distress). It is therefore important to assess not only maladaptive patterns that are implicitly being presented as the status quo within the client, but also these same ineffective patterns within the clinician that may be preventing him or her from addressing these difficulties.

This is not to say that reluctance to use this irreverent communication always reflects the clinician's shortcomings or insecurities. Hesitation to discuss topics that will elicit feelings of anger or shame in the client is prudent, as the clinician should be sure that they are acting in the best interest of the client before they deliberately invoke distress. One of the most effective ways of ensuring that this intervention will be perceived as "benign" is to surround it with validation. In the prior example involving my client's "rage" towards his coach and boyfriend, this took the form of my (WB) saying "I understand why you get angry. I know the missteps I've made that have led you to push me away, and I can see how a similar thing is happening here. I also know that you've later regretted some of these decisions. And I would hate for that to happen again." Here, I was not apologizing for or trying to undo my initial statement. Instead, I was acknowledging that I was giving my client difficult feedback, and in the process consciously causing them to feel distress. Highlighting the maladaptive pattern seemed like one of the most caring things that I could do for my client in this scenario. And so too did acknowledging the pain that the client may have felt in response to my intervention and sharing a rationale for why I was willing to make them feel this distress.

The other side of this dialectic is that it is important for clinicians not to fragilize their clients. DBT clinicians agree not to treat their clients as fragile, because trying to save a client from their distress often prevents an opportunity for new learning. Additionally, any pain highlighted by the clinician has already been lived by the client. The clinician is therefore not so much creating pain as drawing attention to its source. While this intervention may be accompanied by initial discomfort, it also reflects a radical genuineness by the clinician that the client may find validating. Put another way by Linehan in her work with adult BPD clients, but equally relevant to emotionally dysregulated youth, "DBT assumes that borderline patients are both fragile and not fragile; irreverence is directed at patients' nonfragile aspects." (Linehan, 1993, p. 395).

3.2.3 Using a Confrontational Tone

In some ways, using a confrontational tone is an extension of plunging in where angels fear to tread. The clinician uses the same tactic of directing the conversation towards a topic that is discomforting and out of line with social niceties using language that is direct, blunt, and specific. One of my (AM) teen clients gave me a "bullshit" button as a gift when he graduated for me to use with other clients, after he recognized the value of my calling him out many times for his minimizing or denying certain feelings and behaviors. For example, when he said, "my parents don't care if I graduate from HS," or, "my friends don't care if I don't text them back repeatedly," I would simply say "BS. Based on what I know of your parents and your friends they sure as heck care and saying they don't is just a way to reduce your anxiety and guilt!"

The clinician does not try to cushion the impact of their statement through the use of euphemisms or indirect language (e.g., "I wonder if your friends ever see versions of the anger you expressed to your sister, when you locked her out of the house? I know you don't live with them, but your irritation could be coming out other ways.") but instead allows their words to come out unedited, embracing rather than looking to dampen their impact (e.g., "If you treat your friends the way you treat your sister, you won't have any left. And don't say you don't live with them so you can't lock them out. There are many ways to "leave someone in the snow.")

This strategy can apply to any of the clinical scenarios highlighted thus far, where the maladaptive pattern is being endorsed as the status quo either explicitly (verbally) or implicitly (nonverbally). Regardless of the manner in which the client is endorsing this pattern, the clinician can still draw attention to it using language that is forceful and impactful. However, these adjectives draw attention to the primary factor that needs to be considered when considering the use of this strategy: is the pattern severe enough that it warrants a "forceful and impactful" response? For instance, the prior confrontational statement will likely be more effective if the client has lost multiple friendships due to ineffective expressions of anger, rather than if they make an uncharacteristically untoward comment in a moment of distress. Webster's dictionary defines "confrontational" as "feeling or displaying eagerness to fight." It is reasonable to expect the client to experience this kind of tone as somewhat unsettling, if not threatening. Whether or not this response is a warranted and effective way of knocking the client "off their track," or a heavy-handed response to a light problem will be determined by assessing the severity of this maladaptive pattern.

The significant impact of this intervention also draws attention to the difficulty in ensuring that the clinician's words are perceived as "benign." Indeed, this strategy requires the clinician to be confrontational, which by definition involves expressing an openness to conflict. However, the impact of the clinician's message will also be lost if the client perceives the confrontational tone as an unwarranted attack, with no purpose other than causing the client harm. It is therefore necessary to try to set the stage for the intervention to land on benign ground, while also allowing the impact of the confrontational tone to be felt.

One of the most effective strategies is again to surround the confrontational statement with validation. For instance, in the prior scenario, I (WB) could have followed up my prior statement by saying, "I'm giving you this feedback because I like you, and I want others to as well. You're too much fun, too charismatic to be losing relationships left and right. You've got a silver tongue, it's just a little too sharp at times." It is important to note that I am not backing away or apologizing for the prior statement but instead acknowledging its sting and reinforcing my care for and commitment to the client. Dialectically, the message and impact of the confrontational statement need to be allowed, and so too does the fact that this alternative perspective is painful to adopt.

Some might suggest it is helpful for the clinician to establish a strong rapport with the client prior to making use of this intervention to help mitigate the likelihood of the clinician's words being perceived as an attack rather than well-intentioned feedback. The other side of the dialectic, however, is that some teens respond positively to irreverence and "calling their bluff" or "calling bullshit" even in an intake, paradoxically to help build rapport. Thus, we encourage clinicians to remain flexible and not feel rule-bound and necessarily need to wait a certain amount of time before applying this sort of intervention.

3.2.4 Calling the Patient's Bluff

As detailed earlier in this chapter, DBT seeks to strike a balance between acceptance and change, demonstrating support and understanding for clients while also pushing them towards engaging in behaviors that are more in-line with their long-term goals. This act of pushing (as highlighted in the irreverent strategies detailed throughout this chapter) often generates distress within the client, as their current behaviors and beliefs are challenged as being ineffective. It is natural for clients to respond to this distress by pushing back, making statements that function to stop the clinician from pursuing painful topics.

For instance, a client who was weeks away from starting her DBT skills group once told me that although I (WB) "seemed like an ok guy," she would "never participate in that ridiculous group." I had spent weeks trying to build her willingness and motivation for joining (unsuccessfully, it would seem), and I knew it would not be therapeutic to see her without this treatment component. Taking "ok" as a ringing endorsement of our budding rapport, I decided to gamble and leverage our relationship against her willingness to participate in the skills training: "It's a shame because I think you're also 'ok'. And you're right, you'll probably hate the group. I don't know, I guess you just won't come, use up the allowed absences, and then we can say goodbye." The client and I sat in silence until she finally spoke: "I mean, are you at least going to show me where it meets?" She attended the following week, initially begrudgingly.

Calling the patient's bluff differs from previous forms of irreverence, as the setting of the problematic pattern is the therapy room rather than the patient's daily life. Specifically, this intervention is best applied to *problematic patterns of verbal behavior, in which there is an incongruence between the client's words* (i.e., *behaviors) and underlying intentions* (i.e., *cognitions)*. This incongruence causes the client's words to act as red herrings, obfuscating their genuine cognitions and emotions and making it difficult for others to respond appropriately. Calling the patient's bluff seeks to rectify this incongruence, taking what is being stated at face value, thereby blocking the maladaptive function of the behavior.

For instance, we often hear clients state that they want to drop out of treatment during the moments when they seem to need it most. There are an infinite number of reasons why this occurs. The client may be uncertain about their therapists' ability to alleviate their suffering, or their own ability to make use of their therapist's suggestions. They may also fear that the discomfort involved in the process will be unbearable or unrewarding, or feel ambivalent about whether they want to let go of a way of being that has served an important function for them up to this point. However, instead of communicating these thoughts and feelings, they are expressing a tangentially related desire to drop out of treatment. Following this line of thought would bring the clinician farther away from a discussion of these underlying feelings, towards problem solving a scenario that may not occur. Provided that the client is not actually at imminent risk of dropping out of treatment, time spent troubleshooting this topic will only pull the clinician and client away from the painful emotions that preceded this statement.

Of course, this formulation assumes that the client does not actually intend to drop out of treatment. If the assessment of my client's willingness to attend skills group had been inaccurate, or she really did deem me to be not much better than "ok," then my ultimatum may have been met with an early discharge from treatment. In order to effectively call a bluff, one must be sure that the statement is actually a bluff, or at least something that can be reconsidered. This highlights the first component of allowing this intervention to be perceived as "benign," which is that the clinician must have good reason to believe that the client's statements do not reflect their actual intentions. Anecdotal evidence suggests that errors in this area sometimes occur when clinicians are feeling frustrated with their clients and fail to recognize that urges to make an irreverent statement are coming from their own irritation, rather than an accurate assessment of their client. For instance, a particularly frustrated therapist might make the mistake of responding to a client who genuinely does not feel any attachment to therapy by saying "Ok, go ahead, drop out." Here, the urge for irreverence is not originating from the client's problematic pattern of behavior, but instead from the clinician's own distressing emotions or hopeless thoughts.

However, even if the therapist does accurately assess the client's "bluff," they still need to leave the client a way out after the bluff is called. It is provocative to call a client's bluff, as this often involves making an offer that you do not expect them to accept (e.g., "So would you like referrals for a provider who won't make you attend a silly group?"). While an ideal outcome would be for the client to acknowledge the bluff and readjust their focus, this is not always the case due to the potential embarrassment and vulnerability that this can require. A more effective approach is for the clinician to provide the client with a way out, for instance, by saying "Or maybe you could give this a shot? Sometimes I say smart things by accident. Besides, you can always fire me later." It is also important for the clinician to leave a bit of space between calling the patient's bluff and providing them with a way out, so as to allow the impact of this irreverent statement to be felt by the client. In other words, "The secret here is in the timing of calling the bluff and providing the safety net. The meek therapist provides both at once (bluff and net); the cruel, insensitive, or angry therapist forgets the net." (Linehan, 1993, p. 396).

3.2.5   Oscillating Intensity and Using Silence

Conversations are a bit like melodies in that they take on different tones, and with these tones come different expectations of what, when, and how things are said. A conversation about the birth of a child has a different tone than a discussion of the loss of a grandparent, and a joke directed towards a coworker may be appropriate when discussing their impending promotion, but not their impending termination. The ability to assess and respond with the expected tone is one of the ways that people put each other at ease and communicate in ways that feel expected and comfortable.

However, there are also times when what is expected and comfortable is not in the client's best interest. Oscillating intensity and using silence are most effective in these scenarios, where *the emotional tone of the conversation is acting as an obstacle to treatment progress.* For instance, we often find that conversations with clients who are struggling to find the motivation to combat symptoms of depression naturally take on a melancholic tone, with words that are spoken softly and slowly, reflecting the fatigue and hopelessness being discussed. While this parallel between the content and tone of the conversation is understandable, it may not be productive. Although a DBT therapist's words may contain encouragement for fighting against the amotivation that characterizes depression, our tone invites the client to continue engaging with the malaise. We find it beneficial for therapists to oscillate their intensity, altering the delivery to reflect energy, lightness, or playfulness. This could be achieved nonverbally (e.g., changing tone and cadence, or beginning to play catch with the client; we use a foam strawberry or soft mini football that we occasionally toss at clients who are being particularly dour) or verbally, such as by stating, "Geez it's getting dark and damp in here. Downright morose. You ever see that movie, Titanic? This is like the end of Titanic."

The clinician can also change a problematic tone or pattern of interaction through the use of silence. Social norms rarely endorse silence as an appropriate response to a statement or question, which makes it a highly effective way of pulling back from a pattern of interaction that has become unhelpful. The silence puts a sudden stop to the conversation, and invites the client to try a different approach, as their current style of interaction is generating interpersonal discomfort. While this response may not be the final perspective the clinician is hoping the client will adopt, it can help dislodge the conversation from a problematic pattern.

For instance, I (WB) once found myself at an impasse with one of my teen clients, who had not completed her diary card, refused to identify topics she wanted to discuss in therapy, and insisted that she would no longer be using DBT skills outside of session. I do not enjoy feeling stuck in the mud and had urges to once again review the rationale for the diary card that she found so burdensome, suggest difficulties that would be important to discuss in therapy, and convince her that I knew ways of navigating these obstacles. While this intervention was once effective, it had since run its course, having recently been met with counter arguments detailing why DBT was silly, and I was silly for suggesting otherwise. So instead, I fell silent and watched the client with a slight smile. After a few minutes, the client decided she'd had enough of my silence and relented: "What do you want??...Me to do the things?" ("things" being the diary card, agenda, and in-session engagement). "Yes!! Do the things!" I responded. After some hemming and hawing, and a bit more of my aforementioned motivational strategies, my client went on to do the things.

Ensuring that this intervention is experienced as "benign" requires that the tone of the conversation is actually problematic. To oscillate intensity by suddenly becoming flippant and jovial when a client is expressing valid concerns about a loved one's health, or silent if the client shares genuine sadness if this loved one were to pass, is not just ineffective but also deeply invalidating. A less harmful but equally ineffective example of using this strategy might include oscillating intensity or using silence for no discernible reason aside from being irreverent. To return to the prior point about function over form, the irreverent clinician does not make use of these strategies simply because they see the opportunity to do so. Oscillating intensity or using silence without a well-defined purpose is likely invalidating at worst, and unimpactful at best.

3.2.6 Expressing Omnipotence and Impotence

Therapy inherently involves a power differential. Regardless of whether a clinician uses the term "client," "patient," or "consumer," there remains a difference in the assumed expertise in terms of understanding and engendering mental health. This tends to work in favor of the treatment process, with the client acting as the expert on their experiences, and the clinician as the expert on how mental health principles might decrease the frequency and severity of the client's suffering.

This aspect of the status quo is generally favorable, creating a relationship that recognizes the clinician's expertise while remaining collaborative. However, it is also a variable that can be irreverently adjusted if a maladaptive pattern is emerging within treatment. This strategy is often implemented when the patient is stating that the suggested interventions won't work, or that they do not have the mental or physical resources required to carry them out. This could be seen as a *problematic cognitive pattern, in which the client is engaging with beliefs that are not in the interest of their long-term goals.* Both omnipotence and impotence serve the function of jarring this problematic cognitive pattern, the former by suddenly suggesting that the clinician's wisdom is beyond reproach, and the latter by throwing all responsibility for change on to the patient, thereby inviting them to "pick up the rope" as the therapist presents as ineffective and incapable.

For instance, during moments when my (WB) suggested interventions are repeatedly being met with skepticism and hopelessness, I will at times respond with omnipotence ("Look, I'm a smart guy with smart ideas. If you do the things I'm suggesting, things will get better. The skills work. It's the decision of whether or not to use them that gets tricky.") and other times with impotence ("Look, I'm a glorified advice-giver. All I can do is talk at you, and that doesn't seem to be working so I'm out of ideas."). Here, the intention is to change the balance of power within the relationship, throwing all of the weight onto the therapist's back in the first example, and on the client's back in the second.

Ensuring that this strategy is perceived as "benign" is less important than other scenarios, as the intervention is directed at the clinician rather than the client. There is always the risk that this intervention will validate a different problematic cognitive pattern, being the client's belief that the clinician is either insufferably arrogant or incompetent. A strong rapport helps to protect against this interpretation, as it assumes that the client has already established more positive judgments of their provider. That being said, these irreverent strategies can be quite powerful even at intake since they often get the clients' attention in a positive way. In turn, the DBT clinician is seen as different from prior "traditional sounding" therapists they may have seen who, without irreverence being utilized, appear less real or compelling.

3.3   Conclusion

Therapy is an intricate process, in which clinician and client work together to try to understand and address the suffering that brings the client into treatment. It is also a complex and sensitive process, in which the clinician must try to assess and influence an infinite and constantly shifting number of interrelated variables, thereby disrupting patterns that have often taken years to develop. The age of these patterns, and the way that they often serve an important function to the client (i.e., "maladaptive behaviors are often the solutions to problems" (Linehan, 1993, p.99)), can make these well-worn channels difficult to rework. Working with emotionally dysregulated teens, in particular, requires an extra special clinical skill set to engage and retain them in treatment. Irreverence provides a tool to assist in this process and allows a way of causing the client to "jump the tracks" of their unhelpful patterns and begin to approach their distress with new eyes, even as early as the first session. In this chapter, we have sought to outline the process through which this can be achieved: (1) identifying a maladaptive pattern of thoughts, emotions, urges, and behaviors occurring within the client, or between the client and clinician, (2) make use of whichever of the aforementioned strategies most effectively targets the problematic pattern, and (3) do so in a manner that will be perceived as "benign."

Ultimately, these guidelines are intended to provide initial direction on a process that will require significant practice and experimentation. With time, these strategies can become a natural part of the clinical process and help clinicians maneuver around the impasses that obstruct the path between the client and the life they want to live.

References

Cameron, E. L., Fox, J. D., Anderson, M. S., & Cameron, C. A. (2010). Resilient youths use humor to enhance socioemotional functioning during a day in the life. *Journal of Adolescent Research, 25*(5), 716–742.

Erickson, S. J., & Feldstein, S. W. (2007). Adolescent humor and its relationship to coping, defense strategies, psychological distress, and well-being. *Child Psychiatry and Human Development, 37*(3), 255–271.

Führ, M. (2002). Coping humor in early adolescence. *Humor, 15*(3), 283–304.

Geiger, P. J., Herr, N. R., & Peters, J. R. (2019). Deficits in mindfulness account for the link between borderline personality features and maladaptive humor styles. *Personality and Individual Differences, 139*, 19–23.

Horvath, A., Re, A. C., Flückiger, C., & Symonds, D. (2011). Alliance in individual psychotherapy. *Psychotherapy, 48*(1), 9–16.

Keltner, D., Capps, L., Kring, A. M., Young, R. C., & Heerey, E. A. (2001). Just teasing: A conceptual analysis and empirical review. *Psychological Bulletin, 127*(2), 229–248. https://doi.org/10.1037/0033-2909.127.2.229

Kuiper, N. A., Grimshaw, M., Leite, C., & Kirsh, G. (2004). Humor is not always the best medicine: Specific components of sense of humor and psychological well-being. *Humor: International Journal of Humor Research, 17*(1–2), 135–168.

Linehan, M. M. (1993). *Cognitive-behavioral treatment of borderline personality disorder.* Guilford Publications.

Martin, D. J., Garske, J. P., & Davis, M. K. (2000). Relation of the therapeutic alliance with outcome and other variables: A meta-analytic review. *Journal of Consulting and Clinical Psychology, 68*(3), 438–450.

Martin, R. A., Puhlik-Doris, P., Larsen, G., Gray, J., & Weir, K. (2003). Individual differences in uses of humor and their relation to psychological well-being: Development of the humor styles questionnaire. *Journal of Research in Personality, 37*(1), 48–75.

McGraw, A. P., & Warren, C. (2010). Benign violations: Making immoral behavior funny. *Psychological Science, 21*(8), 1141–1149.

Miller, A. L., Rathus, J. H., & Linehan, M. M. (2007). *Dialectical behavior therapy with suicidal adolescents.* Guilford Press.

Rathus, J. H., & Miller, A. L. (2015). *DBT skills manual for adolescents.* Guilford Press.

Chapter 4
Humor with Pediatric Patients

Hara Stephanou, Christina G. Salley, Kelsey Largen, and Becky H. Lois

Keywords Humor · Pediatric psychology · Pediatric medical conditions · Assessment · Intervention · Cultural considerations

4.1 Introduction

Approximately, two million children are hospitalized each year in the United States, and nearly 30% of those occur within freestanding children's hospitals (Leyenaar et al., 2016). Among this group are children living with a chronic health condition who are hospitalized due to complications of their illness or for medical treatment to address disease or symptom management. Chronic pediatric conditions vary widely in severity of symptoms and effects on daily functioning as well as long-term concerns regarding morbidity and mortality. Many children and adolescents with medical conditions face a number of physical challenges including fatigue, pain, reduced or limited mobility, and cognitive impairment. Daily routines may include managing oral medications, overseeing nutritional needs, closely observing symptoms, and participating in physical, occupational, and speech therapies. Children will require outpatient appointments with pediatric subspecialists and

H. Stephanou
St. John's University, Jamaica, NY, USA
e-mail: hara.stephanou15@my.stjohns.edu

C. G. Salley
Department of Child and Adolescent Psychiatry, Hassenfeld Children's Hospital at NYU Langone, New York, NY, USA
e-mail: christina.salley@nyulangone.org

K. Largen
Stephen D. Hassenfeld Children's Center for Cancer and Blood Disorders, Department of Child and Adolescent Psychiatry, New York, NY, USA
e-mail: Kelsey.largen@nyulangone.org

B. H. Lois (✉)
Department of Child and Adolescent Psychiatry, Hassenfeld Children's Hospital at NYU Langone, New York, NY, USA
e-mail: becky.lois@nyulangone.org

R. D. Friedberg, E. V. Rozmid (eds.), *Creative CBT with Youth*,
https://doi.org/10.1007/978-3-030-99669-7_4

43

those needing certain treatments (e.g., chemotherapy for cancer) may have periods of daily outpatient visits or extended inpatient hospital admissions. While the child is the primary focus of care, the condition and its management affect all family members and can be a source of stress for parents and siblings.

Pediatric patients may receive psychosocial support formally through either routine or as-needed referrals. Psychosocial teams may consist of social workers, psychologists, psychiatrists, child life specialists, clowns, and other recreational (e.g., art, music) therapists. These providers are often embedded within pediatric hospital settings and are present to provide psychoeducation, general support, or more targeted therapeutic interventions to patients and their families. These providers address psychosocial concerns including difficulties adjusting to illness, pre-existing or acute emotional or behavioral health challenges, and poor treatment adherence. When psychotherapy is indicated, pediatric psychologists typically draw from evidenced-based treatment modalities (Wu et al., 2014) with Cognitive Behavioral Therapy (CBT) being a commonly applied intervention. Children also benefit from support received through other relationships with nurses, physicians, and other providers (e.g., physical therapists). Even non-clinical staff such as administrative assistants and other essential staff (e.g., housekeeping, maintenance) have opportunities to interact in positive and supportive ways to patients and their families as they travel around the hospital milieu.

4.1.1 The Use of Humor in Pediatric Populations

The Association for Applied and Therapeutic Humor describes the intent of therapeutic humor as "a playful discovery, expression or appreciation of the absurdity or incongruity of life's situations" (aath.org). This definition is compatible with components of CBT, including the use of humorous approaches in Socratic dialogues (Friedberg & McClure, 2015). Furthermore, soliciting worst-case scenarios in an effort to work on decatastrophizing or to propose an exposure exercise can sometimes result in the child realizing their thoughts are so extreme that they are absurd or comical and can elicit some humorous relief in session. While having a serious illness is no laughing matter, the topics of humor and medicine have been paired together for centuries. Humor itself has several components, including a "physiological response (laughter), emotional response (mirth) and/or cognitive response (understanding)" (Sultanoff, 2013 as cited in Dionigi and Canestrari, 2018, p. 2).

The view that laughter and humor have physiological benefits for healthy and ill individuals has been well accepted for many centuries. With regard to theoretical frameworks on the impact of humor on pain (Pérez-Aranda et al., 2018), researchers have come up with a few theories: (1) humor offers a distraction that takes away from the body's pain response (Auerbach et al., 2014); (2) humor aids in cognitive re-appraisal (Kuiper, 2012); and (3) humor provides connections with others (Bell et al., 1986; Sturgeon & Zautra, 2016). In pediatric populations specifically, humor promotes a sense of dignity and normalcy in "dignity robbing conditions" (Francis et al., 1999).

Additionally, there are both historical and cultural references to the use of humor as a potential salve for physical symptoms. Savage et al. (2017) highlight several historical examples describing the use of humor as a medical intervention including Greek physicians who prescribed visits to the hall of comedians for the ill and Native American medicine men who included the use of clowns in their healing approaches. In more recent times, the use of humor to support ill children was popularized by the 1998 film, *Patch Adams*, which was inspired by the real-life story of Dr. Hunter Doherty Adams. Dr. Adams, an American physician, advocates for humor and play as an important element of medical care and connecting with young patients.

Humor and laughter are linked to physical and mental health promotion in these historical references and anecdotally, but researchers have also demonstrated this phenomenon in experimental and laboratory-based studies. Much of the available research stems from studies with adults. Physical benefits described with adult populations include positive effects on the cardiovascular, muscular, respiratory, endocrine, immune, central nervous as well as pain management (Louie et al., 2014; Mora-Ripoll, 2011; Pérez-Aranda et al., 2018).

Fewer studies have addressed the positive physiological effects of laughter and humor for children. However, several studies involving children with medical conditions have addressed common areas of symptom burden such as anxiety, stress, low mood, fatigue, and pain. Within this literature, many studies highlight the benefits of medical clowns who are trained professional performers. Their goal is to use different creative arts mediums (physical comedy, magic, music, etc.) related to medical procedures and medical equipment to decrease procedural-based fear and promote coping, laughter, and mirth during medical events (Stephson, 2017). Otherwise known as "therapeutic clowns" or "clown doctors," they began to more formally establish themselves in hospitals during the late 1980s (Dionigi et al., 2012) and are now commonly integrated within pediatric hospital settings. The positive effects of therapeutic medical clowning are well-documented and much of this work highlights the benefits of clowning for anxiety and pain (Sridharan & Sivaramakrishnan, 2016). For example, in samples of children preparing for surgery, clowning has been demonstrated to reduce preoperative anxiety more effectively than medication and interventions led by clowns have led to increased pain tolerance in children, though this may be via the more direct impact on stress and anxiety (Pérez-Aranda et al., 2018). Additionally, Stuber et al. (2009) found that tolerance for a moderately painful stimulus (the cold pressor task) increased when children were exposed to humorous videos. In a study involving children admitted to an inpatient hospital setting in Columbia, researchers found that salivary cortisol levels, a biological marker of stress, were lower for children who were exposed to a humor intervention when compared to those who were not (Sánchez et al., 2017).

4.2 Assessment of Humor in Pediatric Patients

The way in which patients respond to and use humor depends on a variety of factors. Individual personality traits as well as cultural factors play a role in how individuals will use humor as a coping skill during a stressful situation. In the case of patients with chronic medical conditions, factors such as diagnosis, prognosis, and side effects from the disease or medication may influence openness to humor. All of these factors are important to assess in order to successfully use humor to build rapport or as a stand-alone intervention.

4.2.1 Cultural Factors

An individual's cultural background may impact their perception of what is funny and when humor is appropriate or inappropriate. For example, research has shown that individuals from Eastern cultures are less likely to use humor as a coping strategy than individuals from Western cultures (Jiang et al., 2019) and some research suggests that individuals from the northern United States are more likely to use sarcasm than individuals from the southern United States (Dress et al., 2008). When assessing cultural differences in the use of humor, it is important to consider a broad definition of culture, including consideration of the patient's place of origin, race and ethnicity, and religious beliefs. See Table 4.1 for expert ideas.

4.2.1.1 Humor Assessment in Action: Case Example in Cultural Context

Josiah*, a 14-year-old patient with sickle cell disease, was referred to psychology for concerns with adjustment following bone marrow transplant. While Josiah was born in the United States, his parents were originally from Nigeria and had a different perception of humor. For example, Josiah described his parents as being more serious and noted that there were many references that this patient understood from growing up in the United States that influenced the content of his humor that his parents weren't aware of. For example, Josiah loved rap music and wrote his own

Table 4.1 Expert ideas: cultural assessment of humor questions

1. Was the patient born in the United States or a different country?
(a) If born outside of the United States, what is their immigration history?
(b) If born outside of the United States, are they only here for medical treatment or do they live here permanently?
2. Does this patient need an interpreter to communicate with the medical team?
3. What region of the country are they from?
4. What race and ethnicity does this patient identify with?
5. What religious or spiritual beliefs does this patient have?

songs based on popular beats, many of which contained funny lyrics or situations. Although his parents did not understand this creative outlet, the clinician's receptivity regarding his music allowed them to develop rapport and use this medium as an outlet for his feelings later on in therapy. Knowing the differences between Josiah and his parents' perception of humor allowed the clinician to change style when communicating with Josiah's parents by commenting on shared situations in the moment, such as laughing about the struggles of parenting a teenager or sharing a smile with parents when the clinician and parents were both out of touch with Josiah's interests. By changing styles to meet everyone's needs, the clinician was able to enhance the therapeutic relationship with both the patient and his parents.

It is also important to consider how a clinician's personal background may influence experience of humor. For some clinicians, bringing humor into a session with a patient may feel natural while others may feel reluctant to share their sense of humor in a professional setting. By assessing one's own use of humor, clinicians can understand how to best bring their unique style into a session, for example, by considering how they have used humor in their own lives to cope with difficult situations. See Table 4.2 for expert ideas.

When there are clear cultural differences, humor can be used as a way to bridge the gap between patients and clinicians by acknowledging that although there are differences, one can still create a connection through humor that can help to build rapport and set the groundwork for a therapeutic relationship. In fact, much of the research on the intersection between culture and humor has shown that most cultures have more similarities than differences in the ways that we perceive humor (Schermer et al., 2019). In addition to using one's own cultural background through humor to bridge any cultural differences, a more direct approach might also be appropriate. For example, asking patients and their families directly about what they think is funny and how their culture influences their perception of humor may prove helpful. Clinicians may also consider using more physical humor (e.g., making a funny face or sound, dancing to celebrate a success in treatment) when interacting with pediatric patients that speak a language that is different from their native language. Whether a clinician uses a direct or an indirect approach to assessment of cultural factors, it is always important to come from a place of genuine curiosity and interest, keeping in mind that the understanding of the patient and family's humor may evolve over time as you establish your relationship.

Table 4.2 Expert ideas: personal assessment of humor

1.	How comfortable do I feel using humor in my interactions with patients?
2.	How have I used humor to cope with challenging situations?
3.	What things do I find funny that may not be funny to others who do not share my background?
4.	Is there something uniquely funny about my own culture/upbringing that I could bring into my interactions with this patient?

4.2.2   Individual Factors

There are a number of individual factors that may influence perception of humor in pediatric patients. Some of these factors such as individual personality characteristics and developmental level are true for all children. However, other factors such as diagnosis, prognosis, and current symptoms are unique to this population. One question to consider when assessing humor perception in pediatric patients is when they received the diagnosis. Most patients upon hearing the news that they have been diagnosed with a chronic health condition will likely need some time to adjust and may find jokes and humor insensitive. Another consideration is the nature of the diagnosis. Is this condition something that requires intensive medical intervention? Will the patient's lifestyle be disrupted significantly? Is the disease life-threatening? All of these factors may influence the ways in which a provider may use humor as well as what topics may be sensitive to individual patients because of their diagnosis and the associated complications.

For example, some patients may experience pain due to their condition or may not be alert at all times due to lack of sleep or medication. When patients are experiencing painful complications, they may not be as open to humor as when they are feeling better physically. Assessment of the appropriateness of humor should include consideration of a patient's current medical status. Additional care and sensitivity must be taken for children at end of life. However, studies show that humor can be a useful tool in palliative care in increasing pain tolerance, life-satisfaction, and improving physical and psychological well-being (Linge-Dahl et al., 2018).

4.2.3   Methods for Assessing Humor

Humor assessment will likely look different depending on the pediatric patient population and setting. Formal measures are an option for clinicians when there is ample time or clinicians wish to get an in-depth assessment of humor. For a list of formal measures for assessing humor, please see Table 4.3.

For many pediatric settings, a more informal measure may be more appropriate. For example, in one study, researchers assessed humor by asking participants to write captions for single panel cartoons, add a funny conclusion to a joke, and to include a funny definition for an odd noun-noun pair such as "yoga bank" and "cereal bus" (Nusbaum et al., 2017). This technique could easily be translated when working with pediatric patients as a way to build rapport and learn more about a child's sense of humor. Other informal methods could include using trial and error to see whether a patient responds to a funny prompt. For example, a clinician can blow up a glove with air and place it on their head to see whether they can make a young child laugh during a procedure. If the child laughs or smiles, then the clinician can determine that physical humor is a method that can be used in the future

Table 4.3 Expert ideas: formal measures for assessing humor

Measure	Description	Citations
Humor styles questionnaire	Assesses four different dimensions relating to individual differences in the use of humor; validated in children 11 and older	Fox et al. (2013); Martin et al. (2003)
Humor in our household questionnaire	Asks respondents to answer questions about humor individually and then share with their family members	Eckstein et al. (2003)
State trait cheerfulness inventory	Assesses humor among different mood states including cheerfulness, seriousness, and bad mood; includes parent report	Hofmann et al. (2018)

with this patient. A sample humor assessment measure is included (Fig. 4.1) for review.

Clinicians will also want to continuously assess humor during conversations with patients by paying attention to patient's comments about humor. During the course of treatment for a chronic health condition, a patient may express cognitive distortions around their ability to make jokes or participate in humor that might be appropriate targets for intervention. For example, a patient might say, "My life is miserable. There is absolutely nothing to laugh about." A patient who makes this statement may benefit from introducing cognitive reframing to help change his thoughts to be more accurate. By incorporating humor assessment into a clinician's regular assessment process, clinicians can be better equipped to notice what role humor is playing as well as any opportunities to increase laughter into the patient's life.

Depending on the setting, there may be several psychosocial staff members who are able to carry out a humor assessment. For example, in some outpatient clinics, social workers conduct routine psychosocial assessments for new patients and may be able to incorporate questions about humor into this assessment. Psychologists may use a humor assessment with a new patient referral as a way to build rapport and better understand what techniques may work best. Child Life Specialists, who routinely work with children during medical procedures, may want to ask these questions as a way to understand what might help to increase distraction during a blood draw or finger stick.

Overall, humor assessment in pediatric patients is an important step for better understanding the whole patient. No matter what method is chosen, communication among the interdisciplinary team as to what elicits humor for individual patients and families can improve patient relationships with staff and consequently improve patient care.

Questions for Children	
1.	What is something that makes you laugh?
2.	What is a funny television show you like to watch? Tell me something funny that happened in the show.
3.	What is your favorite funny book? Tell me something funny that happened in the book.
4.	Do you know any silly songs? Can you sing it to me?
5.	Tell me about something funny that happened at school.
6.	Who is the funniest person in your family? Tell me something funny that they did.
7.	Do you know any funny jokes?

Questions for Adolescents	
1.	What is something that makes you laugh?
2.	What is something different about you, your family, or your culture that you think other people would find funny?
3.	How does your culture influence what you think is funny?
4.	Tell me about a funny video or meme that you saw recently.
5.	What is an inside joke that you have in your friend group?
6.	Who is your funniest friend?
7.	Do you ever laugh at yourself?

Humor Prompts	
Make a funny face	Make a silly noise
Wear a funny costume	Watch a funny video
Tell a knock-knock joke	Use medical equipment in a funny way
Observe a child during a clown performance	Play a game of charades where you act out funny characters

Dowling, J.S. (2002). Humor: A coping strategy for pediatric patients. *Pediatric Nursing*, *28*(2).

Fig. 4.1 Humor assessment measure for pediatric patients. Dowling, J.S. (2002). Humor: A coping strategy for pediatric patients. *Pediatric Nursing*, *28*(2)

4.3 Clinical Applications of Humor with Pediatric Patients

Humor interventions have been used in pediatric settings as a complementary intervention and as a therapeutic tool with approaches ranging from therapeutic clowning, magic tricks, strategies for distraction and coping facilitated in collaboration with child life specialists, and creative activities via "artists-in-residence" programs (Bennett et al., 2014; McMahan, 2008). With these approaches integrated in already existing, evidence-based therapies, they promote relaxation and coping with hospitalization, (Consoli et al., 2018), anxiety reduction prior to procedures and medical interventions (Sridharan & Sivaramakrishnan, 2016), and coping with chronic illness management.

4.3.1 Hospital Programs and Staff that Promote Humor

4.3.1.1 Therapeutic Clowning and Magic

> Clowns don't belong in hospitals…Neither do children.- Michael Christensen, Big Apple Circus Clown Care Unit

> The role of a clown and a physician are the same—it's to elevate the possible and to relieve suffering.- Patch Adams

Patch Adams, a medical doctor himself, believes in the importance of a hospital community, which includes integrating humor and laughter as part of culture of medical care (Finlay et al., 2014, p. 596). Similarly, in 1986, the Big Apple Circus in New York City created one of the largest hospital programs pioneered the integration of various performance artists into hospital settings, particularly clown doctors. Since then, this community program has transformed into several free-standing organizations, the largest one being Healthy Humor (healthyhumorinc.org). Healthy Humor is a non-profit organization with performers (magicians, musicians, actors, clown doctors, etc.) trained to use their skills in a hospital environment to promote humor, play, and fun for hospitalized children and their support systems (Christensen, 2020). One of their practices includes "Clown Rounds," which mimics the medical rounds that physicians do in patient rooms as a parody to routine hospital events, such as performing "red nose transplants, kitty-cat scans, chocolate milk transfusions, and funny-bone checks" (Finlay et al., 2014, p. 601).

Therapeutic clowning can provide distraction and/or adaptation, laughter or fun, and may "demystify" medical procedures and events by bringing a sense of familiarity into a medical space (Finlay et al., 2014). Unlike clowns typically associated with circus performances, therapeutic clowns, or "clown doctors," are multi-modal and specifically trained to be mindful of the culture of the medical space, including confidentiality, training on child development, and hygiene. They present with more minimal makeup, usually keeping to funny outfits, a hat, and a traditional clown nose. They may also wear doctor's lab coats. Clowns are trained in non-confrontational approaches, knowing to respect a "no" from patients, using music to draw attention, keeping distance or avoiding eye contact at first, and approaching the child from the side or getting down to the child's height (Koller & Gryski, 2008). While there is an element of performance to a clown doctor visit, it is important to note that the goal is to empower children and give them a sense of control during a hospital stay:

> I'm not there to entertain people. Therapeutic clowning is not about the clown. It's about empowering the children. They don't have any choice over who comes in or out of their room, the doctors who care for them, the illness that they have, or the medications they take. We offer them choices. Always asking permission, we will never go into a room un-invited. If the child says, 'No, I don't want to see you today,' that's great. He can't do that with anyone else. Watson (2008), p. 179

Several children's hospitals have incorporated clown programs, such as "The Laughter League" at Boston Children's Hospital (BC Laughter League Website;

https://www.childrenshospital.org/patient-resources/family-resources/clown-care;
https://laughterleague.org/).

4.3.1.2 Therapeutic Recreation, Child Life, and Creative Arts Therapies

Child life specialists are often on the "front lines" of adjustment and coping in
medical settings, with their work encompassing three major tasks: promoting play
and a sense of normalcy, engaging families and other support systems, and procedural preparation and coping (Child Life Council, 2006). A child life specialist may
meet a child when they are first admitted to offer activities to encourage a sense of
structure throughout the day and behavioral activation, such as participation in a
unit-wide movie night or bingo game, providing board games to a family to pass the
time, or finding ways to celebrate birthdays or commemorate loved ones while still
in the hospital. They are experts in demystifying medical events via play and developmentally appropriate communication of jargon and diagnosis to patients, their
families, siblings, schools, and other support systems (Beickert & Mora, 2017;
Association of Child Life Professionals, 2018; Beer & Lee, 2017; Lerwick, 2016;
Lookabaugh & Ballard, 2018).

While most child life specialists work in hospitals, they may also work in camps
for children with chronic illness, outpatient doctor's offices, and other ambulatory
care centers. Depending on a child's needs, interventions are highly developmentally considered, and may include humor, playfulness, and mirth to ensure consistency in of the largest developmental tasks of childhood: play. For example, a child
life specialist may help a child prepare for chemotherapy port access or a blood
draw by showing the child on a doll first. Child life is often called on for shorter-
term and acute coping interventions, including teaching coping skills such as breathing techniques for relaxation, using ways to ease pain by positioning children for
comfort or using adjunctive tools before a painful shot or IV placement (e.g., a
bee-shaped buzzer that provides gentle vibrations around an injection site in an
effort to reduce pain), and promoting the use of distraction as an evidence-based
procedural pain management technique (Birnie et al., 2017; Bukola & Paula, 2017).
These strategies can potentially decrease the likelihood of adverse events by unnec-
essarily repeating medical procedures (e.g., reinserting an IV or re-doing a blood
draw, decrease in need of sedation prior to imaging). If a child has greater mental
health or developmental needs that would benefit from longer term support, pediatric psychologists work in consultation with child life specialists to implement strategies for longer term coping or behavioral plans.

Creative arts therapies, such as music and art, may be seen as a less intimidating
and invasive way to provide care that is supportive and may reduce distress. They
have been shown to contribute to pain reduction, decreased fatigue, short-term
mood improvements, stress reduction, and reduced symptomatology (Moola
et al., 2020).

4.3.1.3 Psychology

Pediatric psychologists are well-positioned to utilize humor in their work with children and families. As a part of assessment, the psychologist will work to identify patterns in how the child and family may already integrate humor in their lives as well as their openness to utilizing humor as part of their adjustment and coping process. As an intervention tool, there are a few key opportunities where psychologists can use humor. First, utilizing humor as a method to connect to children can be good strategy for initiating communication, building rapport, and gaining trust in the relationship. Younger children may respond well to silly and playful interaction while connecting with adolescents may include the use of sarcasm and wit. Turning aspects of the illness or treatment on their head to highlight the shocking or ridiculous nature of some serious topics (e.g., changes in appearance, decreased independence due to needing assistance with activities of daily living) can be a strategy to acknowledge how unusual the situation must feel for the child. This strategy can validate feelings of disbelief and shock and, in turn, help the child see that the therapist "gets it."

Additionally, cognitive behavioral therapy inherently includes strategies that "pull" for humor. These may include addressing cognitive distortions via playful "thinking traps," confronting social anxiety through in-session exposures such as silly dance moves or initiating funny noises, attempting to change negative emotions through loud, boisterous singing matches with a friend, and many more. Third wave approaches such as dialectical behavior therapy also specifically utilize irreverent approaches to help patients alter their perspectives (Linehan, 1993). Clinicians who typically work from a CBT-based framework should consider how these approaches may be used from a lens of humor in an effort to build rapport and enhance coping.

4.4 Humor Interventions for Pediatric Presenting Problems

Often in pediatric settings, medical team will refer a patient who may appear depressed, sullen, and not engaging with staff during treatment, or for some behavioral concern (what a child may be doing or not doing with regard to treatment goals (Catarozoli et al., 2019). In working with youth with medical conditions, it is important to be mindful that thoughts and feelings surrounding their diagnosis and treatment (e.g., "there is no cure and I will never get better") may in fact be true. Clinicians should be mindful of when to utilize change-based CBT interventions that can incorporate humor (e.g., using medical play/exposure to lessen fear surrounding medical procedures) versus interventions that may use humor as part of acceptance (coping with the potential that a patient will have this condition for the rest of their lives). Several clinical areas ripe for humor intervention are described below, along with case examples to illustrate them in practice.

4.4.1 Psychoeducation/Rapport Building

Psychoeducation is an important component to therapeutic buy-in (Crosling et al., 2009). The use of humor can specifically help with overall comprehension and learning (Hackathorn et al., 2011), as well as decrease defensiveness, enhance therapeutic alliance, and promote trust (Hussong & Micucci, 2021). A rule of thumb when first approaching humor is to direct humor towards factors outside of the child/their family, including humor towards medical staff, treatments, or other events that may be fear-inducing for the child (McGhee & Frank, 2014, p. 161). One of the authors described working with a young client who was referred from the gastroenterology service. There was initially a lot of shame surrounding frequent loose stools. Adding fart noises at the beginning and end of each session as a "hello and goodbye" served as a way to build rapport. This intervention also created expected structure around a session through a shared ritual and took away some of the awkwardness surrounding discussing somatic symptoms by placing the conversation in a "comic frame" (Dziegielewski et al., 2003). The author assisted the patient and team with utilizing this strategy both in the therapy space and during his medical appointments. Another way to incorporate humor may be to use stool shaped emojis to do a mood or symptom check with a patient or play a song/do a dance as a child is able (Adkins, 2018; a Physician Assistant on why he dances with his patients).

4.4.1.1 Humor in Rapport Building: Case Example

Joe,* a 10-year-old Caucasian boy with new-onset diabetes, expressed self-consciousness over what other children in his class would think if his continuous glucose monitor alarmed for out-of-range blood sugar. In discussing how the alarm sounded to his new therapist, Joe thought of other sounds he could think of, from predictable sounds such as a car backing up out of a driveway, to more outlandish examples (e.g., alien spaceship landing from outer space). This discussion helped Joe's connection to his therapist and improved his level of comfort in discussing his feelings about his new diagnosis. This also introduced how to reframe negative automatic thoughts on others' perception of his diabetes management.

4.4.2 Humor as a Coping Skill

Children with a variety of health issues have reported using humor and laughter to cope. They describe strategies such as joking around, making fun of themselves and their limitations, or pranking family members (e.g., Macartney et al., 2014). Research supports a model of stress adaptation among youth with chronic illness, using techniques such as "reappraisal, positive thinking, acceptance, or distraction" (Compas et al., 2012). Humor is also linked with resiliency in youth (Masten, 2001), which supports the idea that incorporating humor-based strategies to reframe thoughts enhances coping (Hilliard et al., 2012). This has been especially highlighted in the pediatric cancer literature where various reports have suggested that a sense of humor enhances coping and adjustment (Dowling & Hockenberry, 2003).

However, benefits of humor are not just for patients. The child's illness is a force that deeply affects parents and siblings and can cause significant distress. Children with chronic medical conditions may also note that they feel as if others treat them as "fragile" or as if they cannot make jokes around them due to the severity of their condition. Research indicates that parents and siblings find humor and laughter to be helpful when it comes to coping with a child's medical condition and that it may help families cope together. For example, qualitative work by Mangelsdorf et al. (2019) describes how one family of a child who had injured his ankle joked that after the child healed they would break his other ankle in order to keep a "handicapped card." Tasker and Stonebridge (2016) interviewed adolescent siblings of youth with cancer who reported that humor and laughter within their families was something they needed in order to cope with the stressful sides of the illness. In other work, parents of children with disabilities who endorse adaptive humor styles such as self-enhancing or affiliative humor report more positive affect and fewer symptoms of depression (Fritz, 2020). The use of humor and joking around has even been described as a strategy that parents use when their child is nearing the end of life (Darlington et al., 2021).

In clinical practice, there is often discussion and planning around a child's "coping kit," used to combat distressing emotions or thoughts. This may include activities for distraction, things that bring comfort, and relaxation. Pain and discomfort can be tied into the "feelings" part of a CBT model for youth with medical and somatic symptoms (Catarozoli et al., 2019). The "rest and digest" response is often taught in the context of relaxation skills and is a natural place to incorporate humorous techniques. For example, a patient can think of different sensory experiences related to a funny memory while doing guided imagery. Humorous anecdotes can be added to create a calming scene (e.g., one young patient imagined beach full of puppies dancing in tutus eating ice cream).

With regard to humor specifically, the idea of a "Laughter First Aid Box" (Schiffman, 2020) promotes coping with difficult medical events throughout the course of illness or a child's hospitalization. Hart and Rollins (2011) suggest similarly creating a "Mirth Aid Kit," a decorative box filled with things that make the child laugh, such as funny cards, comic strips, toys, jokes, and other items. We have created a worksheet (Fig. 4.2) with suggestions for a coping kit that can completed with a therapist or sent home with a family to generate a humor-based coping list. This is meant to be customized to developmental and medical need.

4.4.2.1 Humor as a Coping Skill Case Example 1

Marissa,* a 15-year-old Caucasian female, was born with a congenital heart defect. She required placement of a pacemaker when she was quite young. In later years, she needed an emergency repair of this device, and had since struggled to feel like herself. She entered psychotherapy for support in transitioning back to school, as she felt different than other teenagers. In therapy, she often presented with questions about her identity within a friend group, issues with romantic interests, and worries

<table>
<tr>
<td>

Books that Make Me Laugh

- The Don't Laugh Challenge Books
- Would you rather? Eww! Edition
- Freddie the Farting Snowman
- Diary of a Whimpy Kid books

</td>
<td>

Silly Shows, Movies, and Videos

- Adventure Time
- Nailed It!
- Watching funny dog videos on YouTube

</td>
</tr>
<tr>
<td>

Funny Activities (games, crafts, etc)

- Pie Face
- Pictionary
- The Floor is Lava
- What do you meme? Family Edition
- Throw Throw Burrito
- Don't Make Me Laugh (The Reinvented Charades Party Game)
- Headbands Game (app on my mom's phone)

</td>
<td>

Toys and Tricks that Make me Smile

- Making slime
- Taking test strips and throwing them like confetti
- Putting googly eyes on my emergency snacks
- Making stress balls out of Orbeez

</td>
</tr>
<tr>
<td>

Remember when? List some of your funniest memories!

- When I won the lego-building contest at camp and then my tower toppled over
- When it was pajama day at school and my teacher showed up in cookie monster onesie
- Thinking of my dog dressed up as a school bus for Halloween

</td>
<td>

Other things that make me laugh or smile:

- Getting cool adhesive patches for my Dexcom (sloths and narwahls)
- Reading "The Book with No Words" by BJ Novak to my little cousin and hearing him giggle
- Dressing up my dog in funny outfits

</td>
</tr>
</table>

Fig. 4.2 Case Example: Joe's Humor Coping Kit! (school age child with diabetes)

surrounding school performance and career goals. Marissa sometimes struggled to put her thoughts and feelings into words and would occasionally reference a popular meme or GIF she thought encapsulated her thoughts or feelings. For example, she showed her therapist an image of Kermit the frog flailing his arms with excitement when her romantic interest sent her a text. She later elaborated that Kermit's supposed "frazzled excitement" felt as if she was potentially having an arrythmia and alarming her device, because she struggled to acknowledge how someone so reportedly attractive could potentially like her. The therapist outlined Marissa's use of humor to cope and identify the connection between her thoughts, somatic feelings, and subsequent behaviors in seeking affirmation from others as well as her own assumptions that others may treat her as "fragile" due to having a pacemaker. In subsequent sessions, Marissa's affect towards negative automatic thoughts changed; when she found herself engaging in unhelpful thoughts about what others thought of her medical condition, she would instead laugh and roll her eyes.

4.4.2.2   Humor as a Coping Skill Case Example 2

Gina,* a 13-year-old Asian-American female diagnosed with osteosarcoma, required a surgery to remove a tumor from her leg. Gina had an intellectual disability and often felt scared about working with different staff members, and multiple medical procedures she had to endure, including unexpected events that occurred in the hospital (e.g., longer chemo stays, losing her hair, needing a wound vacuum-assisted closure after her surgery to drain fluid, not returning to school in time). She was referred to psychology to give her and her family some cope-ahead skills for unexpected events, as well as to help find ways for Gina to feel more comfortable with different medical providers. To familiarize her with medical tools and give her a sense of agency over her treatment, Child Life helped Gina create her own medical toolkit, including a "play" stethoscope she would use with the doctor, a joint hammer, and a doll that had her same medical wound. She jokingly shared that she was her surgeon's assistant, and prescribed fake "prescriptions" and care instructions for the medical team. As part of rapport building with her psychologist, Gina made a "headband of the day" during which she cut out different movie characters and funny faces that she liked and stuck them on the headband or paper crown. One day, she cut out pictures of her surgeon and put them on the headband, which gave her and each staff member who came to see her that day a good laugh. This headband activity increased Gina's behavioral activation and helped her to connect with staff members with a conversation starter regarding her interests.

4.4.3 Humor in Medical Play/Exposure

In medical settings, children can encounter unfamiliar items related to medical procedures. It can be helpful to show these items in a different way to familiarize children not only with their function, but to decrease their fear surrounding the item,
similar to traditional exposure therapy. In several evidence-based treatment manuals
(Coping Cat, MATCH ADTC), it is emphasized that sessions should end with an
activity that promotes laughter (e.g., Match ADTC celebrates successes with a
"Leave 'Em Laughing" Activity) to provide reprieve, reinforcement, and levity
from what is often a difficult undertaking for patients. Medical play can be used to
familiarize children with common medical items, such as gauze and gloves. It can
also take away the somewhat intimidating appearance of medical devices and tools.
For example, a child who had an aversion to gloves made a "flower arrangement"
with gloves to be put in her room; another created a "butterfly" with gauze and a
band aid. A syringe can be used to squirt paint for a fun activity that promotes
behavioral activation in the hospital setting, decreased anxiety over unfamiliar or
scary objects, and increased familiarity with a medical tool.

4.4.3.1 Humor in Medical Play/Exposure Case Example

Riley,* a 4-year-old Caucasian male with leukemia, was referred to the psychology team after limited oral intake, resulting in a nasal-gastric tube placement for
supplemental nutrition. Although Riley could still eat by mouth while this tube was
in, Riley was scared to swallow with the tube due to an episode of vomiting after
eating which led to the tube being dislodged. The medical team set a goal for Riley
to increase his oral intake in order to remove the tube altogether; however, he was
afraid of this transition due to his past experience. Child life and psychology worked
together to introduce medical play with toy food, noticing which food Riley gravi-
tated towards. The team created a picnic with these foods, and then incorporated
small portions of real food alongside these foods to take small bites. This served
both as a distraction and as an approach to take away some of the fear involved with
eating. Reinforcement in the form of character stickers the child enjoyed was given
to him, shaping reinforcement with bigger stickers after subsequent bites. Sessions
were timed to coordinate with either the magician or pet therapy dog to add mirth,
levity, and reinforcement after feeding sessions.

In summary, clinicians should strongly consider the utilization of humor as a
primary or adjunctive intervention with pediatric patients. It can enhance therapeutic connection and rapport and optimize coping with conditions or situations that are
out of the patient and family's control.

4.5   Risks and Benefits of Humor Among Medical Providers

As discussed, the use of humor as a mechanism for coping with stressful events may be of significant benefit in pediatric settings. Research has addressed the social functions of humor for staff in various settings (Astedt-Kurki & Isola, 2001;Griffiths, 1998; Sayre, 2001). Despite variability in setting and delivery, findings consistently indicate the importance of humor in improving communication, building relationships, decreasing tension and burn out, and managing emotions (Dean & Major, 2008; Mesmer-Magnus et al., 2012).

However, clinicians using this strategy with their patients may find systemic barriers within their multidisciplinary team members, the team "culture," or the clinic environment. For instance, team members may express concern that the patient, family, or provider is not taking a diagnosis seriously or may not fully understand the severity of a prognosis. They may find it uncomfortable to overhear a provider laughing with a patient or family about changes in the patient's appearance, symptoms, or "gallows humor" during a medical visit. Clinicians who are utilizing humor as a strategy for coping should consider explaining the rationale for this strategy with their team in an effort to decrease discomfort. Providing evidence on the effectiveness of humor in medical treatments and health promotion for stress reduction, pain control, and improved resiliency may prove helpful (Watson, 2011).

Medical teams may also benefit from education on the use of humor to cope and build upon their own resiliency, as humor has been shown to have a positive effect on group cohesion and may be effective in reducing stress in health care workers (Craun & Bourke, 2014; Dean & Major, 2008). However, it is also possible that the strategy could create distance and prevent more serious discussion, particularly in situations where clinicians or medical teams may be attempting to avoid the reality of a patient's diagnosis or prognosis. Further, humor can have a darker side; it can be perceived as aggressive or rude, particularly when offered at the expense of another person (Kuiper et al., 2004). Excessive use of gallows humor, in particular, has been associated with psychological distress (Moran, 2002).

4.6   Conclusion

Evidence suggests that there is an important role for humor in pediatric settings, as it may improve resiliency and coping in patients, families, and staff. There is also considerable evidence that humor may enhance positive life experiences and lead to greater psychological well-being. Clinicians in pediatric settings should strongly consider assessing for humor and utilizing it strategically to promote coping and connection. Medical teams may also benefit from the use of humor to build cohesion and manage the intensity of day-to-day work that can be emotionally challenging. Children and families facing medical conditions require psychosocial support and the opportunity to find humor in even the most scary or unfortunate of situations.

  * All cases are sanitized to ensure confidentiality.

References

Adkins, T. (2018). Why I dance with my patients—Joy is contagious. Retrieved November 30, 2020, from https://www.medpagetoday.com/primarycare/generalprimarycare/75492

Association of Child Life Professionals. (2018). Association of child life professionals position statement on child life practice in community settings. Retrieved December 7, 2020, from https://www.childlife.org/docs/default-source/about-aclp/cbp-on-cl-practice-in-community-settings.pdf

Astedt-Kurki, P., & Isola, A. (2001). Humour between nurse and patient and among staff: Analysis of nurses' diaries. *Journal of Advanced Nursing, 35*, 452–458.

Auerbach, S., Hofmann, J., Platt, T., & Ruch, W. F. (2014). An investigation of the emotions elicited by hospital clowns in comparison to circus clowns and nursing staff. *European Journal of Humour Research, 1*(3), 26–53. https://doi.org/10.5167/uzh-92698

Beer, L. E., & Lee, K. V. (2017). Music therapy and procedural support: Opportunities for practice. *Music and Medicine, 9*(4), 262–268.

Beickert, K., & Mora, K. (2017). Transforming the pediatric experience: The story of child life. *Pediatric Annals, 46*(9), 345–351.

Bell, N. J., McGhee, P. E., & Duffey, N. S. (1986). Interpersonal competence, social assertiveness and the development of humour. *British Journal of Developmental Psychology, 4*(1), 51–55. https://doi.org/10.1111/j.2044-835X.1986.tb00997.x

Bennett, P. N., Parsons, T., Ben-Moshe, R., Weinberg, M., Neal, M., Gilbert, K., et al. (2014). Laughter and humor therapy in dialysis. *Seminars in Dialysis, 27*(5), 488–493.

Birnie, K. A., Chambers, C. T., & Spellman, C. M. (2017). Mechanisms of distraction in acute pain perception and modulation. *Pain, 158*(6), 1012–1013.

Bukola, I. M., & Paula, D. (2017). The effectiveness of distraction as procedural pain management technique in pediatric oncology patients: A meta-analysis and systematic review. *Journal of Pain and Symptom Management, 54*(4), 589–600.

Catarozoli, C., Brodzinsky, L., Salley, C. G., Miller, S. P., Lois, B. H., & Carpenter, J. L. (2019). Necessary adaptations to CBT with pediatric patients. In R. D. Friedberg & J. K. Paternostro (Eds.), *Handbook of cognitive behavioral therapy for pediatric medical conditions* (pp. 103–117). Springer.

Child Life Council. (2006). Child life services. *Pediatrics, 118*(4), 1757–1763.

Christensen, M. (2020). Humanizing healthcare through humor: Or how medical clowning came to be. *TDR/The Drama Review, 64*(3), 52–66.

Compas, B. E., Jaser, S. S., Dunn, M. J., & Rodriguez, E. M. (2012). Coping with chronic illness in childhood and adolescence. *Annual Review of Clinical Psychology, 8*, 455–480.

Consoli, A. J., Blears, K., Bunge, E. L., Mandil, J., Sharma, H., & Whaling, K. M. (2018). Integrating culture, pedagogy, and humor in CBT with anxious and depressed youth. *Practice Innovations, 3*(2), 138.

Craun, S. W., & Bourke, M. L. (2014). The use of humor to cope with secondary traumatic stress. *Journal of Child Sexual Abuse: Research, Treatment, & Program Innovations for Victims, Survivors, & Offenders, 23*(7), 840–852. https://doi.org/10.1080/10538712.2014.949395

Crosling, G., Heagney, M., & Thomas, L. (2009). Improving student retention in higher education: Improving teaching and learning. *Australian Universities' Review, 51*(2), 9–18.

Darlington, A., Randall, D., Leppard, L., & Koh, M. (2021). Palliative and end of life care for a child: Understanding parents' coping strategies. *Acta Paediatrica, 110*(2), 673–681. https://doi.org/10.1111/apa.15429

Dean, R. A. K., & Major, E. (2008). From critical care to comfort care: The sustaining value of humour. *Journal of Clinical Nursing, 17*, 1088–1095.

Dionigi, A., Flangini, R., & Gremigni, P. (2012). Clowns in hospitals. In P. Gremigni (Ed.), *Humor and health promotion* (pp. 213–227). Nova Science Publishers.

Dionigi, A., & Canestrari, C. (2018). The use of humor by therapists and clients in cognitive therapy. *The European Journal of Humour Research, 6*(3), 50–67. https://doi.org/10.7592/EJHR2018.6.3.dionigi

Dowling, J. S., & Hockenberry, M. (2003). Sense of humor, childhood cancer stressors, and outcomes of psychosocial adjustment, immune function, and infection. *Journal of Pediatric Oncology Nursing, 20*(6), 271–292. https://doi.org/10.1177/1043454203254046

Dress, M., Kreuz, R., Link, K., & Caucci, G. (2008). Regional variation in the use of sarcasm. *Journal of Language and Social Psychology, 27*, 71–85. https://doi.org/10.1177/0261927X07309512

Dziegielewski, S. F., Jacinto, G. A., Laudadio, A., & Legg-Rodriguez, L. (2003). Humor: An essential communication tool in therapy. *International Journal of Mental Health, 32*(3), 74–90.

Eckstein, D., Junkins, E., & McBrien, R. (2003). Ha, ha, ha: Improving couple and family healthy humor (healthy humor quotient). *The Family Journal: Counseling and Therapy for Couples and Families, 11*(3), 301–305. https://doi.org/10.1177/1066480703252869

Finlay, F., Baverstock, A., & Lenton, S. (2014). Therapeutic clowning in paediatric practice. *Clinical Child Psychology and Psychiatry, 19*(4), 596–605.

Fox, C., Dean, S., & Lyford, K. (2013). Development of a humor styles questionnaire for children and young people. *Humor: International Journal of Humor Research, 26*, 295–319. https://doi.org/10.1037/t25581-000

Francis, L., Monahan, K., & Berger, C. (1999). A laughing matter? The uses of humor in medical interactions. *Motivation and Emotion, 23*(2), 155–174.

Friedberg, R. D., & McClure, J. M. (2015). *Clinical practice of cognitive therapy with children and adolescents: The nuts and bolts.* Guilford Press.

Fritz, H. L. (2020). Coping with caregiving: Humor styles and health outcomes among parents of children with disabilities. *Research in Developmental Disabilities, 104*, 1–13. https://doi.org/10.1016/j.ridd.2020.103700

Griffiths, L. (1998). Humour as resistance to professional dominance in community mental health teams. *Sociology of Health and Illness, 20*, 874–895.

Hackathorn, J., Garczynski, A. M., Blankmeyer, K., Tennial, R. D., & Solomon, E. D. (2011). All kidding aside: Humor increases learning at knowledge and comprehension levels. *Journal of the Scholarship of Teaching and Learning, 11*(4), 116–123.

Hart, R., & Rollins, J. (2011). *Therapeutic activities for children and teens coping with health issues.* Wiley.

Hilliard, M. E., Harris, M. A., & Weissberg-Benchell, J. (2012). Diabetes resilience: A model of risk and protection in type 1 diabetes. *Current Diabetes Reports, 12*(6), 739–748.

Hofmann, J., Carretero-Dios, H., & Carrell, A. (2018). Assessing the temperamental basis of the sense of humor: Adaptation of the English language version of the state-trait cheerfulness inventory long and standard form. *Frontiers in Psychology, 9*, 2255. https://doi.org/10.3389/fpsyg.2018.02255

Hussong, D. K., & Micucci, J. A. (2021). The use of humor in psychotherapy: Views of practicing psychotherapists. *Journal of Creativity in Mental Health, 16*, 77–94. https://doi.org/10.1080/15401383.2020.1760989

Jiang, T., Li, H., & Yubo, H. (2019). Cultural differences in humor perception, usage, and implications. *Frontiers in Psychology, 10*, 123. https://doi.org/10.3389/fpsyg.2019.00123

Koller, D., & Gryski, C. (2008). The life threatened child and the life enhancing clown: Towards a model of therapeutic clowning. *Evidence-based Complementary and Alternative Medicine, 5*(1), 17–25.

Kuiper, N. A. (2012). Humor and resiliency: Towards a process model of coping and growth. *Europe's Journal of Psychology, 8*(3), 475–491. https://doi.org/10.5964/ejop.v8i3.464

Kuiper, N. A., Grimshaw, M., Leite, C., & Kirsh, G. (2004). Humor is not always the best medicine: Specific components of sense of humor and psychological well-being. *Humor: International Journal of Humor Research, 17*(1/2), 135–168.

Lerwick, J. L. (2016). Minimizing pediatric healthcare-induced anxiety and trauma. *World Journal of Clinical Pediatrics, 5*(2), 143.

Leyenaar, J. K., Ralston, S. L., Shieh, M., Pekow, P. S., Mangione-Smith, R. M., & Lindenaur, P. K. (2016). Epidemiology of pediatric hospitalizations at general hospitals and freestanding children's hospitals in the United States. *Journal of Hospital Medicine, 11*(11), 743–749.

Linehan, M. M. (1993). *Cognitive-behavioral treatment of borderline personality disorder.* Guilford Press.

Linge-Dahl, L. M., Heintz, S., Ruch, W., & Radbruch, L. (2018). Humor assessment and interventions in palliative care: A systematic review. *Frontiers in Psychology, 9*, 890. https://doi.org/10.3389/fpsyg.2018.00890

Lookabaugh, S., & Ballard, S. M. (2018). The scope and future direction of child life. *Journal of Child and Family Studies, 27*(6), 1721–1731.

Louie, D., Brook, K., & Frates, E. (2014). The laughter prescription: A tool for lifestyle medicine. *American Journal of Lifestyle Medicine, 10*(4), 262–267. https://doi.org/10.1177/1559827614550279

Macartney, G., Stacey, D., Harrison, M. B., & VanDenKerkhof, E. (2014). Symptoms, coping, and quality of life in pediatric brain tumor survivors: A qualitative study. *Oncology Nursing Society, 41*(4), 390–398. https://doi.org/10.1188/14.onf.390-398

Mangelsdorf, S. N., Conroy, R., Mehl, M. R., Norton, P. J., & Alisic, E. (2019). Listening to family life after serious pediatric injury: A study of four cases. *Family Process, 59*(3), 1191–1208. https://doi.org/10.1111/famp.12490

Martin, R. A., Puhlik-Doris, P., Larsen, G., Gray, J., & Weir, K. (2003). Individual differences in uses of humor and their relation to psychological well-being: Development of the humor styles questionnaire. *Journal of Research in Personality, 37*, 48–75.

Masten, A. S. (2001). Ordinary magic: Resilience processes in development. *The American Psychologist, 56*, 227–238.

McGhee, P. E., & Frank, M. (2014). *Humor and children's development: A guide to practical applications.* Routledge.

McMahan, S. (2008). Infinite possibility: Clowning with elderly people. *Care Management Journal, 9*(1), 19–24.

Mesmer-Magnus, J., Glew, D. J., & Chockalingam, V. (2012). A meta-analysis of positive humor in the workplace. *Journal of Managerial Psychology, 27*(2), 155–190.

Moola, F. J., Moothathamby, N., Naganathan, M., Curran, C. J., Yerichuk, D., & McPherson, A. C. (2020). A scoping review of music therapy in the lives of children and youth with disabilities and chronic conditions in non-acute medical and community-based settings: A novel consideration for art therapists? *Canadian Journal of Art Therapy, 33*(1), 17–28.

Moran, C. C. (2002). Humor as a moderator of compassion fatigue. In C. R. Figley (Ed.), *Treating compassion fatigue.* New York, NY.

Mora-Ripoll, R. (2011). Potential health benefits of stimulated laughter: A narrative review of the literature and recommendations for future research. *Complementary Therapies in Medicine, 19*, 170–177. https://doi.org/10.1016/j.ctim.2011.05.003

Nusbaum, E. C., Silvia, P. J., & Beaty, R. E. (2017). Ha ha? Assessing individual differences in humor production ability. *Psychology of Aesthetics, Creativity, and the Arts, 11*(2), 231.

Pérez-Aranda, A., Hofmann, J., Feliu-Soler, A., Ramírez-Maestre, C., Andrés-Rodríguez, L., Ruch, W., & Luciano, J. V. (2018). Laughing away the pain: A narrative review of humour, sense of humour and pain. *European Journal of Pain, 23*(2), 220–233. https://doi.org/10.1002/ejp.1309

Sánchez, J. C., Echeverri, L. F., Londoño, M. J., Ochoa, S. A., Quiroz, A. F., Romero, C. R., & Ruiz, J. O. (2017). Effects of a humor therapy program on stress levels in pediatric inpatients. *Hospital Pediatrics, 7*(1), 46–53. https://doi.org/10.1542/hpeds.2016-0128

Savage, B. M., Lujan, H. L., Thipparthi, R. R., & DiCarlo, S. E. (2017). Humor, laughter, learning, and health! A brief review. *Advances in Physiology Education, 41*, 341–347. https://doi.org/10.1152/advan.00030.2017

Sayre, J. (2001). Use of aberrant medical humor by psychiatric unit staff. *Issues in Mental Health Nursing, 22*, 669–689.

Schermer, J. A., Rogoza, R., Kwiatkowska, M. M., et al. (2019). Humor styles across 28 countries. *Current Psychology.* https://doi.org/10.1007/s12144-019-00552-y

Schiffman R. (2020). Laughter may be effective medicine for these trying times. Retrieved December 1, 2020, https://www.nytimes.com

Sridharan, K., & Sivaramakrishnan, G. (2016). Therapeutic clowns in pediatrics: A systematic review and meta-analysis of randomized controlled trials. *European Journal of Pediatrics, 175,* 1353–1360. https://doi.org/10.1007/s00431-016-2764-0

Stephson A. J. (2017, February). Benefits of Medical Clowning: A Summary of the Research. Medicalclownproject.org. Retrieved from https://medicalclownproject.org/wp-content/uploads/2020/04/Benefits-Medical-Clowning-White-Paper-2017-Final.pdf

Stuber, M., Hilber, S. D., Mintzer, L. L., Castaneda, M., Glover, D., & Zelter, L. (2009). Laughter, humor, and pain perception in children: A pilot study. *Evidence-based Complementary and Alternative Medicine, 6*(2), 271–276. https://doi.org/10.1093/ecam/nem097

Sturgeon, J. A., & Zautra, A. J. (2016). Social pain and physical pain: Shared paths to resilience. *Pain Management, 6*(1), 63–74.

Sultanoff, S. M. (2013). Integrating humor into psychotherapy: Research, theory, and the necessary conditions for the presence of therapeutic humor in helping relationships. *The Humanistic Psychologist, 41*(4), 388–399. https://doi.org/10.1080/08873267.2013.796953

Tasker, S. L., & Stonebridge, G. G. S. (2016). Siblings, you matter: Exploring the needs of adolescent siblings of children and youth with cancer. *Journal of Pediatric Nursing, 31,* 712–722.

Watson, S. (2008). Clowning around sets patients at ease. *CMAJ, 179*(4), 313–315.

Watson, K. (2011). Gallows humor in medicine. *Hastings Center Report, 41*(5), 37–45.

Wu, Y. P., Aylward, B. S., & Roberts, M. C. (2014). Cross-cutting issues in pediatric psychology. In M. C. Roberts, B. S. Aylward, & Y. P. Wu (Eds.), *Clinical practice of pediatric psychology* (pp. 32–45). Guilford Press.

Chapter 5
Cognitive Behavioral Play Therapy

Susan M. Knell

Keywords Cognitive behavioral play therapy · Play therapy · Psychotherapy with young children

5.1 Introduction

Cognitive Behavioral Play Therapy (CBPT) integrates cognitive behavioral and play therapies and is based on empirically supported cognitive and behavioral interventions that are incorporated into play. Materials that are appropriate for the child's developmental level are used. By using puppets, stuffed animals, books, and other toys, the therapy is suitable for young children. Modeling allows the therapist to present coping strategies, problem solving, and numerous other interventions to the child via play.

For children to benefit from Cognitive Behavioral Therapy (CBT), it must be adapted for their developmental age. Since pre-operational children are self-centered and concrete by nature, CBT must be modified so that it does not rely on sophisticated language and the use of logic. The theory is the same, namely that our beliefs and thoughts influence our behavior and emotions, the interpretations and perceptions of our environment, and maladaptive beliefs are common in individuals experiencing psychological distress (Beck, 1976). The difference between CBT and CBPT is that interventions are adapted for the developmental level of the child, and largely presented through modeling (Knell, 2009). There is emerging empirical support for the use of CBPT with young (ages 2.5–8 years) children.

S. M. Knell (✉)
Private Practice, Highland Heights, OH, USA

R. D. Friedberg, E. V. Rozmid (eds.), *Creative CBT with Youth*,
https://doi.org/10.1007/978-3-030-99669-7_5

5.2 Foundations

5.2.1 Behavioral Therapy

Behavioral interventions have been shown to be effective with children. These approaches work to modify maladaptive behaviors and identify the factors that reinforce and maintain them. Many behavioral interventions are designed to be implemented by an adult to help a child. However, these interventions can be incorporated into CBPT, so that the child is directly involved with the therapist. The child's direct involvement in change is considered important, particularly in regard to behaviors that are specifically controlled by the child (e.g., eating, elimination). Mastery and control are significant milestones in child development and are considered critical in terms of the child's emerging independence. Whether the therapy is delivered by another adult, or directly implemented with the child in therapy, the therapist tries to identify factors that reinforce and maintain problematic behaviors.

Table 5.1 provides a summary of the behavioral techniques that can be used in CBPT. These include positive reinforcement, shaping, systematic desensitization, stimulus fading, extinction/differential reinforcement of other behavior (DRO), time-out, self-monitoring, exposure with response prevention, activity scheduling, and relaxation training. It is critical that the CB therapist is familiar with these interventions and comfortable using them in play therapy.

5.2.2 Cognitive Therapy

Cognitive therapy was developed as a structured, focused approach to help individuals make changes in their behavior by changing thoughts and perceptions that underly the behaviors. Originally developed as a short-term, present-oriented therapy for depressed adults, the treatment was directed towards changing dysfunctional thinking and behavior (Beck, 1964). Cognitive interventions are effective with children, but often involve more modifications to make them developmentally appropriate. The method of delivering cognitive interventions to children is different than with adults, but the theorical underpinnings are the same (Knell & Dasari, 2011).

The cognitive techniques used through play, provided in Table 5.2, are identifying dysfunctional thoughts, cognitive change strategies/ countering irrational (maladaptive) beliefs, positive self-statements, bibliotherapy, problem solving, and psycho-education.

Table 5.1 Examples of behavioral interventions in CBPT

Positive reinforcement	A puppet who is afraid talk to her teacher gets a sticker for each time she speaks
Shaping	A puppet begins to get closer and closer to talking, and is given a sticker for making utterances, speech sounds, words, and gradually talking. The puppet is getting reinforced for closer and closer approximations (shaping) to talking
Systematic desensitization	A stuffed animal is fearful of the elevator, so systematically goes through the hierarchy (from least to most feared) while simultaneously engaging in relaxing and playful interactions (mutually exclusive with anxiety)
Stimulus fading	A puppet is clingy and upset if father is saying goodnight to her, but able to go to bed easily if mother does the nighttime routine. The mom puppet is gradually faded into the background as dad becomes the parent doing the nighttime routine
Extinction/DRO	A stuffed animal is aggressive with other animals, and does not receive positive reinforcement while aggressive (extinction), but as she exhibits more adaptive behaviors (e.g., playing calmly, sharing) these behaviors are rewarded (DRO)
Time-out	A puppet who is throwing toys at his friends is put in time out away from friends
Self-monitoring	A toy car marks feelings on a scale from frowning to smiling to express his feelings
Exposure/response prevention	A stuffed animal is afraid to use the toilet because she might fall in is gently held on the toilet (exposure) while not being allowed to fall in (response prevention)
Activity scheduling	A puppet who is withdrawing from others is engaged in activities
Relaxation training	A puppet is taught to do deep breathing and practices it with the therapist and other puppets

Table 5.2 Examples of cognitive interventions in CBPT

Identifying dysfunctional thoughts	A puppet draws pictures in a notebook or otherwise records feelings about particular situations
Cognitive change strategies/countering maladaptive beliefs	A puppet says that no one likes her because she was teased. The puppet is taken through the process of examining this, talking about her friends, and how they feel about her, exploring reasons, and trying to make friendships with other puppets
Positive self-statements	A stuffed animal who is afraid to talk in class is helped to make positive statements, "I can talk to my friends"; "It will be nice to talk with them"
Bibliotherapy	A puppet who has divorced parents is read a book about another puppet in that situation
Problem solving	A stuffed animal who is struggling going back and forth between his divorced parents, talks out loud about how he could do this; strategies are discussed and explored
Psychoeducation	A puppet is guided through matching feeling faces with words for those emotions

5.2.3   Integration of Behavior and Cognitive Therapies

It is important to know and understand how behavioral and cognitive interventions can be used and incorporated into CBPT. Once the practitioner is familiar with these interventions, the next step is understanding how they can be incorporated into play. Integrating CB interventions into play communicates concepts without complex verbalizations. Knell and her colleagues have demonstrated such communication through play (Dasari & Knell, 2015; Knell, 1993a, b, 1994, 1997, 1998, 1999, 2000, 2009; Knell & Moore, 1990; Knell & Ruma, 1996, 2003; Knell & Dasari, 2006, 2009).

The clinical efficacy of CBPT (Knell, 1993a) can be expressed by six specific characteristics:

1. Involves the child in therapy through play. So, the child is an active participant, and the problems of resistance and lack of compliance can be more easily addressed. In addition, the therapist can address the child's problems directly, rather than through a parent or significant adult.
2. Focuses on the child's thoughts, feelings, fantasies, and environment. By paying attention to the child's world, the therapist acknowledges that the people, places, and activities the child experiences play a critical role in the development and maintenance of behaviors.
3. Proposes a strategy, or strategies, for the development of adaptive thoughts and behaviors that can help the child deal with situations and feelings. One goal is for the child to replace maladaptive beliefs with more positive adaptive thoughts in order to better cope.
4. It is a structured, directive, and goal-oriented therapy rather than open-ended. Mainly, the therapist works with the child and the family to set goals and helps them work towards achieving these goals.
5. Involves the use of empirically demonstrated techniques. Modeling is one of the most important techniques (Bandura, 1977), and can be easily implemented using puppets and dolls, or other toys. Quite simply, the therapist (via puppets/dolls/toys) models specific behaviors for the child, so that the child observes concrete examples. This, in fact, responds to the need for concrete and non-verbal demonstrations, particularly when addressing children of preschool age.
6. CBPT allows empirical control of treatment, so that both empirically supported treatments can be used, and in situations where possible, the treatment can be empirically studied.

5.2.4   Modeling

Modeling exposes the child to someone or something (e.g., character in a book, stuffed animal, or a toy) that serves as a model and demonstrates adaptive behaviors and coping strategies. According to Bandura (1969, 1976, 1977), modeling is regulated by interrelated subprocesses such as attention, retention, motoric reproduction, and reinforcement. These processes account for the acquisition and maintenance of observational learning or modeling. Considerable research has demonstrated how people quickly reproduce the actions, attitudes, and emotional responses exhibited by models (Bandura & Walters, 1963; Bandura, 1969; Flanders, 1968). Preschool children are able to induce abstract concepts from cognitive models and to generalize those concepts to unfamiliar tasks (Zimmerman & Lanaro, 1974).

In CBPT, modeling is applied through various tools such as puppets, therapeutic books, storytelling, and movies. For example, a puppet might verbalize problem solving skills, as the therapist speaks at every step: Providing an auditory stimulus and a concrete example for the observing child. At the same time, the therapist can comment out loud and address the issues raised by the puppet. Or, through storytelling, the child has the opportunity to learn models of positive and adaptive behavior through identification with the characters of the story.

A good example of modeling in CBPT is with a 5.5-year-old Terry[1] (first described in Knell & Moore, 1990; Knell, 1993a). Terry refused to use the toilet for bowel movements and was resistant to all parental efforts to finish his "toilet training." After an assessment, a stuffed bear who "pooped his pants" was introduced to Terry. Terry's reactions to the bear in play provided assessment information for the therapist and were used to develop the intervention. The therapist had the bear going through a similar contingency management program as the child (implemented for the child by the parents). In sessions, the bear received stickers, stars, and praise for appropriate toileting and non-soiled pants. The bear expressed maladaptive cognitive beliefs about his toileting which were designed to be like the child's expressed thoughts, and were gradually shaped to be more positive, adaptive self-statements. Thus, the bear's "treatment" was modeled for Terry, who interacted with the bear, and gradually began to exhibit more positive coping skills and toileting behaviors in sync with the bear's behavior and expressed thoughts. Modeling is the main way in which cognitive and behavioral interventions are demonstrated for the child. When one tries to enhance skills, a coping model is often used. Coping models display less than ideal skills and then gradually become proficient. This is contrasted with a mastery model, where the goal behavior is immediately exhibited. For example, a mastery model stops hitting/exhibits calm behavior, whereas a coping model begins to bring hands in to his body, holds them together, and says out loud things that will help with "gentle hands." Modeling is improved by the use of coping models (Bandura & Menlove, 1968; Meichenbaum, 1971). Although there is no clear information regarding when mastery models might be better than coping models, we do know that any type of modeling can be enhanced by positive reinforcement of the model for appropriate/desired behavior and use of models with whom the child identifies (e.g., by age, race, gender, etc.).

---

[1] This and all subsequent case examples have been scrubbed of any identifiable information.

5.2.5 Structured vs. Unstructured Play

One of the difficult aspects of CBPT for many therapists is how to manage structured vs unstructured play. The goal is to have a balance of both, with structured play possibly leading to more goal-directed activities and unstructured play, where the child brings spontaneous materials to the session. Often the more structured play can be incorporated into the session in a way that is mostly seamless. Examples might be reading a psychoeducational book while characters are enacting being in school, incorporating CB interventions into family play which the child has initiated, but where the therapist has characters introduce such interventions.

CBPT with Terry (encopretic child discussed in the previous section) provides good examples of structured and unstructured play in treatment. Although Terry was engaged and interested in the play, he likely would not have been as involved if therapy had been exclusively structured around the bear's encopresis. The therapist was able to engage Terry by introducing structure into his unstructured play. For example, the therapist introduced the bear as having difficulty "pooping on the potty" (identifying dysfunctional thoughts and behavior), helping the bear work his way, both behaviorally and verbally through using the toilet (exposure/response prevention; countering maladaptive cognitive beliefs), reinforcing the bear for his efforts (positive reinforcement), and ultimately having the bear model appropriate toilet use. These were all structured interventions that were interwoven into Terry's play with the bear and other stuffed animals.

5.2.6 Developmental Issues

CB interventions rely on sophisticated cognitive abilities (e.g., abstract thinking, hypothesis testing), and it is reasonable to question the young child's ability to participate in CBT. However, there is much evidence to suggest that children's ability to understand such interventions can be facilitated by providing them through more developmentally appropriate, accessible means. As such, the therapist can capitalize on the child's abilities, and use play and modeling through play as primary means to communicate some of the more complex CB interventions.

For example, in CBPT with a child who feels no one likes her, a puppet says, "no one likes me" and describes how she is teased. Through play, the puppet "examines" this belief by talking about her friends, and how they feel about her, exploring reasons, and trying to make friendships with other puppets. The therapist can voice some of the alternative explanations for the peers (e.g., Another puppet saying, "My mom was yelling at me, so I was mean to you"; "I teased you because I wish I had that backpack, it's nicer than mine" or other explanations that are derived from the information gathered from the child, parents, and teachers).

5.3 Treatment Description

The CBPT therapist attempts to:

1. Focus on the child's strengths and abilities, rather than weaknesses—play is the child's natural and developmentally appropriate means of communication, so that utilizing play as a communication with the therapist is a logical and natural modality.
2. Focus on experiential interventions that can be incorporated into play, rather than relying on complex verbal skills. When interventions are acted out with toys, the verbal component reinforces the intervention. In these situations, the child does not need to rely on understanding the verbal intervention or be able to express him/herself verbally.
3. Encourage and facilitate language development so that the child learns to describe experiences and emotions. Children are encouraged to learn to associate behaviors with feelings and to express feelings in more adaptive, language-based ways. For example, the child can understand that she is angry and can express that feeling in words (i.e., "I'm angry") rather than behavior (i.e., yelling or hitting). In moving to a more verbal mode of expression, the child can acquire a sense of control and mastery, as well as receive positive feedback from adults around them. For example, if the child is better able to use his words for feelings, and aggressive behavior begins to diminish, he will be showing mastery over those aggressive behaviors and will (hopefully) receive positive feedback for his calmer demeanor (thus reinforcing words rather than aggressive acts). In the previous case example, when Terry would become aggressive with the bear, it was possible to facilitate language development around his feelings, with statements such as, "I think you are angry because the bear…".

CBPT usually takes place in a playroom with traditional toys, art supplies, and books. (See Appendix 10.1 in Knell & Dasari, 2011 for a list of a well-stocked CBPT playroom). There are times when specific anxieties or phobias are best treated outside of a typical playroom, so that they can be approached in vivo. For example, working with a child with an elevator phobia would likely be done both in the playroom and with the therapist in and around a variety of elevators. A fear of being outside, because of bugs, would be better treated in a natural environment, and not in a playroom.

5.3.1 Stages

CBPT is divided into several phases (Knell, 1999), described as the introductory/orientation, assessment, middle, and termination stages.

5.3.2   Introductory/Orientation

The initial interview usually takes place with parents, without the child present, where the therapist gathers a history and background. Additionally, the therapist will help the family know how to prepare the child for the first session. The therapist uses a variety of means, including interviews with parents, bibliotherapy, and structured tasks to explain the therapeutic process to the child. Therapeutic objectives are also identified at this stage (Knell, 2009), and the role of parents and other significant adults are clarified. Parental work is typically an integral part of child assessment and treatment. The therapist can work directly with parents to help them manage child behaviors and establish treatment goals. Knell (1994) points out that although most of the CBPT's work is with the child, the therapist typically continues to schedule regular meetings with parents to support them and work with them towards the achievement of goals.

5.3.3   Assessment

Assessment always takes place at the beginning of treatment, but in many ways is an ongoing process. The therapist aims to define the concerns and develop a treatment plan. The parent interview is used as part of the assessment. In addition to the comprehensive history and background obtained, information is gathered regarding the parental perception of the problem and what has been tried to alleviate the issues. The assessment may also include parent report inventories (e.g., Child Behavior Checklist, Achenbach, 1991), and teacher information obtained via interview and/or teacher report forms (e.g., Teaching Rating Form (TRF)).

When the child is first seen, assessment may include more formal assessment (See Gitlin-Weiner et al., 2000 for such scales), observation of the child's verbalizations and play, and informal measures (e.g., The Puppet Sentence Completion task; Knell, 2018, 1992, 1993a; Knell & Beck, 2000) or therapist-created measures. During this stage, the therapist can collect baseline data (e.g., frequencies of behaviors), if appropriate. During the assessment phase, it is important to gather information regarding maladaptive thoughts that the child may have. These are often obtained via parent report, and through the child's verbalizations during play.

5.3.4   Middle

After a treatment plan is developed, therapy focuses on reinforcement of adaptive behaviors, in efforts to increase the child's self-control and sense of accomplishment, along with teaching the child more appropriate responses to dealing with specific situations. Depending on the presenting problem, the therapist chooses the most appropriate cognitive and behavioral interventions while engaging the child via play. The interventions must be evaluated carefully, with as much specificity as possible related to the intervention and the child's specific problems/concerns. Caregivers are often involved in the treatment. They may be taught the principles of CBPT, positive reinforcement/ time out, and other approaches to increase the desired behaviors.

The intermediate stage of therapy focuses on interventions to help the child develope adaptive responses to problems, circumstances, and stress factors. Interventions during this phase are often aimed at shifting negative thoughts and beliefs as well as adopting positive self-statements. These traditional cognitive interventions are adapted through tools that do not depend on the use of language, such as expressive arts, bibliotherapy, and semi-structured puppet play (Knell, 1998). Bibliotherapy is particularly useful in CBPT and can involve both published books and books that the child and therapist work on together. The characters in books can function as the model for the child, exhibiting coping skills and demonstrating how to make things better. Additionally, the book may normalize a situation for a child (e.g., "There are so many kids who are dealing with the divorce of a parent, they've written a book about it"). In non-published writings, children might draw pictures of their feelings or tell stories about a child or an animal who shares similar fears. The child observes models of behaviors and coping skills through a character, or interactive dialogue with a puppet (played by the therapist). There are many modes of conveying the CBT aspects of treatment to the child; limited only by the creativity and flexibility of the therapist. The therapist and the child work together to understand the fears and anxieties shared by the puppet and the child to develop affirmations and positive behaviors to help the child.

Towards the end of therapy, the therapist aims to help the child generalize what has been learned in therapy and to bring this "wisdom" back into the natural environment. The child will need to maintain these adaptive behaviors after treatment ends, and therefore promoting generalization should be part of the therapy. Therapy should also be geared to help prevent relapse (Meichenbaum, 1985). This often involves anticipating high risk or difficult situations that might arise and preparing the child and family for dealing with such situations.

5.3.5 Termination

The child and family should be prepared for the end of therapy. As treatment approaches its conclusion, the child may be dealing with feelings associated with losing the therapeutic relationship. The therapist should reinforce the positive changes that the child has made and organize therapy with the conclusion in mind. Generalization and response prevention, which may be introduced in the middle stages of therapy, are a primary focus in the termination phase. Flexibility is usually key. The therapist can gradually decrease therapy appointments with intermittent sessions, rather than having an abrupt end. During these occasional sessions, the therapist's focus should be on strengthening the learning that has been accomplished. Obviously, any new problems or concerns that arise during this time can be addressed.

5.4   Clinical Applications

By definition, CBPT is playful and there are really no limits to how an individual practitioner can approach each individual child. Play therapists are often, by nature individuals who enjoy getting down on the floor and playing with young children, and as such often capitalize on their own energy, humor, joyfulness, and ability to be "child-like" (in a good way!) Lowenstein (2016) described how creative, play-based activities, when presented within the context of a therapeutic relationship can enhance CBPT's effectiveness. Knell and Dasari (2009) describe a detailed approach for implementing and integrating CBPT into clinical practice.

Therapists may have favorite toys, but it is always important to choose toys that the child enjoys. A favorite toy in the playroom is often a magic wand. Shaking the wand, making a wish, expressing magical thoughts are all things that the therapist can use in positive ways. The child can make a wish at the end of the session which can be an important window into the child's fears and hopes. With parents, the therapist may inquire, "If I had a magic wand that really worked, what would you wish for, for your child?" Again, this may provide important insight into the family's wishes and hopes for their child.

Puppets are another favorite and have been used by play therapists since the early days of play therapy (Woltmann, 1940; Irwin, 1985). Although much of the play therapy literature focuses on puppets, some children do not enjoy them, and it is important to let the child influence the choice of toys. Toy cars and stuffed animals can easily be used as if they were puppets, and therapists need not do much adaptation to make any toy "work" in the CBPT setting.

Children will often identify with certain characters, like superheroes or positive cartoon characters. By integrating these characters and what they stand for into the play, the child can have a clear model of making good choices and doing positive things. The nature of the characters and how they are "super" is critical. Unfortunately, for many young children, characters with over- the -top strength and power, are not helpful models. For example, a child dealing with the struggle between right and wrong can begin to incorporate the powerful, at times aggressive stance of many of the traditional superheroes. This child may try to exert his own strength in negative, aggressive ways. Most play therapists have experienced children bringing strong characters into the playroom, and using them in negative ways (e.g., "I will squash you"; "I am going to kill you").

Sometimes it is important to consider alternatives to these all powerful/all- knowing superheroes. Rescue Heroes is an older (1999–2002) animated series (based on a toy line of the same name, later a movie, currently rebooted on YouTube) in which rescue personnel tried to save lives around the world from human -made and natural disasters. Calls for help came through a command center where team members (including both male and female rescuers) were dispatched to handle such situations. Personal disagreements were sometimes included, such that the group would demonstrate how to handle conflicts in a positive way. One of the most positive aspects of this series was that the characters were not exhibiting unnatural strength and prowess, but rather using their skills (e.g., as paramedics, firefighters) to "do good." This can be juxtaposed against some of the larger-than-life characters, such as Superman and Batman, the archetypal superheroes. Introducing Rescue Heroes or other positive characters can be critical for some children.

5.5 Case Examples

5.5.1 Clark

Clark was a 6-year-old boy referred because of behavioral issues in his private school classroom. At school, he was often non-compliant and defiant. He had difficulty separating from the parent who brought him to therapy, and often wanted to include his parents in his play. His play frequently portrayed good guys versus bad guys, with lots of violence and killing. His parents noted that they curtailed such play at home. When guided to make better choices, Clark stated that violence was good. This was counter to the messages he was getting at home. His behavior was often silly (in a negative way) and contrary. As therapy progressed, Clark used some of these themes to address issues. For example, he created a circus, in which there were many characters, representing a range of good behaving and problematic characters. As part of the circus, various individuals encouraged others to make positive choices and discourage (e.g., extinguish) negative/aggressive acts. The therapist would encourage various characters when they made positive choices by adding a high five, labeled praise about what they had done, or in some other way behavioral and verbally reinforce adaptive behaviors. Clark leaned towards the powerful characters to determine what direction the play should take, where the therapist encouraged calmer, more appropriate characters. Including the parents in his play, at various times, allowed Clark to involve them in the scenarios he created. A turtle puppet, who could slip into its shell, was used as part of the circus, as the turtle was shy (a term that Clark often used to identify himself) and did not always want to participate in circus activities. The therapist, and later Clark, guided the turtle in slowly feeling more comfortable interacting with the others. Often, the therapist would add positive self-statements for the turtle (e.g., "It feels good to join the others," "It might be scary at first, but I am happy when I join the circus activities"). Later in therapy, when Clark was struggling with "good sportsmanship" in real life, the play often involved games between the therapist and Clark, where he would "teach" good sportsmanship to one of his toys that was observing the game.

This case example shows that CBPT can be quite playful, and that the therapist can use the child's scenarios and issues to encourage characters (models) for the child to exhibit more adaptive and appropriate behaviors. The circus was Clark's idea and came from his spontaneous play. Introducing calmer, more adaptive behaviors to the characters was initiated by the therapist.

5.5.2   Walker

Walker was a 9-year-old boy diagnosed with OCD. His obsessions were extreme and often associated with violence, sexuality, and destruction. The family first consulted a child psychiatrist, and Walker was prescribed medication and CBPT. Walker had a difficult time discussing his obsessions, which he described as "part of his brain being himself, trying to control things, and the other part being controlled by negative forces." In his book, "Talking back to OCD," March (2007) describes how children can take control of their obsessive thoughts and fight back against their compulsive behaviors. His CBT approach to helping children with OCD, described earlier in March and Mulle (1998), puts them in charge of fighting the "bully" in their head. He suggests empowering children in many ways, including giving their OCD a nickname, and countering its maladaptive intrusive thoughts. Because of Walker's interest in war planes, and love of Mexican food, the therapist encouraged him to draw war planes dropping bombs on his obsessions. Walker pretended to be in charge of flying the planes, and ultimately dropping the bombs. He was encouraged to come up with a nickname for the powerful pilot, whom he labeled "General Salsa." General Salsa would drop bombs on the negative, intrusive thoughts. Walker could then write some of the obsessions on a piece of paper, and posing as General Salsa, stomp on the pages, and rip them up. The power and control that these acts provided helped Walker begin to "chase away'" his obsessions. Similarly, General Salsa would crush the compulsive behaviors and help Walker decrease the urges to act out these behaviors.

Walker used the "power" of General Salsa to begin to fight back against negative and intrusive obsessions. By using things that he loved (e.g., War planes, Mexican food), we helped Walker take on the powerful role in talking back to his obsessions.

5.6   Empirical Support for CBPT

A small, but growing body of research considers Cognitive Behavioral Play Intervention (CBPI) with young children. These interventions are not considered to be psychotherapy per se, but they incorporate a standardized three session protocol based on CBPT principles. This work was first introduced in Pearson's (2008) study utilizing CBPT for a non-clinical example of young children. In her study, teachers reported significantly higher hope and social competence in and fewer anxiety/withdrawal responses in children who received a CBPI intervention.

Fehr reported on the use of CBPI with children with sleep difficulties (Fehr et al., 2016), anxious feelings (Russ & Fehr, 2016) and adjustment in siblings of children with cancer (Fehr et al., 2017). There are also ongoing studies using CBPT with school adjustment and with siblings of children with Autism Spectrum Disorder (ASD) (Personal communication, Fehr, 2020). Although not specifically psychotherapy, these studies are some of the first to empirically support CBP techniques and strategies.

The importance of this preliminary work suggests that CBPI can be used to improve children's adjustment. Given that it is short term (usually three sessions), administered individually or in groups, and targeting both non-clinical and clinical populations, it is an important contribution to the field.

From the perspective of actual psychotherapy, there is strong empirical support for the effectiveness of play therapy with young children (PT-Bratton & Ray, 2000; Bratton et al., 2005; Davenport & Bourgeois, 2008; LeBlanc & Ritchie, 2001). Many of the previous studies did not differentiate among the various theoretical orientations to PT. Given the differences among approaches to PT (e.g., non-directive vs. directive), it is important to utilize as much specificity as possible to understand the findings related to CBPT with young children.

Research has demonstrated that CBT with older children and adolescents is efficacious for a variety of psychological diagnoses (e.g., Compton et al., 2004; Weisz & Kazdin, 2010). Much less research exists when using CBT with young children (under the age of 8) or when integrating CBT with play therapy (e.g., CBPT).

Case reports have described effective adaptations of CBT with younger children (Scheeringa et al., 2007; Miller & Feeny, 2003) although most of these studies do not have a play component. A meta-analysis reviewed studies of CBT with young children (Reynolds et al., 2012). They found that children 4–8 years old, who received CBT displayed better outcomes than no intervention or wait list control children. When compared with 9–18-year-old children, the effectiveness of CBT was not as robust as with the younger population. It seems likely that adding a play component to CBT would increase its effectiveness, but this has not been demonstrated.

Introducing more developmentally appropriate interventions, particular ones that are play based, should increase the effectiveness of CBT protocols as currently used with older children. Trauma Focused Cognitive Behavioral Therapy (TF-CBT), developed by Cohen and colleagues (e.g., Cohen et al., 2000, 2012), is an empirically based intervention used to help children and adolescents recover from trauma. Drewes and Cavett (2012) have developed a CBT intervention that integrated TF-CBT with play for young children.

Knell and colleagues have provided many examples of case reports with CBPT and young children. Presenting problems include: Anxiety (Knell, 1993a, 2000; Dasari & Knell, 2015; Knell & Dasari, 2016,), Behavioral Problems (Knell, 2000), Divorce (Knell, 1993a; Knell, 2003), Fears and phobias (Knell, 1993a; Knell & Dasari, 2006, 2009), Selective Mutism (Knell, 1993a, b; Knell & Dasari, 2011),

Separation Anxiety (Knell, 2000, Knell & Dasari, 2006), Toileting issues and encopresis (Knell & Moore, 1990; Knell, 1993a), and Sexual abuse (Ruma, 1993; Knell & Ruma, 1996, 2003).

One extremely important aspect in understanding any CBPT study involves the use of the term CBPT (which is often applied to studies that do not use a truly CB approach to PT). CBPT is a specific intervention that delivers empirically supported CB techniques using play as the medium. Many researchers are using the term as a catch-all for child therapy that incorporates specific goals and includes play. Given that there is no CBPT manual, there are a wide range of studies that have been labeled CBPT. Many do not truly capture the nature of CBPT and might best be called something else. The term CBPT should be used to describe child psychotherapy, utilizing play, that incorporates cognitive and behavioral interventions. The goals should be psychological in nature (e.g., not purely educational or academic) and should be only used to describe work done by a licensed mental health professional with appropriate training.

Another important consideration is the age range. Even though play is appropriately used with older children, studies of CBPT focusing on children over age 8 years are better categorized as CBT rather than CBPT (Although consideration of intellectual disability should be considered. Thinking of the developmental, rather than chronological age of the child will be critical in cases with older children. For example, a study by Kahveci (2017) used CBPT with a 14-year-old girl with Down syndrome and intellectual disability).

There are some studies that showed improvement after CBPT for children with externalizing behavior problems (Akbari & Rahmati, 2015; Zare & Ahmadi, 2020; Ashori & Bidgoli, 2018) and nighttime fears (Ebrahimi-Dehshiri & Mazaheri, 2011). Several of these studies are published in Arabic, with only an English abstract, making them fairly inaccessible to non-Arabic speaking individuals.

A number of studies described the use of CBPT in group settings with various populations. Included were children with inadequate social skills (Ashori & Yazdanipour, 2018), learning disabilities (Azizi et al., 2018), intellectual disabilities (Bana et al., 2017), self- esteem and social anxiety (Atayi et al., 2018), autism spectrum disorder (Rafati et al., 2016), loneliness and need for self-efficacy (Hadipoor & Akbari, 2017) and externalizing problems in street and working kids (Ghodousi et al., 2017). Although each of these studies documented improvement based on being in a CBPT (vs control) group, it is difficult to truly understand the actual treatments used. Most of these studies do not describe the treatment beyond the broad label of CBPT. Others describe treatment that does not really fall within the rubric of CBPT. For example, Bana et al. (2017) developed play modules, where each session was based on tasks like matching, improving fine motor skills, etc. Although self-esteem improvement was included as a goal of the hands-on skills, the treatment was not geared towards emotional and behavioral improvement, per se. CBPT, by definition, is a psychotherapy approach, not a means of promoting motor skills, cognitive functioning, etc. Furthermore, the children in the Bana et al. study were 8–12 years, which makes them older than the "target" age for CBPT.

Clearly, there is much need for further research in CBPT. Given the current empirical support for use of CBT with older children (ages 9 years and above) and play therapy (ages 3–8 years old) and many successful case studies using CBPT, it seems likely that the play component of CBPT may increase the effectiveness of CBT with younger children.

Future research should be designed to empirically study the use of CBPT with young children with a variety of presenting problems. A clear, concise definition of what constitutes CBPT (ideally a manual, which has yet to be developed) will be critical as a foundation for this research.

5.7 Conclusions

CBPT is a directive therapy focused on improving child behavior and the maladaptive thinking that may exacerbate such behavior. Knell (2009) observes that "cognitive distortions in very young children may be appropriate from the point of view of development, but maladaptive" (p. 119). It is for this reason that the term "maladaptive" seems more appropriate for use with children, as contrasted with the term "irrational" largely used with adults. CBPT focuses on shifting such maladaptive beliefs and cognitive biases and on strengthening adaptive thinking and behavior. The clinical implications of CBPT are based on the correspondence between the level of development of the child and the complexity of the intervention, emphasize the strengths of the child, and reduce the focus on complex linguistic tasks. It is empirical, encourages the development of language regarding feelings, helps the child to develop the correspondence between behaviors and feelings, and encourages the expression of maladaptive behaviors in more adaptive ways.

Finally, cognitive behavioral play therapy interventions are adapted to a child's developmental age. The modality is used as a means of communicating and teaching evidence-based techniques indirectly and as engagingly as possible to young children.

References

Achenbach, T. (1991). *Manual for the child behavior checklist/4–18 and 1991 profile*. University of Vermont, Department of Psychiatry.

Akbari, B., & Rahmati, F. (2015). The efficacy of cognitive behavioral play therapy on the reduction of aggression in preschool children with attention-deficit/hyperactivity disorder. *Journal of Child Mental Health, 2*(2), 93–100.

Ashori, M., & Bidgoli, F. D. (2018). The effectiveness of play therapy based on cognitive-behavioral model: Behavioral problems and social skills of pre-school children with attention deficit hyperactivity disorder. *Journal of Rehabilitation, 19*(2), 102–115. https://doi.org/10.32598/rj.19.2.102

Ashori, M., & Yazdanipour, M. (2018). Investigation of the effectiveness of group play therapy training with cognitive- behavioral approach on the social skills of students with intellectual disability. *Journal of Rehabilitation, 19*(3), 262–275.

Atayi, M., Razini, H. H., & Hatami, M. (2018). Effect of cognitive- behavioral play therapy in the self-esteem and social anxiety of students. *Journal of Research and Health, 8*(3), 278–285.

Azizi, A., Drikvand, F. M., & Sepahvandi, M. A. (2018). Effect of cognitive-behavioral play therapy on working memory, short-term memory and sustained attention among school-aged children with specific learning disorder: A preliminary randomized controlled clinical trial. *Current Psychology, 39*, 2306–2313.

Bana, S., Sajedi, F., Mirazaie, H., & Rezasoltani, P. (2017). The efficacy of cognitive behavioral play therapy on self esteem of children with intellectual disability. *Iranian Rehabilitation Journal, 15*(3), 235–242.

Bandura, A. (1969). *Principles of behavior modification*. Holt, Rinehart & Winston.

Bandura, A. (1976). Social learning theory. In J. T. Spence, R. C. Carson, & J. W. Thibaut (Eds.), *Behavioral approaches to therapy* (pp. 1–46). General Learning Press.

Bandura, A. (1977). *Social learning theory*. Prentice Hall, Englewood Cliffs.

Bandura, A., & Menlove, F. L. (1968). Factors determining vicarious extinction of avoidance behavior through symbolic modeling. *Journal of Personality and Social Psychology, 8*, 99–108.

Bandura, A., & Walters, R. H. (1963). *Social learning and personality development*. Holt, Rinehart & Winston.

Beck, A. (1964). Thinking and depression: II. Theory and therapy. *Archives of General Psychiatry, 10*, 561–571.

Beck, A. (1976). *Cognitive therapy and emotional disorders*. Meridian.

Bratton, S., & Ray, D. (2000). What the research shows about play therapy. *International Journal of Play Therapy, 9*(1), 47–88. https://doi.org/10.1037/h0089440

Bratton, S. C., Ray, D., Rhine, T., & Jones, L. (2005). The efficacy of play therapy with children: A meta-analytic review of the outcome research. *Professional Psychology: Research and Practice, 36*(4).

Cohen, J. A., Mannarino, A. P., Berliner, L., & Deblinger, E. (2000). Trauma-focused cognitive behavioral therapy for children and adolescents: An empirical update. *Journal of Interpersonal Violence, 15*(11), 1202–1223.

Cohen, J. A., Mannarino, A. P., & Deblinger, E. (Eds.). (2012). *Trauma focused CBT for children and adolescents: Treatment applications*. Guilford Press.

Compton, S. N., March, J. S., Brent, D., Albano, A. M., Weersing, V. R., & Curry, J. (2004). Cognitive-behavioral psychotherapy for anxiety and depressive disorders in children and adolescents: An evidence-based medicine review. *Journal of the American Academy of Child and Adolescent Psychiatry, 43*(8), 930–959.

Dasari, M., & Knell, S. M. (2015). Cognitive-behavioral play therapy for anxiety and phobias. In H. G. Kaduson & C. E. Schaefer (Eds.), *Short term play therapy for children* (3rd ed., pp. 25–52). Guilford.

Davenport, B. R., & Bourgeois, N. M. (2008). Play, aggression, the preschool child, and the family: A review of literature to guide empirically informed play therapy with aggressive preschool children. *International Journal of Play Therapy, 17*(1), 2–23.

Drewes, A. A., & Cavett, A. M. (2012). Play applications and skills components. In J. A. Cohen, A. P. Mannarino, & E. Deblinger (Eds.), *Trauma-focused CBT for children and adolescents: Treatment applications* (pp. 105–123). Guilford Press.

Ebrahimi-Dehshiri, V., & Mazaheri, M. A. (2011). Efficacy of cognitive-behavioral play therapy in reducing children's night-time fears. *Journal of Behavior Science, 5*(3), 253–259.

Fehr, K., Russ, S., Anderson, J., Leigh J. K., Cousino, M. (2017). Application of a cognitive-behavioral play intervention to pediatric populations: A pilot study for siblings of children diagnoses with cancer. In C. Sieberg (Chair), Behavioral interventions for pediatric health conditions: Results from prospective studies. Symposium presented at the annual meeting of the Association for Behavioral and Cognitive Therapies, San Diego, CA.

Fehr, K., Russ, S., & Ievers-Landis, C. (2016). Treatment of sleep problems in young children: A case series report of a cognitive-behavioral play intervention. *Clinical Practice in Pediatric Psychology, 4*(3), 306–317.

Flanders, J. P. (1968). A review of research on imitative behavior. *Psychological Bulletin, 69,* 316–337.

Ghodousi, N., Sajedi, F., Mirzaie, H., & Rezasoltani, P. (2017). The effectiveness of cognitive-behavioral play therapy on externalizing behavior problems among street and working children. *Iranian Rehabilitation Journal, 15*(4), 359–366.

Gitlin-Weiner, K., Sandrund, A., & Schaefer, C. (2000). *Play diagnosis and assessment* (2nd ed.). Wiley.

Hadipoor, S., & Akbari, B. (2017). Effectiveness of cognitive behavioral play therapy on self-efficacy and loneliness of primary school students with learning difficulties. *Middle Eastern Journal of Disability Studies, 7,* 64. Retrieved from https://jdisablistud.org/article-1-741-en.html

Irwin, E. C. (1985). Puppets in therapy: An assessment procedure. *American Journal of Psychotherapy, 39*(3), 389–400.

Kahveci, G. (2017). Cognitive behavioral play therapy in behavior consultation treatment: Making behavior changes from the inside out in down syndrome. *International Journal of Humanities and Education, 3*(2), 297–321.

Knell, S. M. (1992). The puppet sentence completion task. Unpublished manuscript.

Knell, S. M. (1993a). *Cognitive behavioral play therapy.* Jason Aronson.

Knell, S. M. (1993b). To show and not tell: Cognitive-behavioral play therapy in the treatment of elective mutism. In T. Kottman & C. Schaefer (Eds.), *Play therapy in action: A casebook for practitioners* (pp. 169–208). Jason Aronson.

Knell, S. M. (1994). Cognitive-behavioral play therapy. In K. O'Connor & C. E. Schaefer (Eds.), *Handbook of play therapy* (Advances and innovations) (Vol. 2, pp. 111–142). Wiley.

Knell, S. M. (1997). Cognitive-behavioral play therapy. In K. O'Connor & L. Mages (Eds.), *Play therapy theory and practice: A comparative presentation* (pp. 79–99). John Wiley and Sons.

Knell, S. M. (1998). Cognitive-behavioral play therapy. *Journal of Clinical Child Psychology, 27,* 28–33.

Knell, S. M. (1999). Cognitive-behavioral play therapy. In S. W. Russ & T. Ollendick (Eds.), *Handbook of psychotherapies with children and families* (pp. 385–404). Plenum.

Knell, S. M. (2000). Cognitive-behavioral play therapy with children with fears and phobias. In H. G. Kaduson & C. E. Schaefer (Eds.), *Short term therapies with children* (pp. 3–27). NY: Guilford.

Knell, S.M. (2003). Cognitive-Behavioral Play therapy. In C. E. Schaefer (Ed). *Foundations of Play therapy.* (pp 175–191). NY: Wiley.

Knell, S. M. (2009). Cognitive behavioral play therapy: Theory and applications. In A. Drewes (Ed.), *Blending play therapy with cognitive behavioral therapy: Evidence-based and other effective treatments and techniques* (pp. 117–133). Wiley.

Knell, S. M. (2018). Puppet sentence completion task. In A. A. Drewes & C. E. Schaefer (Eds.), *Puppets in play therapy: A practical guidebook* (pp. 59–73). Routledge Press.

Knell, S. M., & Beck, K. W. (2000). Puppet sentence completion task. In K. Gitlin-Weiner, A. Sandgrund, & C. E. Schaefer (Eds.), *Play diagnosis and assessment* (2nd ed., pp. 704–721). Wiley.

Knell, S. M., & Dasari, M. (2006). Cognitive-behavioral play therapy for children with anxiety and phobias. In H. G. Kaduson & C. E. Schaefer (Eds.), *Short term therapies with children* (2nd ed., pp. 22–50). Guilford.

Knell, S. M., & Dasari, M. (2009). CBPT: Implementing and integrating CBPT into clinical practice. In A. Drewes (Ed.), *Blending play therapy with cognitive behavioral therapy: Evidence-based and other effective treatments and techniques* (pp. 321–352). Wiley.

Knell, S. M., & Dasari, M. (2011). Cognitive-behavioral play therapy. In S. W. Russ & L. N. Niec (Eds.), *Play in clinical practice: Evidence-based approaches* (pp. 236–263). Guilford.

Knell, S. M., & Dasari, M. (2016). Cognitive behavioral play therapy for anxiety and depression. In L. A. Reddy, T. M. Files-Hall, & C. E. Schaefer (Eds.), *Empirically based play interventions for children* (2nd ed., pp. 77–94). American Psychological Association.

Knell, S. M., & Moore, D. J. (1990). Cognitive-behavioral play therapy in the treatment of encopresis. *Journal of Clinical Child Psychology, 19*(1), 55–60.

Knell, S. M., & Ruma, C. D. (1996). Play therapy with a sexually abused child. In M. Reinecke, F. M. Dattilio, & A. Freeman (Eds.), *Cognitive therapy with children and adolescents: A casebook for clinical practice* (pp. 367–393). Guilford.

Knell, S. M., & Ruma, C. D. (2003). Play therapy with a sexually abused child. In M. A. Reinecke, F. M. Dattilio, & A. Freeman (Eds.), *Cognitive therapy with children and adolescents: A casebook for clinical practice* (2nd ed., pp. 338–368). Guilford.

LeBlanc, M., & Ritchie, M. (2001). A meta-analysis of play therapy outcomes. *Counseling Psychology Quarterly, 14*, 149–163.

Lowenstein, L. (2016). *Creative CBT interventions for children with anxiety*. Champion Press.

March, J. S. (2007). *Talking back to OCD*. Guilford Press.

March, J. S., & Mulle, K. (1998). *OCD in children and adolescents: A cognitive-behavioral treatment manual*. Guilford Press.

Meichenbaum, D. A. (1971). Examination of model characteristics in reducing avoidance behavior. *Journal of Personality and Social Psychology, 17*, 298–307.

Meichenbaum, D. A. (1985). *Stress inoculation training*. Pergamon Press.

Miller, A. M., & Feeny, N. C. (2003). Modification of cognitive-behavioral techniques in the treatment of a five year-old girl with social phobia. *Journal of Contemporary Psychotherapy, 33*, 303–319.

Pearson, B. L. (2008). Effects of a cognitive behavioral play intervention on children's hope and school adjustment. Ph.D. thesis, Department of Psychology, Case Western Reserve University.

Rafati, F., Pourmohamadreza-Tajrishi, M., Pishyareh, E., Mirzaei, H., & Biglarian, A. (2016). Effectiveness of group play therapy on the communication of 5-8 year old children with high functioning autism. *Journal of Rehabilitation, 17*(3), 200–211.

Reynolds, S., Wilson, C., Austin, J., & Hooper, L. (2012). Effects of psychotherapy for anxiety in children and adolescents: A meta-analytic review. *Clinical Psychology Review, 32*(4), 251–262.

Ruma, C.D. (1993). Cognitive-behavioral play therapy with sexually abused children In Knell, S.M. Cognitive behavioral play therapy. (pp. 199–230). : Jason Aronson.

Russ, S., & Fehr, K. (2016). The use of pretend play to overcome anxiety in school age children. In A. Drewes & C. Schaefer (Eds.), *Play therapy in middle childhood* (pp. 77–95). American Psychological Association.

Scheeringa, M., Salloum, A., Arnberger, R. A., & Weems, C. F. (2007). Feasibility and effectiveness of cognitive-behavioral therapy for posttraumatic stress disorder in preschool children: Two case reports. *Journal of Traumatic Stress, 20*(4), 631–636. https://doi.org/10.1002/jts.20232

Weisz, J. R., & Kazdin, A. E. (Eds.). (2010). *Evidence-based psychotherapies for children and adolescents* (2nd ed.). The Guilford Press.

Woltmann, A. G. (1940). The use of puppetry in understanding children. *Mental Hygiene, 24*, 445–458.

Zare, M., & Ahmadi, S. (2020). The effectiveness of cognitive behavior play therapy on decreasing behavior problems of children. *Applied Psychology, 1*(3), 18–27.

Zimmerman, B. J., & Lanaro, P. (1974). Acquiring and retaining conservation of length through modeling and reversibility cues. *Merrill-Palmer Quarterly, 20*(3), 145–161.

Chapter 6
Incorporating Play into Cognitive Behavioral Therapy for Youth

Alayna L. Park and Rachel E. Kim

Keywords Cognitive behavioral therapy · Play · Therapy adaptation · Youth mental health · Common elements

6.1 Incorporating Play into Cognitive Behavioral Therapy for Youth

Psychotherapy is widely considered to be both a science and an art. There are thousands of clinical trials and hundreds of efficacious psychotherapy protocols for addressing a variety of youth social, emotional, and behavioral problems (Chorpita et al., 2011). These evidence-based treatments significantly improve youth well-being and functioning and outperform usual care delivered in public sector mental health settings (Weisz et al., 2013). At the same time, common or non-specific factors, such as therapeutic alliance, therapist expertise, therapist style (e.g., warmth, respect, empathy), and trust between a client and their therapist, substantially contribute to client outcomes (Huibers & Cuijpers, 2015). These findings suggest that children, adolescents, and families enrolled in mental health services may benefit from psychotherapy that is informed by the extensive evidence base and that explicitly attends to ways for promoting a positive client experience.

A. L. Park (✉)
Department of Psychology, University of Oregon, Eugene, OR, USA
e-mail: alaynap@uoregon.edu

R. E. Kim
Judge Baker Children's Center, Boston, MA, USA
e-mail: rkim@jbcc.harvard.edu

A promising approach for balancing the science and art of psychotherapy is to use psychotherapy practices that are supported by research evidence but to adapt the script for delivering those practices, as needed, based on the characteristics of the client and context (Chorpita & Daleiden, 2014; Kendall & Frank, 2018; Lau, 2006). The use of play is a natural strategy for adapting the youth psychotherapy process in a way that promotes a positive client experience. It is often easier and more comfortable for youth to express themselves through play than through oral or written dialogue (e.g., Ray et al., 2013). Play can also facilitate rapport building, psychological defusion (e.g., viewing specific thoughts and behaviors as problematic rather than viewing oneself as problematic), and knowledge and skill acquisition (Beidas et al., 2010; Briggs et al., 2011; Lieneman et al., 2017). Additionally, play can be enjoyable for both clients and their therapists.

In this chapter, we describe how to incorporate play into Cognitive Behavioral Therapy (CBT), an evidence-based treatment for many youth social, emotional, and behavioral problems. First, we provide an overview of CBT. Next, we propose a general process for incorporating play into CBT. We then offer ideas for delivering common CBT practices through the use of play. We conclude this chapter with a discussion of considerations for incorporating play into CBT with diverse clients and contexts.

6.2   Overview of Cognitive Behavioral Therapy (CBT)

CBT is one of the most widely researched and practiced psychosocial interventions for promoting youth well-being and functioning. More than 200 randomized clinical trials demonstrate the efficacy of CBT for treating youth anxiety, depression, disruptive behavior, eating problems, substance use, and traumatic stress (Chorpita et al., 2011; PracticeWise, 2020). CBT is a treatment family of time-limited (i.e., usually between 6 and 20 sessions), present-oriented, skills-based interventions that focus on the relationships between thoughts, feelings, and behaviors (Beck, 2011; Bunge et al., 2017). In CBT, clients initially learn to identify their thoughts (i.e., the words or images that pop into their mind), feelings (i.e., their emotions and/or physiological sensations), and behaviors (i.e., what they say or do). For example, in a situation where Alex sees a friend at the grocery store and waves, but Alex's friend does not wave back, Alex may have the thought, "My friend does not like me," experience the emotion of sadness and the physiological sensations of feeling cold and shaky, and then enact the behavior of ignoring a message sent by their friend later that day. Once clients are able to identify their thoughts, feelings, and behaviors, they are taught cognitive and behavioral skills for effectively responding to distressing situations, under the premise that changing an unhelpful thought or behavior will lead to more adaptive thoughts, feelings, and behaviors. Returning to the previous example, if Alex practices the cognitive skill of restructuring unhelpful thoughts to be more accurate, then they may generate the thought, "My friend did not see me," feel indifferent about the situation, and engage in an enjoyable conversation when their friend messages them later. Alex may also practice relaxation skills to soothe any physiological feelings of distress after their friend does not return their greeting, which may allow Alex to respond effectively to the situation rather than react emotionally. As another option, Alex may practice engaging in prosocial behavior, such as sending a friendly response to their friend's message, which may promote feelings of camaraderie and warmth, as well as test and potentially disprove their negative automatic thought.

6.3 Process for Incorporating Play into CBT

Play is commonly featured in youth CBT and other evidence-based treatment protocols. For instance, the *Coping Cat* program, an evidence-based treatment for child anxiety, recommends the use of fun activities, particularly in the first session, to build rapport, cultivate trust, and promote client engagement in their mental health treatment (Beidas et al., 2010). As another example, the developers of trauma-focused CBT (TF-CBT) suggest scheduling periodic free play or nondirective play during sessions to reward clients' willingness to engage in difficult work and to help clients regulate their emotions (Briggs et al., 2011). In Parent–Child Interaction Therapy (PCIT), caregivers play with their child and receive real-time coaching from their therapist on how to increase their child's positive behaviors (e.g., compliance, prosocial behaviors) and decrease their child's negative behaviors (e.g., temper tantrums, aggressive behaviors) (Lieneman et al., 2017). Additionally, many social skills programs call for children and adolescents to play games in small groups to learn and refine skills related to reading social cues, perspective taking, and social problem solving (Laugeson & Park, 2014).

Although many youth psychotherapy protocols encourage the use of play, there are not always clear guidelines on how to do this, or therapists may wish to incorporate play in ways other than what is specified in the protocol. To provide some guidance, we propose the following process for incorporating play into CBT:

1. *Develop an evidence-informed treatment plan.* There is an extensive evidence base on efficacious psychotherapies for children, adolescents, and families (Chorpita et al., 2011), so it seems efficient and logical to leverage it. There are dozens of youth CBT protocols that can be used to inform which psychotherapy practices therapists choose to implement with their clients. We have also included sample treatment plans featuring psychotherapy practices supported by research evidence in Fig. 6.1.
2. *Identify your session objective.* What do you want to accomplish in your next session? What do you want your client to learn? What skill do you want them to strengthen? Identifying a clear session objective will help you use play in a way that bolsters rather than detracts from your client's psychotherapy experience.
3. *Prepare a play activity for meeting your session objective.* We offer some ideas of play activities for delivering common CBT practices in the next section. If you

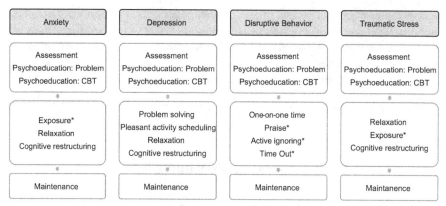

Note: *Practice is not described in this chapter but is commonly featured in evidence-based treatments for the corresponding problem area.

Fig. 6.1 Sample treatment plans. Note: *Practice is not described in this chapter but is commonly featured in evidence-based treatments for the corresponding problem area

Table 6.1 Examples of developmentally-appropriate activities

Activity	2–7 years old	7–13 years old	13–17 years old
Art	Finger painting, molding Play-Doh, drawing and coloring with crayons or washable markers	Drawing and coloring with colored pencils or glitter pens	Drawing and coloring with colored pencils or paint
Games	Playing Candy Land, Go Fish, Uno	Playing Connect Four, Jenga, Exploding Kittens	Playing Scrabble, Taboo, card games
Sports	Running, hopping or skipping, throwing and catching	Playing soccer, dancing, jumping rope	Playing baseball/softball, basketball, bowling
Toys	Playing with giant building blocks, dolls or trucks, simple jigsaw puzzles	Playing with Legos, Rubik's cube	Playing with Legos, 3-D puzzles

are creating your own play activity, consider whether your session objective will be best accomplished through structured or unstructured play (e.g., Bratton et al., 2009). Structured play works well for assessing presenting problems and skill competency, promoting self-expression, and teaching psychosocial concepts and skills. Unstructured play works well for building rapport, trust, and psychological safety. Choosing a developmentally appropriate activity that your client will likely find enjoyable is advised (e.g., an activity that they do with their friends) (see Table 6.1 for a list of developmentally appropriate arts and crafts activities, toys, games, and sports).

4. *Play!* Everyone involved is likely to have a more positive experience if you engage in the play activity with your client rather than simply observe them. If a solitary play activity is chosen, try to model the activity before asking your client to engage in the activity, provide enthusiastic descriptions or commentary of

their play, and look for opportunities to praise their use of skills during the play activity.

5. *Evaluate whether the activity was successful and adapt as needed.* Following the play activity, we encourage you to reflect on whether the session objective was achieved. Did the activity strengthen the client's understanding or use of the skill you were targeting? Did the client seem engaged in the session? Did the client seem to enjoy the play activity? If the answer to any of these questions is "no," then consider repeating steps 2–5 of this process with an adapted play activity.

6.4 Common CBT Practices and Play

There are several psychotherapy practices that are commonly featured in youth CBT protocols. In this section, we provide brief descriptions of some of these practices, as well as ideas for using play in practice delivery.

6.4.1 Assessment and Rapport Building

Assessment is typically the first procedure of any psychosocial intervention. This procedure involves gathering information about the youth's strengths, social, emotional, and academic functioning, and presenting problem. In addition to gathering information that will inform the case conceptualization (i.e., how the youth's thoughts, feelings, and behaviors contribute to their distress), a primary aim of assessment is to promote client engagement (Becker et al., 2018).

Accordingly, both unstructured and structured play can facilitate assessment. As a client and therapist get to know each other, they may engage in unstructured play (e.g., drawing or playing with building blocks) while the therapist casually asks the client questions about their family, friends, hobbies, favorite subject in school, and so forth. Unstructured play can also provide valuable information about the client's social functioning (e.g., Does your client interact with you as they play? Does your client offer to share?). Once some rapport is established, structured play can be very informative. For example, a therapist can ask a client to draw a picture of their family and then describe their relationship with each family member. This activity may provide insights into the client's social supports, as well as any potentially negative and unhelpful beliefs the client may hold (e.g., "My brother hates me"). Structured play can also provide helpful information about the client's compliance with requests from adults and ability to transition from one task to another. As an example, a therapist may ask to be handed a toy that the child client is playing with and may note the child's willingness to hand over the toy. This observation can help the therapist conceptualize the client's strengths and challenges and inform the treatment plan (e.g., if the client refuses to hand over the toy, then it may be beneficial to incorporate psychotherapy practices for addressing noncompliance into the treatment plan).

6.4.2 Psychoeducation about the Problem

The goal of providing psychoeducation about the problem is to promote a shared understanding of the client's social, emotional, or behavioral concerns. Psychoeducation about the problem usually involves normalizing the problem, dispelling any misconceptions, and providing information about what causes and maintains the problem (Becker et al., 2018). Increasing the client's understanding of the problem can help validate their experiences, enhance their engagement in psychotherapy, and even reduce symptomatology (Martinez et al., 2017). That said, it is easy for psychoeducation to become didactic.

Play enhances the process of psychoeducation by making it more interactive and enjoyable. One fun activity is to have a client envision and draw themselves as a superhero and their problem as a villain. The villain's abilities should be based on the nature of the problem (e.g., puts self-critical thoughts in others' minds; makes others feel down), with their power being fueled by stressful situations (e.g., the client being bullied at school or getting a bad grade on a test). The superhero's powers should initially be based on the client's strengths but grow as the client learns more cognitive and behavioral skills. This activity aims to create psychological distance between the client and their problem and instill hope that they will be able to better manage their problem with the help of psychotherapy.

As another example, psychoeducation about anxiety can be provided using the red light, green light game. Specifically, anxiety can be likened to an alarm system: just like a fire alarm warns us about a potential fire, feelings of anxiety warn us about potential danger. However, sometimes our anxiety alarm goes off when there is no danger—similar to how a fire alarm sometimes goes off when there is no fire (i.e., sound a false alarm). To help clients understand this concept, a therapist may brainstorm a series of situations that are cause for a real alarm, false alarm, or no alarm. For example, for a client who experiences social anxiety, a situation that may be cause for a real alarm is being bullied on the playground, a situation that may prompt a false alarm is hearing peers laughing at another student's silliness while the client asks a question in class, and a situation that may not necessitate an alarm is speaking with a sibling. As another example, for a client who experiences separation anxiety, a situation that may be cause for a real alarm is becoming separated from their caregiver at the zoo, a situation that may prompt a false alarm is being in a different room than their caregiver at home, and a situation that may not necessitate an alarm is playing with their caregiver. Within the context of the red light, green light game, the client can be instructed to run from the starting line when the therapist mentions a situation that is cause for a real alarm, walk when the therapist mentions a situation that may raise a false alarm, and stop when the therapist mentions a situation that is not cause for any alarm.

6.4.3 Psychoeducation about CBT

Psychoeducation about CBT is usually provided early in psychotherapy before starting to teach cognitive and behavioral skills. Psychoeducation about CBT aims to enhance the client's knowledge about CBT, specifically how CBT can help address the client's social, emotional, and behavioral concerns. This involves teaching the client that their thoughts, feelings, and behaviors are inter-related and that intervening on any one of these components can help the client respond to distressing situations more effectively.

An initial but crucial step of this work is to teach the client how to identify their thoughts, feelings, and behaviors. To build this skill, a therapist could brainstorm a list of thoughts (e.g., "I'm a loser," "I'm dumb," "No one likes me"), feelings (e.g., sad, scared, angry), and behaviors (e.g., watching TV, sleeping, yelling at a caregiver). The therapist could then set up a ball toss game, where the therapist reads a thought, feeling, or behavior from the list and instructs the client to toss the ball into the appropriately labeled bucket (e.g., if the therapist says, "mad," then the client should toss the ball into the bucket labeled "feelings").

To help a client understand the relationships between thoughts, feelings, and behaviors, a therapist may ask a client to draw a four-square comic—where the first square depicts a situation, the second square depicts a thought, the third square depicts a feeling, and the last square depicts a behavior. See Fig. 6.2 for an example.

Case Example. Lilah[1] is a 9-year-old, Mexican American girl. Lilah was referred for individual psychotherapy by her parents for frequent complaints of boredom, bouts of crying, low energy, and negative commentary about herself, such as "It's my fault when my parents argue" or "Other kids don't want to be friends with me because I'm boring." After starting the rapport building process, assessing the presenting problem, and identifying the family's treatment goals, Lilah's therapist determined that Lilah could benefit from CBT for depression and collaboratively developed a treatment plan with the family. Lilah's therapist introduced the connection between thoughts, feelings, and behaviors and decided to use play to reinforce this concept. Lilah's therapist set session objectives of (a) enhancing Lilah's ability to distinguish between thoughts, feelings, and behaviors; (b) building Lilah's insight into how thoughts, feelings, and behaviors are inter-related; and (c) improving Lilah's mood through engaging in a fun activity. To achieve these session objectives, Lilah's therapist planned a game of "CBT baseball," where each base represented thoughts, feelings, and behaviors. Lilah and her therapist played CBT baseball at a local park, but this game could be played in a traditional psychotherapy room with each corner representing a base. Lilah's therapist "pitched" by stating an example situation that would exacerbate negative mood. To advance bases, Lilah was tasked with providing an example of a thought, feeing, and behavior. Lilah was prompted to nominate a more adaptive thought or behavior to run to home base. As innings progressed, Lilah's therapist used example situations that were increasingly

---

[1] This case example is a composite of several clients, and the name has been changed.

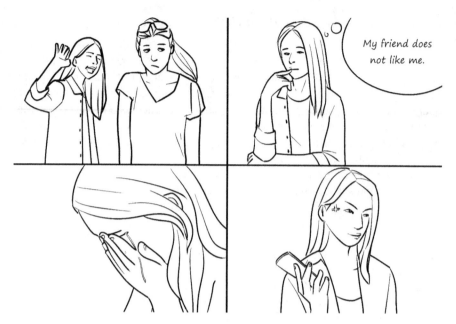

Fig. 6.2 Comic depicting the relationships between thoughts, feelings, and behaviors. (CC BY 4.0 Alayna Park)

similar to the challenges reported by Lilah and her parents during their assessment. In early innings, Lilah struggled to differentiate between thoughts and feelings (e.g., labeling sadness as a thought). Following some gentle correction from her therapist, Lilah began to distinguish between thoughts and feelings. She also presented as increasingly engaged and incrementally happier as the game progressed—indicating that CBT baseball was successful in achieving the therapist's session objectives.

6.4.4 Self-monitoring

Self-monitoring is a skill in which the client tracks a target behavior or the intensity of a target emotion over time. For example, a therapist may request that a caregiver document the number of temper tantrums that their child throws each week. As another example, a therapist may ask a client to rate how sad they feel on a scale ranging from 0 (not at all sad) to 10 (extremely sad) at the beginning of each psychotherapy session. Self-monitoring yields valuable information about a client's treatment progress and is associated with positive client outcomes at post-treatment (Borntrager & Lyon, 2015). Since ratings of emotional intensity are subjective, clients should create their own rating scale (e.g., thermometer, dial, or color gradient), with behavioral, physiological, and/or cognitive benchmarks that are meaningful to them. Please see Fig. 6.3 for an example. Therapists may reinforce the practice of

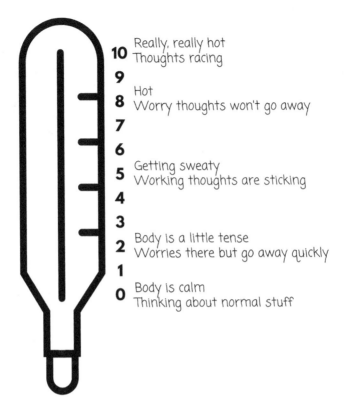

Fig. 6.3 Sample anxiety self-monitoring rating scale. (CC BY 4.0 Rachel Kim)

monitoring behaviors or emotions through play. For example, a therapist can prompt a client to rate their mood, then engage the client in a quick game, and afterwards direct the client to re-rate their mood, with the expectation that the client's mood would improve because of playing the game.

6.4.5   Cognitive Restructuring

Cognitive restructuring aims to help clients challenge negative or unhelpful beliefs and generate more realistic alternative thoughts. This skill usually involves teaching a client how to identify the words or images that pop into their mind, examine evidence for and against those thoughts, and then brainstorm an alternative interpretation that is more accurate, complete, and balanced. In one example, a client challenges their negative and unhelpful beliefs by pretending to be a detective and identifying other possible ways of interpreting ambiguous situations. Returning to the example where Alex waves to their friend who does not wave back, possible interpretations include: "My friend does not like me"; "My friend is mad at me";

"My friend did not see me"; "My friend did not recognize me"; "My friend was distracted"; and so forth—with some thoughts promoting more helpful feelings and behaviors than others. To reinforce a more accurate, complete, and balanced interpretation, a therapist could instruct the client to draw two four-square comics. The first comic should depict an ambiguous situation, unhelpful automatic thought, and consequent, usually maladaptive, feelings, and behaviors (please see Fig. 6.2). The second comic should depict the same ambiguous situation, helpful interpretation, and consequent, often adaptive, feelings, and behaviors (please see Fig. 6.4). These comics can help the client not only internalize the alternative interpretation but also reinforce the relationships between thoughts, feelings, and behaviors.

6.4.6 Pleasant Activity Scheduling

Pleasant activity scheduling (i.e., a primary component of behavioral activation) inherently involves play. This behavioral skill is based on the notion that engaging in enjoyable activities improves mood. Pleasant activity scheduling involves having a client identify pleasurable activities (e.g., activities that have been fun for the client in the past, involve spending time with a friend, or involve helping others), schedule a day and time to do the activity, and monitor their mood before, during, and after the activity. Activity ideas for young children include playing with

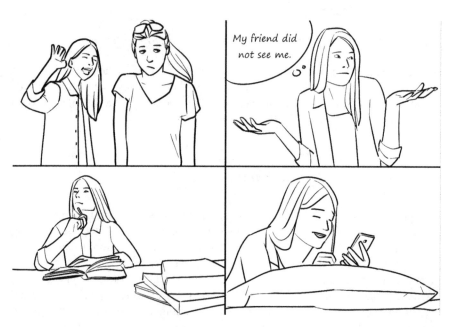

Fig. 6.4 Comic depicting feelings and behaviors following a restructured thought. (CC BY 4.0 Alayna Park)

building blocks, drawing or painting, and partaking in dance parties. Activity ideas for adolescents include playing sports, cooking or baking, and volunteering at a local animal shelter. Clients are encouraged to schedule pleasurable activities for days in between psychotherapy sessions and/or in a psychotherapy session to highlight the relationship between feelings and behaviors.

Relatedly, therapists can schedule a fun activity for the last 5–10 min of psychotherapy sessions to positively reinforce a client's participation and, if needed, to help a client regulate their emotions after a difficult session (e.g., a session where a client's trauma history is discussed). End of session play should be unstructured, such as shooting basketball hoops, drawing or coloring, playing a quick card or board game, or watching lighthearted videos.

6.4.7 Problem Solving

Problem solving aims to teach a client how to solve problems more effectively. This skill involves identifying a problem, brainstorming a list of possible solutions, assessing the potential benefits and consequences of each of these solutions, implementing the solution perceived to be the best, and evaluating the effectiveness of that solution. Oftentimes, therapists teach problem solving through worksheets; however, therapists can easily demonstrate these steps through playful activities. For example, a therapist may propose a problem of needing to place a ball into a bucket without using their hands. The therapist and client may then brainstorm possible solutions (e.g., holding the ball with their elbows, bouncing it off their head), discuss the potential of each solution, and iteratively enact proposed solutions until one is successful.

6.4.8 Relaxation

There are a variety of relaxation skills that therapists can teach to children and adolescents to reduce physiological sensations of distress. If a client reports feeling muscle tension, then a therapist may employ progressive muscle relaxation. Progressive muscle relaxation involves tensing and relaxing muscle groups one at a time until the client feels a sense of calm. A therapist may use fun metaphors when teaching progressive muscle relaxation, such as directing the client to pretend that they are a turtle retreating into (and out of) their shell to tense (and relax) shoulder muscles. Please see Table 6.2 for a list of fun metaphors for progressive muscle relaxation.

Diaphragmatic breathing or "belly breathing" is another relaxation skill that therapists can teach playfully. Diaphragmatic breathing involves taking slow, deep breaths from one's diaphragm to counteract the quick, short breaths that one typically takes when distressed. A therapist may illustrate this relaxation skill by asking

Table 6.2 Playful instructions for progressive muscle relaxation

Muscle group	Tensing instructions
Feet	"Curl your toes, like your shoes are too tight"
Legs	"Stomp your feet, and press them into the ground"
Stomach	"Pretend that a baby elephant is passing you in the hallway and suck in your stomach so that they can get by"
Chest	"Puff out your chest, like a bird"
Hands	"Ball your hands into fists and pretend that you are squeezing all of the juice out of a lemon"
Arms	"Flex your biceps and show me your muscles"
Shoulders	"Raise your shoulders and pretend that you are a turtle going into your shell"
Jaw	"Open your mouth as wide as you can, like a cat yawning"
Forehead	"Raise your eyebrows as high as you can, like you are really surprised"

their client to pretend that they are inflating and deflating a balloon in their belly by taking slow, deep breaths in through their nose and exhaling through their mouth. This relaxation skill can also be taught through imagining that one is blowing on a steaming cup of hot chocolate to cool it or having a client practice blowing bubbles, where short and fast breaths produce a stream of small bubbles and slow and steady breaths produce a single large bubble.

6.4.9 Social Skills

Social skills training aims to provide children and adolescents with concrete skills for developing healthy relationships. This psychotherapy practice involves skills for communicating effectively (e.g., entering a conversation, listening, taking turns speaking), asserting one's needs, taking another's perspective, and exhibiting prosocial behaviors (e.g., sharing toys with others). Children and adolescents are often taught social skills in small groups to allow for in-vivo practice. For example, youth may practice several social skills through an informal game of catch. By initiating a game of catch with a couple of group members, the remaining youth can practice joining the game. They may practice their verbal and nonverbal communication skills as they indicate who they plan to throw the ball to next. Youth may also practice prosocial behaviors, such as passing the ball to different group members or praising other group members for a "good throw" or "good catch." If social skills are to be practiced in a small group, then group rules should be established at the outset (e.g., therapist will pre-assign groups; score will not be kept; aggressive behavior will not be tolerated). Children and adolescents should also be encouraged to use previously learned cognitive and behavioral skills to manage their emotions and behaviors as they practice their social skills (e.g., generating adaptive thoughts if they were not thrown the ball as often as they would have wanted).

6.4.10 Maintenance

Maintenance refers to the practice of reviewing a client's treatment progress and brainstorming ways to maintain treatment gains. This involves discussing the client's progress toward achieving treatment goals, reviewing cognitive and behavioral skills covered in psychotherapy, identifying and planning for challenges that may interfere with continued skill use, and expressing confidence in the client's ability to cope with problems on their own, including recognizing if or when it may be helpful to re-enroll in psychotherapy. Maintenance is typically done during the final sessions of an episode of psychotherapy. To reinforce client's cognitive and behavioral skills learned in psychotherapy, a therapist can set up a game where the client must choose which skill(s) to use in various situations. For example, a therapist may write all of the skills covered in psychotherapy on a whiteboard, then state various situations, and ask the client to tag the skill(s) that can help them in each situation (e.g., the client would be expected to tag the relaxation skill if the therapist states the situation of experiencing stomachaches before a big test). As another idea, if the client was directed to draw themselves as a superhero and their problem as a villain at the start of psychotherapy, then a fun activity may be to ask the client to re-draw themselves and their problem at the end of psychotherapy.

6.4.11 One-on-One Time

Play is also a promising avenue for teaching caregivers skills for managing their child's behaviors and promoting family well-being and functioning. One-on-one time, or special play time, refers to a 5- to 15-min period of time each day where a caregiver plays with their child to increase attachment, promote prosocial behaviors, and decrease the frequency of destructive or aggressive behaviors. One-on-one time is beneficial for younger children, particularly those with disruptive behavior problems. During one-on-one time, caregivers are encouraged to praise their child's appropriate behavior (e.g., "I'm proud of you for sharing your crayons"), reflect appropriate speech (e.g., responding to a child's comment that they drew a cat by saying "you *did* draw a cat"), imitate appropriate play (e.g., "I'm going to draw a cat, just like you"), describe appropriate behavior (e.g., "You are putting your crayons back after using them"), and enjoy time with the child (e.g., "I'm having fun drawing together") (e.g., Eyberg & Funderburk, 2011). Caregivers are also taught to ignore inappropriate behaviors (e.g., screaming, making demands, refusing to play or to share toys, playing roughly with toys), avoid giving commands (e.g., "Let's draw a dog now"), avoid asking questions (e.g., "What are you drawing?"), and avoid criticizing (e.g., "That's not what a cat looks like"). Although many of these parenting skills should be applied beyond one-on-one time, play provides a natural opportunity for caregivers to practice these skills while building a warm and secure relationship with their children.

Case Example. Noah[2] is a 5-year-old, non-Hispanic, White boy. Noah was referred for individual psychotherapy by his mother, Betty, for frequent temper tantrums at home, noncompliance with adult requests at home and school, and repeated physical aggression (i.e., kicking and hitting) towards family members. After completing an initial assessment, the family's therapist determined that Noah and Betty could benefit from behavioral parent training for disruptive behavior and collaboratively developed a treatment plan with the family. The family's therapist introduced one-on-one time skills to Betty and decided to use play to reinforce her skill use. To achieve this session objective, the family's therapist planned for Noah and Betty to play with building blocks (i.e., one of Noah's favorite unstructured play activities) while the family's therapist observed their interaction and provided discreet coaching on Betty's use of one-on-one time skills. As Noah and Betty played, the family's therapist noticed that Noah often knocked down structures that Betty built and that Betty would consequently become upset and make comments such as, "You're being mean," and "Why can't you be nice like your brother?" The family's therapist coached Betty to ignore Noah's destructive behaviors and to continue building her own structures while subtly watching for Noah to resume appropriate behavior (e.g., adding more blocks to his own structures) to immediately praise (e.g., "You're doing a good job building that truck"). To provide Betty with additional opportunities to practice her one-on-one time skills, the family's therapist continued to coach Betty as she and Noah played for the next several sessions. At the beginning of each session, the family's therapist prompted Betty to report the number of temper tantrums from the previous week; and at the close of each session, the family's therapist privately rated Betty's use of one-on-one time skills. After six sessions of one-on-one time coaching, the family's therapist noted a decrease in the number of Noah's temper tantrums and an increase in Betty's use of one-on-one time skills. The family's therapist considered this activity to be a success, topped with Betty reporting that she and Noah have been having fun building towns during one-on-one time at home.

6.5   Multicultural Considerations

When incorporating play into your psychotherapy sessions, it is important to consider the family's cultural norms, beliefs, and values. Families differ in their worldviews about the importance of play in child development (e.g., European-American caregivers tend to view play as more important for physical, cognitive, and social development than Asian-American caregivers; Parmar et al., 2004). There are diverse conceptualizations of appropriate play activities (e.g., European-American families engage in more pretend play than Argentine, French, and Japanese families; Roopnarine & Davidson, 2015; Asian-American caregivers are more likely to

---

[2] This case example is a composite of several clients, and the names have been changed.

engage their children in preacademic activities, such as number games, than European-American caregivers; Parmar et al., 2004). Caregiver involvement in play also varies by culture (e.g., approximately 60% of mothers in the United States report playing with their children compared with 24% of mothers in India and 7% of mothers in Guatemala; Roopnarine & Davidson, 2015). Additionally, cultures have distinct play settings (e.g., youth in the United States commonly get together for play dates in each other's homes, whereas youth in Korea commonly hang out in the community; Yoo et al., 2014). Furthermore, humor perception and usage differ across cultures (e.g., "knock-knock" jokes are common in the United States, whereas "panda jokes" are common in Hong Kong; Shum et al., 2019). Accordingly, therapists should ask about the family's established play activities at the outset of psychotherapy. For example, what does the client do for fun? Who participates in those fun activities with the client? When and where do those fun activities take place? Using this information, therapists can craft play activities in collaboration with the family to increase the likelihood that play will not only promote therapeutic skill acquisition but will also align with the family's cultural norms, beliefs, and values. For instance, therapists may consider initially recommending 5 min (rather than 15 min) of one-on-one time for caregivers who usually engage in little to no play with their children, while challenging caregivers who frequently play with their children to incorporate multiple one-on-one time skills (e.g., praising desired behaviors, reflecting respectful speech, and imitating appropriate play).

It is also important to consider the family's resources, especially when assigning therapeutic play activities outside of sessions. For instance, when scheduling pleasant activities for the client to complete for homework, therapists should consider activities that are free or low-cost, such as drawing or coloring, cooking or baking, going for a walk, visiting the local library during story time, or attending a concert in the park. Similarly, one-on-one time can involve inexpensive toys and games, such as engaging in pretend play, building structures with Play-Doh, or playing a game of catch. Another consideration is the common expectation for adolescents in low-income families to contribute through working a part-time job or babysitting younger siblings. When working with a client who is balancing multiple roles, then it can be beneficial to schedule time for the client to practice their cognitive and behavioral skills, including their engagement in mood-boosting pleasant activities. Relatedly, caregivers working multiple jobs, night shifts, or extended hours can plan therapeutic play activities in short but frequent increments (e.g., 5 min each weekday) or can consider involving other family members in therapeutic play activities (e.g., teaching older siblings to praise a child client's appropriate play).

6.6 Telehealth Considerations

Telehealth, or the use of videoconferencing or other information and communication technologies to support the delivery of mental health services, has become increasingly prevalent over the past two decades (Perle & Nierenberg, 2013)—most prominently during the COVID-19 outbreak (Zhou et al., 2020). There is a rapidly growing literature on telehealth applications and effectiveness (e.g., Boydell et al., 2010; Goldstein & Glueck, 2016; Myers et al., 2008; Nelson & Patton, 2016), which is outside of the scope of this chapter to summarize. However, we offer the following considerations regarding incorporating play into CBT via telehealth. One consideration is that the family will often attend telehealth sessions from their home—allowing the therapist to teach the family cognitive and behavioral skills in a naturalistic environment, which may lead to greater skill generalization. The therapist can also capitalize on resources available in the family's home, such as teaching one-on-one time by having the child and caregiver play with the child's own toys or promoting social skills by having the child practice trading information with their siblings.

One disadvantage of telehealth is that the caregiver rather than the therapist will often need to prepare the play activity for the session. Therefore, telehealth sessions require play activities to be planned in advance and coordinated with the caregiver prior to session. Another option is for the therapist to consider online games. For example, the popular videoconferencing platform, Zoom, has a whiteboard feature that allows the therapist and client to draw together. Since many online games are open to the public and/or may contain mature content, we recommend that therapists preview any online games before playing with their clients. A final consideration is that engaging clients via telehealth may be more difficult than in-person psychotherapy. For instance, youth, particularly younger children, are unlikely to remain attentive for an entire telehealth session. Accordingly, therapists should consider interspersing brief play activities throughout the telehealth session, such as having periodic stretch breaks or dance breaks.

6.7   Conclusion

Incorporating play activities into CBT for youth can benefit both client experience and outcomes. Through strategic design and implementation, play can facilitate rapport building (e.g., gathering information about the client's presenting problem while coloring together), boost mood (e.g., playing an enjoyable game of catch to highlight the relationship between feelings and behaviors), and promote CBT knowledge and skill acquisition (e.g., teaching parents to praise their child's positive behaviors during unstructured play time). Play is part of the art of psychotherapy, which when merged with the science behind CBT, can promote the well-being and functioning of youth and families in need.

References

Beck, J. S. (2011). *Cognitive behavior therapy: Basics and beyond*. Guilford.

Becker, K. D., Boustani, M., Gellatly, R., & Chorpita, B. F. (2018). Forty years of engagement research in children's mental health services: Multidimensional measurement and practice elements. *Journal of Clinical Child and Adolescent Psychology, 47*, 1–23.

Beidas, R. S., Benjamin, C. L., Puleo, C. M., Edmunds, J. M., & Kendall, P. C. (2010). Flexible applications of the coping cat program for anxious youth. *Cognitive and Behavioral Practice, 17*, 142–153.

Borntrager, C., & Lyon, A. R. (2015). Client progress monitoring and feedback in school-based mental health. *Cognitive and Behavioral Practice, 22*, 74–86.

Boydell, K. M., Volpe, T., & Pignatiello, A. (2010). A qualitative study of young people's perspectives on receiving psychiatric services via televideo. *Journal of Canadian Academy of Child and Adolescent Psychiatry, 19*, 5.

Bratton, S. C., Ceballos, P. L., & Ferebee, K. W. (2009). Integration of structured expressive activities within a humanistic group play therapy format for preadolescents. *Journal for Specialists in Group Work, 34*, 251–275.

Briggs, K. M., Runyon, M. K., & Deblinger, E. (2011). The use of play in trauma-focused cognitive-behavioral therapy. In *Play in clinical practice: Evidence-based approaches* (pp. 168–200). Guilford Press.

Bunge, E. L., Mandil, J., Consoli, A. J., & Gomar, M. (2017). *CBT strategies for anxious and depressed children and adolescents: A clinician's toolkit*. Guilford.

Chorpita, B. F., & Daleiden, E. L. (2014). Structuring the collaboration of science and service in pursuit of a shared vision. *Journal of Clinical Child and Adolescent Psychology, 43*, 323–338.

Chorpita, B. F., Daleiden, E. L., Ebesutani, C., Young, J., Becker, K. D., Nakamura, B. J., Phillips, L., Ward, A., Lynch, R., & Trent, L. (2011). Evidence-based treatments for children and adolescents: An updated review of indicators of efficacy and effectiveness. *Clinical Psychologist, 18*, 154–172.

Eyberg, S. M., & Funderburk, B. (2011). *Parent-child interaction therapy protocol*. PCIT International.

Goldstein, F., & Glueck, D. (2016). Developing rapport and therapeutic alliance during telemental health sessions with children and adolescents. *Journal of Child and Adolescent Psychopharmacology, 26*, 204–211.

Huibers, M. J. H., & Cuijpers, P. (2015). Common (nonspecific) factors in psychotherapy. In *The encyclopedia of clinical psychology* (pp. 1–6). American Cancer Society.

Kendall, P. C., & Frank, H. E. (2018). Implementing evidence-based treatment protocols: Flexibility within fidelity. *Clinical Psychologist, 25*, e12271.

Lau, A. S. (2006). Making the case for selective and directed cultural adaptations of evidence-based treatments: Examples from parent training. *Clinical Psychologist, 13*, 295–310.

Laugeson, E. A., & Park, M. N. (2014). Using a CBT approach to teach social skills to adolescents with autism spectrum disorder and other social challenges: The PEERS® method. *Journal of Rational-Emotive & Cognitive-Behavior Therapy, 32*, 84–97.

Lieneman, C. C., Brabson, L. A., Highlander, A., Wallace, N. M., & McNeil, C. B. (2017). Parent-child interaction therapy: Current perspectives. *Psychology Research and Behavior Management, 10*, 239–256.

Martinez, J. I., Lau, A. S., Chorpita, B. F., Weisz, J. R., & Health, R. N. (2017). Psychoeducation as a mediator of treatment approach on parent engagement in child psychotherapy for disruptive behavior. *Journal of Clinical Child and Adolescent Psychology, 46*, 573–587.

Myers, K. M., Valentine, J. M., & Melzer, S. M. (2008). Child and adolescent telepsychiatry: Utilization and satisfaction. *Telemedicine and e-Health, 14*, 131–137.

Nelson, E. L., & Patton, S. (2016). Using videoconferencing to deliver individual therapy and pediatric psychology interventions with children and adolescents. *Journal of Child and Adolescent Psychopharmacology, 26*, 212–220.

Parmar, P., Harkness, S., & Super, C. M. (2004). Asian and euro-American parents' ethnotheories of play and learning: Effects on preschool children's home routines and school behaviour. *International Journal of Behavioral Development, 28*, 97–104.

Perle, J. G., & Nierenberg, B. (2013). How psychological telehealth can alleviate society's mental health burden: A literature review. *Journal of Technology in Human Services, 31*, 22–41.

PracticeWise. (2020). PracticeWise evidence-based youth mental health services literature database. Retrieved from https://www.practicewise.com/pwebs_1/index.aspx

Ray, D. C., Lee, K. R., Meany-Walen, K. K., Carlson, S. E., Carnes-Holt, K. L., & Ware, J. N. (2013). Use of toys in child-centered play therapy. *International Journal of Play Therapy, 22*, 43–57.

Roopnarine, J. L., & Davidson, K. L. (2015). Parent-child play across cultures: Advancing play research. *American Journal of Play, 7*, 228–252.

Shum, K. K. M., Cho, W. K., Lam, L. M. O., Laugeson, E. A., Wong, W. S., & Law, L. S. (2019). Learning how to make friends for Chinese adolescents with autism spectrum disorder: A randomized controlled trial of the Hong Kong Chinese version of the PEERS intervention®. *Journal of Autism and Developmental Disorders, 49*, 527–541.

Weisz, J. R., Kuppens, S., Eckshtain, D., Ugueto, A. M., Hawley, K. M., & Jensen-Doss, A. (2013). Performance of evidence-based youth psychotherapies compared with usual clinical care: A multilevel meta-analysis. *JAMA Psychiatry, 70*, 750–761.

Yoo, H. J., Bahn, G., Cho, I. H., Kim, E. K., Kim, J. H., Min, J. W., Lee, W. H., Seo, J. S., Jun, S. S., & Bong, G. (2014). A randomized controlled trial of the Korean version of the PEERS® parent-assisted social skills training program for teens with ASD. *Autism Research, 7*, 145–161.

Zhou, X., Snoswell, C. L., Harding, L. E., Bambling, M., Edirippulige, S., Bai, X., & Smith, A. C. (2020). The role of telehealth in reducing the mental health burden from COVID-19. *Telemedicine and e-Health, 26*, 377–379.

Chapter 7
Playful Approaches to CBT with Aggressive Children

Eva L. Feindler and Alexandra Mercurio Schira

Keywords Emotion regulation · Anger · Aggression · Cognitive behavioral therapy · Play therapy · Bibliotherapy · Preschool

7.1 Emotion Competence and Regulation in Young Children

Emotional competence is a noteworthy concept in children's development. Children must gain mastery over understanding the meaning of emotions before expressing and regulating emotions. In 2000, Saarni proposed a model of emotional competence which emphasized cognitive and social moderators including awareness of one's own emotions, the skills to discern the emotions of others, and the capacity to cope adaptively with difficult emotions (Saarni, 2000; Suveg et al., 2007). One aspect of emotional competence is emotional knowledge or understanding. Pons and Harris (2000) developed the Test of Emotion Comprehension (TEC) to assess the hypothesized domains of emotional understanding. These domains have improved our understanding about how to guide youth through learning and understand the function and impact of their emotions. These domains are recognition of emotions, based on facial expressions; the comprehension of external emotional causes; impact of desire on emotions; emotions based on beliefs; memory influence on emotions; possibility of emotional regulation; possibility of hiding an emotional state; having mixed emotions; contribution of morality to emotional experiences.

E. L. Feindler (✉)
Clinical Psychology Doctoral Program, Brookville, NY, USA
e-mail: eva.feindler@liu.edu

A. M. Schira
Ridgewood, NY, USA

© The Author(s), under exclusive license to Springer Nature Switzerland AG 2022
R. D. Friedberg, E. V. Rozmid (eds.), *Creative CBT with Youth*,
https://doi.org/10.1007/978-3-030-99669-7_7

While youth must learn to understand their emotions, they must also master inhibitory control, the ability to inhibit or suppress salient thought processes or behaviors that are not relevant to the goal or task at hand (Carlson & Wang, 2007). Mostly develop this control mechanism during the preschool years, but if children do not develop these skills, they are left with poor inhibitory control and become easily frustrated and prone to reactive aggression.

Finally, the concept of emotion regulation (ER) has been emphasized in both the developmental and clinical literature. ER refers to the regulation of the experience of an emotion first by monitoring one's expressive behavior (Carlson & Wang, 2007). Then as an internal modulation of triggered emotions via the application of various behavioral and cognitive strategies (Cole & Jacobs, 2018). Explicit awareness of emotion regulation strategies emerges between ages 3 and 5 years. Then, over the preschool period, children acquire a new range of skills such as theory of mind, the capacity to inhibit a dominant response and the process of cognitive reappraisal (Sala et al., 2014). This crucial emotion regulation strategy requires that the child changes their ways of thinking about an emotional trigger in order to regulate their response. Overall, a review of available research indicates a universal acceptance of the idea that understanding one's emotional life is a central component of children's socio-emotional competence and adjustment.

7.2 Anger and Aggression in Young Children

Some aggression is normative in early childhood and generally declines during the transition to elementary school. Coinciding with language acquisition and increased expressive vocabularies, children between the ages of 2 and 5 years tend to rely less on physical forms of aggression and more on verbal abilities for emotional expression (Wilson & Ray, 2018). However, children who are persistently aggressive are at greater risk for poor academic and interpersonal outcomes (Evans et al., 2019). Aggressive behavior problems in young children are one of the most frequent referral issues for clinicians and since early patterns may predict later antisocial behaviors, early interventions are fundamental (Robson et al., 2020). Many risk factors that lead to the development of anger and aggression problems have been identified. These include a difficult or uninhibited temperament, deficiencies in affect regulation and social information processing, hostility biases and misappraisals, and poor problem-solving skills. Contextual risk factors have focused on parents who provide harsh discipline, poor monitoring, and inconsistent contingency management (Feindler, 1995). Finally, coercive patterns of family interactions and the absence of positive parenting behaviors are also influential in the development and maintenance of aggressive behavior patterns.

Emotion regulation, the ability to manage anger and frustration, influences the development of cognitive and social skills necessary for prosocial functioning. Young children who exhibit aggressive behaviors most likely experience intense levels of negative affect and have few internal coping skills to manage their emotions. Children struggling with their self-regulatory processes often lack the ability to control their feelings and emotions and therefore may display aggressive behaviors out of impulse. High impulsiveness most commonly characterizes conflicts related to self-regulation and aggression. Very young children often express aggression through impulsive acts related to their feelings of anger, frustration, and the like (Wilson & Ray, 2018). Further, empathy and self-regulation are identified components of aggression that theoretically contributes to a child's inhibition and expression of aggressive acts. A child's ability to experience and demonstrate empathy is directly related to his or her ability to take on the emotional experiences of another and thus is largely connected to regulation of aggressive behavior (Wilson & Ray, 2018).

Within a cognitive behavioral theoretical model, anger is viewed as a subjective experience which can vary in intensity and duration and which emerges across various interpersonal contexts. Anger expression, which includes the ability to show it outwardly, to suppress it deliberately or to cope with it actively, varies between individuals (Sukhodolsky et al., 2004). Anger as one of the many emotions that children learn to master is a complex emotional construct composed of physiological, cognitive, and behavioral components. For young children, the link to aggressive behavior is fairly common and most children learn to control their aggression and express their emotional experience in a socially competent fashion. However, there are significant numbers of children who fail to achieve skills of emotional regulation and impulse control who will then need clinical intervention as early patterns of aggressive behavior tend to remain stable across time. Therefore, early intervention is advised for youth who display aggressive tendencies, have little impulse control, or have difficulty understanding emotions.

During the past 10 years, there has been a proliferation of cognitive behavioral anger management intervention programs. Based on the understanding that children's aggressive behaviors are the outcome of poor emotion regulation and self-control, programs have been developed to remediate these deficits. Social information processing theory indicates that children's emotions and subsequent actions (in this case anger and aggression) are regulated by the way they perceive, process, and /or mediate environmental/interpersonal events. Their experiences of frustration and anger are related to identifiable deficits and distortions in this cognitive processing sequence as well as deficits in problem-solving and appropriate anger expression skills. Thus, each child will need to learn ways to manage their subjective emotional experience, to reframe his or her cognitive appraisals of events and to respond to provocation in an effective prosocial manner (Feindler & Gerber, 2008). Yet, teaching young children coping skills and emotion regulation strategies is no easy feat. Play activities offer clinicians an accessible way to connect and work with younger children to improve their emotion regulation.

7.3 The Role of Play

Children's pretend play has long been proposed as a mode of social interaction that enhances the development of emotion regulation (Hoffmann & Russ, 2012). Pretend play provides children with a unique environment in which to practice and master social and emotional skills. According to Fein (1989) pretend play, by transcending literal meaning, provides a context to process, manifest, and modify experiences involving high levels of emotional arousal. Themes and stories acted out in play help to teach display rules about emotions, such as when and how to express anger as well as model aspects of modulating emotions (Hoffmann & Russ, 2012). Clearly, play is a learning mode for young children and should be incorporated into clinical interventions. Abstract forms of play allow for the processing of emotion reactions, attuning of motivational states, and enhanced understanding of interpersonal interactions (Peterson & Flanders, 2005). Many aggressive young children have difficulty playing imaginatively and instead release their aggressive impulses by acting out during play: hitting, throwing, breaking, biting, etc. Further, they seem to have difficulties engaging in rich or complex play and in coordinating symbolic play themes (Landy & Menna, 2001).

Opinions vary as to the availability of aggressive toys in clinical settings when working with young aggressive children. Some therapists see the use of toys such as the punching bag or Bobo doll, as necessary to a child's behavioral expression of emotion and underlying conflict (Trotter et al., 2003), while others see aggressive toys as possibly harmful. Schaefer and Mattei (2005) in their review of catharsis and children's aggression concluded that "when adults permit and encourage children's release of aggression in play, the children are likely to maintain this behavior at its original level or actually increase it" (p. 107). Therefore, many therapists incorporate the use of structured play to teach children numerous affect expression and regulation skills as well as teach children how to control aggressive impulses. Drewes (2008) concluded that the use of the Bobo doll and other aggressive toys is not effective and recommended alternative expressive material as providing a more constructive and perhaps symbolic means to express emotions. Unfortunately, little recent research comparing these cathartic strategies with other play therapy strategies when working with young aggressive children has been reported.

Instead, we recommend that child therapists work with age-appropriate toys, games, and books while implementing intervention strategies. Knell (2009, and this volume) has described an elegant but practical way to blend play therapy and cognitive behavior therapy for effective work with young children. Table 7.1 includes a list of anger management themed books and YouTube programs for young children to help with a bibliotherapy component as well. In *Appendix B,* there are several supplemental anger management intervention ideas that can be blended into clinical work with young children along with the Turtle Magic Intervention described next.

Table 7.1   Child-friendly resources

Books:
Alber, Diana: A Little Spot of Anger (2019) (30 pages)
Bang, Molly: When Sophie Gets Really, Really Angry (2004) (4–6 years) (40 pages)
Bartlein, Kate: Lennon Bruce Fire Breather (2019) (28 pages)
Boyd, Melissa: B is For Breathe: The ABCs of Coping with Fussy and Frustrating Feelings (2019) (4–6 years) (32 pages)
Crary, Elizabeth: I'm Furious (1994) (34 pages)
Dahl, Michael: Little Monkey Calms Down (2014) (20 pages)
Gaither, Jennifer: I Can Yell Louder! (2020) (48 pages)
Graves, Sue: I Hate Everything (2013) (28 pages)
Green, Agnes: Today I'm a Monster (2017) (42 pages)
Green, Andi: The Very Frustrated Monster (2016) (72 pages)
Herman, Steve: Train Your Angry Dragon (2018) (44 pages)
Huebner, Dawn: What To Do When Your Temper Flares (2007) (88 pages)
Kurtzman-Counter, Sam & Schiller, Abbie: When Miles Got Mad (2013) (30 pages)
Lite, Lori & Stasuyk, Max: Angry Octopus: An Anger Management Story introducing active progressive muscular relaxation and deep breathing (2019) (30 pages)
Madison, Linda: The Feelings Book (Revised): The Care and Keeping of Your Emotions (2013) (104 pages)
Maude Spelman, Cornelia: When I Feel Angry (2000) (Board Book) (24 pages)
Mayer, Mercer: I Was So Mad (2000) (24 pages)
Meiners, Cheri: Cool Down and Work Through Anger (2010) (40 pages)
Schiller, Abbie: Sally Simon's Super Frustrating Day (2013) (30 pages)
Verdick, Elizabeth: Calm Down Time (2010) (Board Book) (24 pages)
Viorst, Judith: Alexander and the Terrible, Horrible, No Good, Very Bad Day (1972) (32 pages)
Movies:
Inside Out
Frozen
The Incredible Hulk
TV Shows:
Daniel Tiger: Anger episode
Sesame Street: *Sticks learns to deal with his anger*
YouTube:
A Little Spot of Anger: https://www.youtube.com/watch?v=ptDqMeAcn9w
When Sophie Gets Really, Really Angry: https://www.youtube.com/watch?v=dNfd8WFDBAY
B is For Breathe: The ABCs of Coping with Fussy and Frustrating Feelings: https://www.youtube.com/watch?v=sEmlKSlZzNo
Little Monkey Calms Down: https://www.youtube.com/watch?v=5Yj6pWEsqBU
I Hate Everything: https://www.youtube.com/watch?v=9F_wnrNtD58
Today I'm a Monster: https://www.youtube.com/watch?v=xUwlVR72Zpg
The Very Frustrated Monster (2016): https://www.youtube.com/watch?v=MaVEAtEJd7E
Train Your Angry Dragon: https://www.youtube.com/watch?v=0Z637pUJx2I
When Miles Got Mad (2013): https://www.youtube.com/watch?v=37Nv68AdrWo

(continued)

Table 7.1 (continued)

When I Feel Angry (2000): https://www.youtube.com/watch?v=mEMWNjIHL_U
I Was So Mad (2000): https://www.youtube.com/watch?v=xec0MvTNegc
Angry Octopus: An Anger Management Story introducing active progressive muscular relaxation and deep breathing: https://www.youtube.com/watch?v=6PxfJC_89Lk&t=153s
Calm Down Time (2010): https://www.youtube.com/watch?v=j6Ik72R2rjc
Alexander and the Terrible, Horrible, No Good, Very Bad Day: https://www.youtube.com/watch?v=w6HhKlpp7ok
Board/Tabletop Games:
Trouble
Jenga
Operation
Sorry
Don't Wake Daddy
Don't Break the Ice
Connect 4

7.4 Turtle Magic

7.4.1 Turtle Magic Intervention Program Description

Turtle Magic Intervention (TMI) is a short-term therapeutic treatment program originally developed for preschool-aged children informed by tenets of cognitive behavioral play therapy (CBPT). CBPT is based on the cognitive theory of emotional disorders and is designed to be developmentally appropriate for children for a range of presenting problems (Knell, 2009). TMI was originally designed as a pilot treatment for preschool-aged children who demonstrated marked externalizing problems and aggressive behavior in their classroom (Schira, 2018). TMI may be used as a psychoeducational emotion regulation program with young children.

The TMI program aims to teach children the skills necessary to identify and express their emotions, regulate their emotional responses by implementing coping skills, and solve problems in a developmentally appropriate way. TMI may be utilized in an individual or group format. TMI is designed as a nine-session treatment program with sessions lasting approximately 30 min. After the eight core sessions, a ninth "booster" session is administered approximately 1 month later.

7.4.2 About Turtle Magic

The Turtle Magic Intervention was developed to be used in conjunction with the short therapeutic storybook, *Turtle Magic,* that highlights the core anger management components (Feindler, 2009). The protagonist in the story, Timmy Turtle, struggles to adjust to school and get along with his peers, and can be seen engaging in aggressive and impulsive behaviors. In the story, Timmy Turtle receives a recommendation from the Wise Old Turtle to use his shell as a calm space to relax and consider other possible solutions to a conflict (Feindler, 2009). The phrase "doing a turtle" involves "(a) recognizing anger as it swells, (b) interrupting the swell and pulling inside, (c) taking a few deep breaths and thinking about how to solve the conflict, and (d) returning to the scene and implementing a possible solution" (Feindler, 2009, p. 409). These skills can be applied on the individual level or with group related problems that provoke frustration in young children. Through *Turtle Magic*, children enhance their narrative abilities and therefore, view multiple perspectives on a situation and further develop their empathy (Feindler, 2009).

7.4.3 TMI Treatment Description

All meetings begin with the welcome song and discussion of the session agenda. The welcome song, described later in the TMI manual, outlines the rules for whole body listening with behavioral descriptions for their eyes, ears, voices, and bodies. Songs and choreographed body movements are playful and engaging ways to orient children to the sessions. Each week the child learns and practices target coping skills. The fundamental coping skills of TMI include relaxation, positive self-talk, and problem-solving. The TMI lessons are designed to progressively build on one another with ample opportunities for review and practice. Throughout each session, the therapist and child refer to the *Turtle Magic* (Feindler, 1991) storybook to identify and emphasize the skills being learned; the child will also role-play the story content using accompanying animal puppets and other play materials. Children engage in structured activities and games along with peers and the therapist to increase skill generalization. At the end of each session, the child receives a small prize and is awarded a skill badge based on the session's target skill (e.g., Emotion Badge, Relaxation Badge).

Each of the nine TMI treatment sessions is divided into four components:

1. **Welcome/ Check-In**	The therapist welcomes participants and sings the Welcome Song. The therapist facilitates an emotion check-in e.g., "How are you feeling today?" Next, the therapist reviews the session agenda with the child/ group, including a preview of the skill to be learned together
2. **Fun & Learning**	Each week the child/group will learn a new skill and engage in activities and games aimed at practicing the learned skills
3. ***Turtle Magic* story**	After the skill is explained and modeled, the child/group will read the *Turtle Magic* storybook about a young turtle named, Timmy Turtle, who struggles to adjust to school and get along with his peers, and often engages in aggressive and impulsive behaviors. The children will be instructed to identify the learned skill in the storybook and role-play the skill using animal puppets and play props

4. **Reinforcement**	At the end of each session, the children receive a small prize and are awarded a badge based on the session content and skill learned (e.g., Emotion Badge, Relaxation Badge)

The following list outlines the materials needed for all the TMI sessions:
- *Turtle Magic* storybook: (Feindler, 1991) available online from author.
- Puppets (2 minimum): Turtles, one big, one small (Folkmanis Turtle Hand Puppet)
- To Do/Done Checklist: DIY (suggested white board, pen/paper)
- Whole Body Listening Cue Cards https://lessonpix.com/materials/1090565/Picture+Cards
- Stickers, prizes, and badges
- Emotion visual cue cards: happy, sad, angry, excited, surprised, scared
- Handheld Mirror
- Props and toys: *Pizza, Stop Sign, Microphone, Thought Bubble*
- Freeze Dance Song: https://www.youtube.com/watch?v=2UcZWXvgMZE
- Timmy Turtle problem-solving pages
- Additional animal puppets
- Yoga mat (optional)

The Turtle Magic Intervention- Individual and Group Manual (Fig. 7.1), available below, is available for application with young children in both individual and group formats. The suggested group size is between three and five group participants. Therapists are encouraged to have materials prepared before the session and to structure each session using the four-component outline: Welcome/Check-in, Fun & Learning, Turtle Magic Story, and Reinforcement.

7.4.4 Brief Review of Evidence for Turtle Magic Intervention

Schira (2018) conducted a single-subject, pilot study of TMI to examine the effectiveness and feasibility of the treatment program with three children at a special education preschool who were identified as exhibiting aggressive behaviors. Participants enrolled in the pilot study were 3 years old at the start of treatment. Eligibility was determined based on a T-score of 65 or above on the *aggressive problems* subscale, a T-score of 65 or above on the *oppositional defiant problems* subscale, or a T-score of 60 or above on the *externalizing problems* subscale on the Caregiver-Teacher Report Form for Ages 1 ½ to 5 (C-TRF; Achenbach & Rescorla, 2001). Evaluation of TMI treatment fidelity was coded using video-recorded treatment sessions implemented by a trained mental health professional. Within-participant analyses focused on comparing the subscale T-scores obtained from the C-TRF at three time points: pre (baseline), post (after completion of study), and at 4-month follow-up. Data collected from the C-TRF suggested that Child 1 displayed no significant change from pre- to post-assessment; however, at follow-up assessment, the teacher reported a significant decrease in all three subscales. Child 2 and 3, on the other hand, demonstrated an increase in problematic behaviors from

TURTLE MAGIC INTERVENTION- INDIVIDUAL & GROUP MANUAL
Alexandra Mercurio Schira, Psy.D.

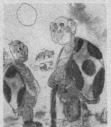

SESSION 1: Therapy Induction

The first session of the TMI program begins with an induction to the therapeutic program including: an explanation of the program rationale, review of therapist and/or group confidentiality agreement, establishing the lesson agenda, and learning a welcome song about whole body listening rules. The child is also introduced to the *Turtle Magic* storybook themes, characters, and concepts.

Materials: Turtle Magic storybook, Puppets (2), To Do/Done Checklist, Whole Body Listening Visual Cue Cards, Reward stickers/prizes and Skills badge

Welcome/ Check-in

Introductions and Building Rapport:

Welcome Song: [sung in key of *Frere Jacques* nursery rhyme. Therapist should point to the corresponding body part when singing the welcome song.]
Lyrics: "Eyes are watching, Ears are listening, Voices Quiet, Body Calm…This is how we listen, This is how we listen, At group time, At group time."

Fun & Learning

Therapist Introduction:
- The therapist introduces him/herself to the child and explains the agenda for the session and future sessions.
  - *"We will meet 8 times! We'll get to have fun and do cool stuff like read books, play games, and practice learning new things!"*
- The therapist explains that their job is to help the child:
  - Learn about their bodies and feelings
  - Practice learning how to take care of themselves/feel good
  - Solve problems
- Therapist explains child roles:
  - Learn new things and practice in a safe space together with the therapist

Fig. 7.1 Turtle Magic Intervention—Individual & Group Manual

pre- to post-assessment, although these behaviors improved at follow-up assessment (Schira, 2018). Overall, researchers found that there was an improvement in teacher-reported prosocial behaviors from baseline to follow-up and that the treatment was implemented with high fidelity.

      ○ Earn prizes for their work
   ● Therapist explains confidentiality:
      ○ This is a protected, safe space.
         ■ *"We want to feel safe together and practice trying new things. What is said in the session/group, stays in the session/group."*
         ■ Therapist introduces: To Do/ Done checklist for the session using visual aid.

Turtle Magic Story

● Read *Turtle Magic*
● Read the story interactively, stopping to pause and reflect on the different parts of the story that appeal to the child.
● Map out story using puppets
    "We're going to read a story and this puppet is going to help us read it!"
    "What would you do? How would you respond in this situation?"
    Role play with puppets (and/or other group members).

Reinforcement

Prize/Badge and Wrap-Up:
● Child receives Participation badge and picks from prize box

SESSION 2: Emotions

The second session is aimed at teaching the child to identify six core emotions and understand why emotions are important. In this lesson, the child learns that emotions help humans communicate about their wants and needs. Emotions are an everyday part of life, and we can usually tell how someone is feeling by looking at their faces or bodies to get some clues. Emotions also have a range of intensity- feelings can be big or small.

Additional Materials: Emotion Visual Cue Cards, Mirror

Welcome/ Check-in

Welcome Song
Recap
● Introduction for sessions and therapist/children role
    ▪ *"Remember I'm here to help you learn about your bodies and feelings, teach you how to solve problems, and play games with you."*

Fun & Learning

● Introduce Emotions/Feelings
Activities and games aimed at increasing emotional knowledge:
   ○ <u>Emotion visual cue cards:</u> Have child identify 6 core emotions - Happiness, Sadness, Fear, Anger, Surprise, Disgust
    ▪ *"What feeling is this? How do you know? What might make someone have that feeling?"*

Fig. 7.1 (continued)

An adaptation to TMI was Turtle Magic Intervention for Groups (TMI-G) of young children was developed by Pazmino Koste (2021). Interventions in small groups of children offer increased opportunities for in vivo role-plays of frustration eliciting situations as well as the practice of emotion regulation and social skills with peers. The first study of TMI-G was to examine the treatment acceptability of o Check yourself out: using handheld mirrors, children can practice making feeling faces with therapist or each other (i.e., personal mirrors or passing around shared mirror)

   o *Intensity of emotions-big and small emotions
     ▪ This may be incorporated if children are focused and capable.
     ▪ *"You might feel a little angry if you had to wait your turn in a game or you might feel really scared if you couldn't find your adult at the playground."*

Turtle Magic Story
- Read *Turtle Magic* for connection to and emphasis of emotions - using emotion cards for visual recognition task
     ▪ *"Remember Timmy Turtle? Let's see if we can find any of the feelings we talked about today in the book."*
     ▪ *"How does Timmy's face look? Why would he be angry? What did he do when he was angry?"*
   o Child(ren) can hold the puppets and act out the emotions while reading story
- Normalize and provide psychoeducation about the nature of emotions and aggressive behavior
     ▪ *"Everyone has feelings – grown-ups, teachers, children. Sometimes it helps to know how we are feeling to know what we are going to do about it."*
   o Expand with examples to generalize
     ▪ *"I feel sad when I lose a game or get hurt on the playground."*
     ▪ Role play and play with puppets

Reinforcement
Badge/ Prize and Wrap-Up:
- Child receives Emotion/Feeling badge and picks prize from box

SESSION 3: Relaxation Strategies

In the third session, the child learns about body awareness and how to recognize when their body feels relaxed versus tense. The child will practice body clench/release techniques such as being a robot (tense, stiff) and wiggly worm (loose, relaxed) or uncooked spaghetti (tense, stiff) and cooked spaghetti (loose, relaxed). The child will also learn deep breathing exercises which can be aided using visual props and toys, including a pizza to smell and blow on hot pizza or cake prop to practice blowing out candles on a birthday cake. The child will also learn yoga poses, such as the turtle pose from the *Turtle Magic* storybook, when Timmy learns to tuck inside his shell. The child will then read *Turtle Magic* and role play with puppets and practice shifting from wiggly worm to the turtle pose.

Additional Materials: Pizza or Cake prop/toy, yoga mat (optional)

Fig. 7.1 (continued)

TMI-G for children with aggressive behaviors and emotion dysregulation. Further, this study examined whether the type of professional degree, years of experience as a school practitioner, or the type of school setting participants are employed would impact acceptability of TMI-G. Knowing the predictors associated with treatment

Welcome/ Check-in

Welcome Song
Recap:
- *"We talked about emotions & feelings last time"-* refer to emotion cue cards
Emotion Check in:
- Have children identify how they are feeling- referring to emotion cards
- Expand emotional vocabulary- *"How does each emotion feel in your body? Why do we have emotions?*
  - o Emotions tell people things. - *"For example, a baby who is crying might want a snack or might have a dirty diaper."*

Fun & Learning

Fun and Learning Activity:
Today we are going to use our bodies ...
- Introduce Relaxation- *"This is how your body feels when it is calm, and you are feeling good and safe."*
- Body awareness physical practice (Robot/Lego vs. wiggly worm, uncooked spaghetti vs. cooked spaghetti)
  - ▪ *"Let's see how your body feels when you are a robot! Lego character! Wiggly worm!"*
  - o Deep breathing: Model taking big inhale and exhale (incorporate images such as fresh flowers, pizza, birthday cake and candles)
  - o Turtle pose (child practices tucking into shell and taking deep breaths)
- Incorporate body awareness and how it connects to emotions
  - o *"When you are calm, your body is relaxed, and you feel safe and happy. If you get upset, try to relax your body to help you feel good again."*
- Read *Turtle Magic* for reference and practice doing Turtle pose
  - o Use puppets and play to act out turtle pose while reading story
  - o *"Remember Timmy? What pose does Timmy do?" "He uses the turtle pose to stay calm and peaceful."*
- Role play with puppets and practice shifting from wiggly worm to turtle pose (i.e., your friend will tag you to do the turtle pose!

Turtle Magic Story
- Read *Turtle Magic* for connection to and emphasis of emotions - using emotion cards for visual recognition task
  - ▪ *"Remember Timmy Turtle? Let's see if we can find any of the feelings we talked about today in the book."*
  - ▪ *"How does Timmy's face look? Why would he be angry? What did he do when he was angry?"*
  - o Child(ren) can hold the puppets and act out the emotions

Reinforcement
Badge/ Prize and Wrap-Up

Fig. 7.1 (continued)

acceptability will help identify who would likely benefit from access to and training in TMI-G, which could foster engagement with the program. Finally, school practitioners were asked their opinion if TMI would be better implemented in an

- Child receives Turtle Pose badge and picks from prize box

SESSION 4: Stop and Freeze

In the fourth session, the stop/freeze skill is introduced and reinforced with the use of a stop sign as a visual prop. Active practice of behavioral inhibition is key for targeting impulsivity. The child will engage in activities, such as the freeze dance game and Simon Says, for practicing the skill. The therapist and child will read *Turtle Magic* and identify how Timmy uses the stop/freeze skill, thinks about his problem, uses his turtle pose to keep calm, and goes back into play with his peers calmly.

Additional materials: Stop sign prop

Welcome/ Check-in
Welcome Song
Emotion Check in:
- Have children identify how they are feeling referring to 6 emotion cards or visual cues
  - *"How are you feeling today? Remember emotions tell people things. How would I know you are sad? Show me in the mirror. What made you feel sad today?"*
- Expand emotional vocabulary- "how does each emotion feel?"
- Emotions tell people things
Recap:
- Review Relaxation and incorporate cues for relaxation using imagery, puppets, and props--- use body tension/relaxation to help identify how child is feeling
  "Show me Robot (or Lego)! Show me Wiggly Worm!"

Fun & Learning
Fun and Learning Activity:
- Introduce Stop/ Freeze Skill- after children have learned how to recognize how their body feels relaxed versus tense, begin to introduce the Stop/Freeze skill. Children should practice inhibiting their behaviors and vocalizations.
- Play freeze dance game and Simon Says for skill practice
  - Take turns being "Simon", use the stop sign prop

Turtle Magic Story
- Read *Turtle Magic* and refer to the stop/freeze skills Timmy uses
  - *"Timmy stops/freezes, thinks about his problem, goes into his shell, gets peaceful, and goes back into play."*
  - Reference stop sign prop in story, incorporate stop sign into play

Reinforcement
Badge/ Prize and Wrap-Up:
- Child receives Freeze Pose badge and picks from prize box

Fig. 7.1 (continued)

individual, group format, or other, and if preschool-aged children would benefit from the intervention.

Participants for this study included 92 licensed/certified school psychologists, licensed clinical and master social workers, school counselors, and guidance

SESSION 5: Self-Talk

The fifth session focuses on self-talk and identifying what the child can say to themselves when getting ready to calm down so they can solve a problem. A visual teaching tool, such as a microphone, will be used to reinforce this skill. The child will refer to the self-talk pages in *Turtle Magic* and identify how Timmy uses positive self-talk to calm himself.

Additional Materials: Microphone toy/prop, Thought bubble printout/prop

Welcome/ Check-in
Welcome Song
Emotion Check in
Stop and Freeze - play song, practice skill
Recap:
- Review Stop/Freeze skill- practice impulse control games (i.e., Freeze Dance, Simon Says)

Fun & Learning
Fun and Learning Activity:
- Introduce positive self-talk: positive statements and phrases that the child can say to themselves to feel better, slow down, and think of positive coping thoughts to deal with a situation.
- Visual teaching tool - using thought bubble and microphone prop
  o *"It's hard to wait, but I can do hard things"*
  o *"It's not my turn, but I am working on sharing so everyone can have fun"*
  o *"I don't want to stop, but I will play again soon."*
- Role play positive self-talk - use puppets, thought bubbles, and microphone prop
  o Incorporate thought bubble props with puppets (model thinking, feeling, doing process with puppets)
    ▪ e.g., (Thinking) Sally the fox thought, "I wanted to use the paints during choice time."
      (Feeling) She feels disappointed and sad she cannot use the paints.
      (Doing) Sally will try building with blocks instead today. She makes a big castle tower with her blocks.

Turtle Magic Story
- Read *Turtle Magic* and refer to self-talk pages (p. 7)
    ▪ *"How does Timmy use this skill? Point out the times he is talking to himself!"*
      Child(ren) may use microphone prop to demonstrate Timmy's self-talk

Reinforcement
Badge/ Prize and Wrap-Up:
- Child receives Self-Talk badge and picks from prize box

Fig. 7.1 (continued)

counselors who worked with children between the ages of 3 and 12 years old at preschools and elementary schools in the United States. Participants were recruited to read a case vignette of three aggressive preschoolers, followed by the TMI-G treatment description and then complete self-report questionnaires to assess for

<u>**SESSION 6: Problem Solving**</u>

The sixth session introduces problem solving and uses a visual problem-solving chart to teach the three steps: stop, breathe (three deep breaths), and think ("what else can I do?"). The child will play out various problems and solutions using animal puppets. *Turtle Magic* will be read, and the child will be asked to identify how Timmy uses his skills to solve his problems.

Additional Materials: Extra puppets (animals, people), Problem Solving visual

Welcome/ Check-in

Welcome Song
Emotion Check in
Stop and Freeze practice (song, Simon says)
Recap:
- Recap positive self-talk: this is what I can say to help me feel better.
"Timmy, keep trying. You can do this!" (Use microphone prop)

Fun & Learning

Fun and Learning Activity:
- Introduce Problem Solving: ways we figure it out, come up with an answer or plan for a problem or challenge
    - Include 3 steps and method for problem solving (include visual 3 steps)

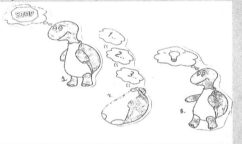

  - 1. Stop
  - 2. Breathe-Take three deep breaths
  - 3. Think-What else can you/I do?
- Play out problems and solutions in group - can use additional animal puppets

Turtle Magic Story
- Read *Turtle Magic* and refer to self-talk pages (p.7)
    - *"How does Timmy solve his problems?"*
- Child(ren) may use microphone prop, thought bubbles, turtle pose, etc. to demonstrate Timmy's problem-solving

Fig. 7.1 (continued)

treatment acceptability of the *Turtle Magic Intervention-Group*. Scores on the Treatment Evaluation Inventory-Short Form (TEI-SF, Newton & Sturmey, 2004) range from 9 to 45, with higher scores indicating greater acceptance of a given treatment. A total TEI-SF score of 27 indicates moderate acceptability of a treatment

Reinforcement
Badge/ Prize and Wrap-Up:
- Child receives Problem solving badge and picks from prize box

SESSION 7: Skills Recap

The seventh session is a skills recap session during which the therapist reviews relaxation strategies, self-talk, and problem solving. Each skill is reviewed and practiced using games and learning activities previously introduced.

Welcome/ Check-in
Introduction
Welcome Song
Emotion Check in
Stop and Freeze
Recap:
- Recap positive self-talk: This is what I can say to help me feel better.
  - *"Alex, keep trying. You can do this!"*
    - Use microphone prop

Fun & Learning
Fun and Learning Activity:
Review relaxation & deep breathing
- Robot vs. Wiggly Worm: Bodily sensations give us clues about how we feel
  - *"When you are calm, your body is relaxed, and you feel safe and happy. If you get upset, try to relax your body to help you feel good again."*
- Deep breathing with Pizza, Flower, Birthday cake

Self-talk
- Thought bubbles
  - Microphone [*If you feel angry you can help yourself. You can tell yourself to calm down:" It's okay. I can wait."*]

Problem solving
  - Review behavioral cues:
    - Solidifying sequence of 3 steps to problem solving:
      1. Stop
      2. Deep Breath
      3. Think about problem, think what else I can do?

Turtle Magic Story
- Read *Turtle Magic* in context of all cues and skills.

Fig. 7.1 (continued)

intervention. Results from the present study indicate that participants found TMI-G to be above moderate acceptability (Mean = 33.77, SD = 3.90) for children with aggressive behaviors and emotion dysregulation. Correlations were used to determine the relations between treatment acceptability and type of professional degree,

Reinforcement

Prize/Badge & Wrap-up:
- Child receives Turtle Skills badge and picks from prize box
- Prepare for final session- Termination discussion

SESSION 8: Termination and Putting It All Together

The final core session, Session 8, focuses on termination and recapping the skills learned in the context of the *Turtle Magic* storybook.

Welcome/ Check-in

Welcome Song
Emotion Check in
Termination Discussion
- *"This is the last time we will meet together for a while and learn with Timmy Turtle."*

Fun & Learning

Fun and Learning Activity:
- Putting it all together to RECAP all skills and concepts
  - Emotions, Relaxation, Freeze, Self-Talk, and Problem Solve

Turtle Magic Story

- Review *Turtle Magic* Story, skills, and cues

Reinforcement

Badge/ Prize and Wrap-Up
- Child receives the Turtle Magic badge and picks from prize box

SESSION 9: Booster Session

After four weeks, the child meets for a booster session during which time they review the skills learned throughout the sessions (Emotions, Relaxation, Freeze, Self-Talk, and Problem Solve).

Welcome/ Check-in

Welcome Song: "Eyes are watching, Ears are listening, Voices Quiet, Body Calm…This is how we listen, This is how we listen, At group time, At group time." (With whole body visual cues)

Emotion Review & Check in:
  - Emotion visual cue cards: identifying 6 core emotions: Anger, Disgust, Fear, Happiness, Sadness, Surprise

Fig. 7.1 (continued)

years of experience as a school practitioner, type of school setting, racial and/or ethnic background most prevalent amongst students, and geographical region in the US. No significant correlations were found. School practitioners were also asked if they believed TMI would be better implemented in an individual format, group format, or other. Of the participants, 65.1% indicated TMI would be better

    o Check yourself out: use a handheld mirror, children can practice making feeling faces.
    o *Intensity of emotions- this may be incorporated if child is focused and capable

Fun & Learning

Fun and Learning Activity:
Let's see how well you remember Timmy Turtle and all the things we learned and practiced together.

  • Putting it all together to RECAP all skills and concepts
    o Emotions: Recap 6 core emotions and what our feelings help us to do
    o Relaxation: Calm body and nice thoughts about ourselves keep us feeling good and safe.

Turtle Magic Story

  • Read *Turtle Magic* and refer to self-talk pages
    ▪ *"How does Timmy solve his problems?"*
    o Child(ren) may use microphone prop, thought bubbles, turtle pose, etc. to demonstrate Timmy's problem-solving steps

Reinforcement

Badge/ Prize and Wrap-Up:
  • Child receives Booster Turtle Magic badge and picks from prize box

Fig. 7.1 (continued)

implemented in a group format, while 10.8% preferred TMI for individual therapy. Additionally, 24.1% of participants selected "other" and provided short answer responses including TMI as a combination of individual and group therapy, and TMI as a classroom intervention. Of the school practitioners who completed this study, 94% believed preschool-aged children would benefit from TMI, while 6% did not believe it would be appropriate.

   Since the TMI approach is so new, there has been limited research on its efficacy for young children. The single-subject pilot study (Schira, 2018) with three aggressive preschoolers indicated teacher observed changes in the right direction at follow-up. Excellent treatment implementation fidelity was also determined for each session of the TMI manual. Since the treatment acceptability study completed by Pazmino Koste (2021) indicated strong acceptability ratings from school mental health practitioners, the logical next step would be to examine treatment outcomes with small groups of children. The small group format was highly endorsed by these school practitioners and we would also recommend adding parent pre-post assessments to future program evaluations.

7.5   Summary

Incorporating play materials, games, stickers/badges, and stories, the *Turtle Magic Intervention* described in this chapter is based upon the integration of cognitive behavioral concepts and play therapy approaches as a promising treatment of young children with anger and aggression problems. The nine sessions of *Turtle Magic Intervention,* implemented either individually or in a small group, are engaging and enjoyable for young children and can be easily implemented in school or community settings. Tables 7.1 and 7.2 include child-friendly resources and additional anger management strategies that can be included to extend treatment and/or to supplement the TMI protocol. Although outcome results on TMI are currently limited, the treatment program seems highly acceptable to mental health professionals working with young and aggressive children.

Table 7.2 Supplemental anger management play strategies for kids

1. *Anger in my body:* Where does anger live in your body? Using an outline of a body, have the child draw where the anger lives inside them Examples: "anger explodes out of my hands, I hit or break things", "anger comes from my mouth, I yell and say mean things", "anger lives in my brain, I think mean thoughts about others"
2. Symbolize your anger: Draw what it looks like, personify it, give it a name or use a character: it is important for children to see their angry feelings as outside of themselves and therefore able to be worked through and managed Examples of fictional characters: *Draco Malfoy* (Harry Potter), *Scar* (Lion King), *Sid* (Toy Story), Regina George (Mean Girls)
3. Playful breathing exercises:
• Blowing out birthday candles. Ask child to put all 10 fingers up, breath in and smell the flavored cake, and have them blow out the candles (fingers) as slow as they can
• Five finger breathing: Trace your hand breathing. Hold up one hand taking long deep inhales when tracing upward and slowly exhaling when moving down the finger
• Elsa breathing. Take the biggest and longest breath possible through the nose and slowly blow out of the mouth creating an amazing ice sculpture!
• Rainbow breathing. Start at the bottom of the red arch and inhale on the way up the rainbow, exhaling on the way down, adding as many colors as they'd like

(continued)

Table 7.2 (continued)

4. 5 Point Rating Scale (Buron & Curtis, 2003): Use 5-point rating scale teach feelings and intensities concepts. Rate the different levels of target feelings (i.e., anger, worry, sadness). Use different feeling words to expand emotional vocabulary. Can expand to incorporate body sensations, thoughts, or strategies to use at each level

5		**Angry** I've lost control. I'm not listening Anymore. I could hit, kick or bite. I need a quiet place to calm down.	
4		**Overwhelmed** Everything is too hard. I'm losing control and need to leave the environment I'm in. Give me space	
3		**Frustrated** I'm not getting it, I'm showing signs of stress I should take a break now.	
2		**Anxious** Trying to stay focused, but having a hard time staying on task Use calming strategies now	
1		**Happy** Ready and willing to Work	

5. *Trigger tracker* (identify typical triggers for angry feelings): have child write down triggers encountered in their day, as well as how affected they were (use scale 1–5)
   - Being told "no"
   - Getting teased
   - Being Left out
   - Losing a game/turn
   - Fight with a friend
   - Bad dream/poor sleep
   - Hungry
   - Bad grade on a test
   - Forgot homework

(continued)

Table 7.2 (continued)

6. *Make an Anger Iceberg:* Explain that most of the iceberg is underwater and cannot be seen clearly. Anger works much in the same way. We may be able to see angry behaviors, but what it is underneath anger can give us important information about how it starts and how we can resolve it. Can use this along with the trigger tracker

7. *Quiet corner:* Provide a quiet, calm corner for the child to use when they need a break. Build it with blankets, squishable toys, books, sensory fidgets, feelings poster, coping phrases basket

References

Buron, K. D., & Curtis, M. (2003). *The incredible 5-point scale: Assisting students with autism spectrum disorders in understanding social interactions and controlling their emotions responses.* Autism Asperger Publishing Company.

Carlson, S. M. & Wang, T. S. (2007). Inhibitory control and emotion regulation in preschool children. *Cognitive Development, 22,* 489–510.

Cole, P. M., & Jacobs, A. E. (2018). From children's expressive control to emotion regulation: Looking back, looking ahead. *European Journal of Developmental Psychology, 15*(6), 658–677. https://doi.org/10.1080/17405629.2018.1438888

Drewes, A. A. (2008). Bobo revisited: What the research says. *International Journal of Play Therapy, 17*(1), 52. https://doi.org/10.1037/1555-6824.17.1.52

Evans, S., Frazer, A., Blossom, J., & Fite, P. (2019). Forms and functions of aggression in early childhood. *Journal of Clinical Child & Adolescent Psychology, 48*(5), 790–798. https://doi.org/10.1080/15374416.2018.1485104

Fein, G. G. (1989). Mind, meaning, and affect: Proposals for a theory of pretense. *Developmental Review, 9*(4), 345–363. https://doi.org/10.1016/0273-2297(89)90034-8

Feindler, E. L. (1991). *Turtle magic.* Unpublished manuscript available at eva.feindler@liu.edu.

Feindler, E. L. (1995). Ideal treatment package for children and adolescents with anger disorders. *Issues in Comprehensive Pediatric Nursing, 18*(3), 233–260. https://doi.org/10.3109/01460869509087272

Feindler, E. L. (2009). Playful strategies to manage frustration: The turtle technique and beyond. In A. A. Drewes (Ed.), *Blending play therapy with cognitive behavioral therapy: Evidence-based and other effective treatments and techniques* (pp. 401–422). Wiley.

Feindler, E. L., & Gerber, M. (2008). Chapter 6. TAME: Teen anger management education. In C. W. LeCroy (Ed.), *Handbook in evidence-based treatment manuals for children and adolescents* (pp. 139–169). Oxford University Press.

Hoffmann, J., & Russ, S. (2012). Pretend play, creativity, and emotion regulation in children. *Psychology of Aesthetics, Creativity, and the Arts, 6*(2), 175. https://doi.org/10.1037/a0026299

Knell, S. M. (2009). Cognitive behavioral play therapy: Theory and applications. In A. A. Drewes (Ed.), *Blending play therapy with cognitive behavioral therapy: Evidence-based. and other effective treatments and techniques* (pp. 401–422). Wiley.

Landy, S., & Menna, R. (2001). Play between aggressive young children and their mothers. *Clinical Child Psychology and Psychiatry, 6*(2), 223–239. https://doi.org/10.1177/1359104501006002005

Newton, J. T., & Sturmey, P. (2004). Development of a short form of the treatment evaluation inventory for acceptability of psychological interventions. *Psychological Reports, 94*(2), 475–481. https://doi.org/10.2466/pr0.94.2.475-481

Pazmino Koste, E. (2021). Turtle Magic intervention: A group based intervention for aggressive preschoolers, a treatment acceptability study. (Unpublished doctoral dissertation). Long Island University Post.

Peterson, J. B., & Flanders, J. L. (2005). Play and the regulation of aggression. In R. E. Tremblay, W. W. Hartup, & J. Archer (Eds.), *Developmental origins of aggression* (pp. 133–157). The Guilford Press.

Pons, F., & Harris, P. (2000). *Test of emotion comprehension—TEC*. University of Oxford.

Robson, D. A., Allen, M. S., & Howard, S. J. (2020). Self-regulation in childhood as a predictor of future outcomes: A meta-analytic review. *Psychological Bulletin, 146*(4), 324–354. https://doi.org/10.1037/bul0000227

Saarni, C. (2000). Emotional competence: A developmental perspective. In R. Bar-On & J. D. A. Parker (Eds.), *The handbook of emotional intelligence: Theory, development, assessment, and application at home, school, and in the workplace* (pp. 68–91). Jossey-Bass.

Sala, M. N., Pons, F., & Molina, P. (2014). Emotion regulation strategies in preschool children. *British Journal of Developmental Psychology, 32*, 440–453. https://doi.org/10.1111/bjdp.12055

Schaefer, C. E., & Mattei, D. (2005). Catharsis: effectiveness in children's aggression. *International Journal of Play Therapy, 14*(2), 103–109. https://doi.org/10.1037/h0088905

Schira, A. M. (2018). Turtle magic intervention: A cognitive-behavioral play therapy treatment for aggressive preschool children, a pilot study (Unpublished doctoral dissertation). Long Island University Post.

Sukhodolsky, D. G., Kassinove, H., & Gorman, B. S. (2004). Cognitive-behavioral therapy for anger in children and adolescents: A meta-analysis. *Aggression and Violent Behavior, 9*(3), 247–269. https://doi.org/10.1016/j.avb.2003.08.005

Suveg, C., Southam-Gerow, M. A., Goodman, K. L., & Kendall, P. C. (2007). The role of emotion theory and research in child therapy development. *Clinical Psychology: Science and Practice, 14*(4), 358–371. https://doi.org/10.1111/j.1468-2850.2007.00096.x

Trotter, K., Eshelman, D., & Landreth, G. (2003). A place for Bobo in play therapy. *International Journal of Play Therapy, 12*(1), 117. https://doi.org/10.1037/h0088875

Wilson, B. J., & Ray, D. (2018). Child-centered play therapy: Aggression, empathy, and self-regulation. *Journal of Counseling & Development, 96*(4), 399–409. https://doi.org/10.1002/jcad.12222

Chapter 8
Playful CBT with Children Diagnosed with OCD

Jennifer Herren, Elena Schiavone, Anna Charlton Kidd, and Briana A. Paulo

Keywords Exposure and response prevention (ERP) · Cognitive behavioral therapy (CBT) · Play therapy · Obsessive-compulsive disorder (OCD) · Children · Pediatric OCD

8.1 Introduction

Obsessive-compulsive disorder (OCD) is a heterogeneous psychiatric condition characterized by unwanted, intrusive thoughts (obsessions) and repetitive or ritualized behaviors (compulsions) aimed to reduce distress associated with obsessions (American Psychiatric Association, 2013). OCD impacts individuals across development, including young children and adolescents. Pediatric OCD is often

J. Herren (✉)
Pediatric Anxiety Research Center, Bradley Hospital and Department of Psychiatry and Human Behavior, Warren Alpert Medical School of Brown University,
East Providence, RI, USA
e-mail: jennifer_herren@brown.edu

E. Schiavone
Florida International University, Miami, FL, USA
e-mail: eschi018@fiu.edu

A. C. Kidd
Department of Psychology and Neuroscience, Baylor University, Waco, TX, USA
e-mail: Anna_Kidd1@baylor.edu

B. A. Paulo
Department of Applied Psychology, Bouvé College of Health Sciences, Northeastern University, Boston, MA, USA
e-mail: paulo.b@northeastern.edu

R. D. Friedberg, E. V. Rozmid (eds.), *Creative CBT with Youth*,
https://doi.org/10.1007/978-3-030-99669-7_8

associated with functional impairment, disruption to developmental gains, and chronicity, making early intervention key (Albert et al., 2019; Fineberg et al., 2019). Family-based cognitive behavioral therapy (CBT) using exposure and response prevention (ERP) is a well-established and efficacious behavioral treatment for pediatric OCD with treatment response rates ranging between 64.7 and 100% in clinical trials (Freeman et al., 2018). Efficacy for family-based CBT using ERP extends to young children, ages 3–8 (Freeman et al., 2014; Lewin et al., 2014), and exposure-based CBT for OCD has been found to be effective when transported into community settings (Torp et al., 2015). ERP involves actively approaching anxiety-provoking stimuli while not engaging in any rituals or safety behaviors. Exposures may include facing actual in vivo situations, imaginal content, or distressing physical sensations (interoceptive exposures). For example, if a client with OCD experiences contamination-related obsessions and performs mental counting rituals, an effective exposure might involve the client touching a surface perceived to be contaminated (i.e., doorknob), focusing on the distress caused by that activity, and resisting the urge to count.

ERP is rooted in behavioral theory of both classical and operant conditioning. OCD symptoms are thought to be maintained through a negative reinforcement cycle, with rituals or avoidance behaviors being reinforced by providing temporary relief from distress. ERP aims to disrupt this cycle by eliminating avoidance and escape behaviors (e.g., rituals). Two main theories have emerged to explain the effectiveness of ERP: inhibitory learning (Craske et al., 2008; Craske et al., 2014) and habituation (Foa & Kozak, 1986; Benito & Walther, 2015). In both models, exposure to anxiety-provoking stimuli is necessary and is believed to directly facilitate a corrective experience through extinction learning; however, the processes thought to promote learning differs between the two models (Himle, 2015). The habituation model emphasizes exposure procedures that facilitate a natural decrease in anxiety over time (Foa & Kozak, 1986; Benito & Walther, 2015). The inhibitory model focuses on exposure procedures that create new expectations about what will happen when the feared stimulus is encountered such as a feared outcome not occurring or the ability to tolerate one's distress (Craske et al., 2008). Clinical applications discussed in this chapter are based upon the tenets of extinction learning that are broadly relevant to both theoretical models.

This chapter has a special emphasis on integrating play when delivering ERP. Integrating play into exposures can make them more tolerable and fun, which in turn may increase a child's engagement. More specifically, play is used strategically to foster a child's: (a) willingness to complete exposures, (b) engagement throughout exposures, and (c) favorable perception of treatment. Additionally, creating space for silliness and humor allows the child to have a different experience with a feared stimulus than they might have anticipated, which is a key tenet of the inhibitory learning approach (Craske et al., 2014). As a child's sustained engagement with exposure stimuli is essential to learning from an exposure, the benefits of play are particularly powerful to a child's treatment gains. It is important to be mindful of the *function* play has on an exposure. Depending on how play is used, it may detract from exposure (e.g., distract the child from the worries or distress the child is meant to face in the exposure) or enhance it (e.g., facilitate the child's engagement with their worries or distress). For example, simply playing a card game likely distracts from the targeted fear (i.e., detracts from the exposure) if the game does not relate to or trigger the core fear. Simple and quick modifications (e.g., contaminating the game, changing the rules of the game), however, changes the card game to target a fear. Examples of play-based exposures will be discussed with an emphasis on engaging a target fear.

Techniques in this chapter are described generally for a pediatric population but therapists should consider the developmental level of their own clients and tailor the intervention accordingly. For more detailed information on delivering CBT for pediatric OCD, consider reviewing *Treating OCD in Children and Adolescents* (Franklin et al., 2019).

8.2 Clinical Applications for Pediatric OCD

8.2.1 Providing Psychoeducation

Psychoeducation is an important foundation of treatment and is used throughout the course of treatment as needed. This early stage of therapy is a great opportunity for therapists to illustrate key concepts in a playful, engaging, and relatable manner. Primary components of psychoeducation outlined below typically include information about OCD, orientation to and rationale for ERP, and externalizing of OCD. General information about OCD (e.g., prevalence rates, nature of OCD) can be individually tailored based on a family's understanding of OCD. It is important to clarify any misconceptions during this part of treatment and to make clear that OCD is not the child or family's fault. The International OCD Foundation (2020) provides helpful online resources, including brochures and fact sheets that can be used to guide this discussion with families.

8.2.1.1 Our Body's Alarm System

Describing the body's innate fear response as a natural alarm system is a helpful metaphor for explaining how OCD functions in the brain and why ERP works. Below is an example of how this could be explained to a family.

> Example: Explaining the Alarm "Many people think of anxiety as bad, but anxiety is meant to be a helpful emotion. Anxiety is our body's natural alarm system. Just like a smoke detector would go off if there was a fire, our body's anxiety alarm alerts us when there is danger. For instance, if a tiger walked into the room right now our anxiety alarm would go off telling us to get away

instead of trying to pet the tiger! This is called a 'true alarm' and it keeps us safe from danger. Sometimes, however, people's alarms can become very sensitive—the volume is turned way up—and their alarm goes off when it doesn't need to. For example, this would be the case if after a kitten walked into the room your anxiety alarm went off telling you to run away or if a smoke detector went off when toast was burnt but there was no fire. These are called 'false alarms.' They feel just like true alarms even though there isn't any danger. Essentially, OCD takes over this alarm system. Rituals or compulsions can be thought of as specific ways you've learned to turn off this alarm. The ritual makes you feel better in the moment but leads to more rituals in the future. We want to help you turn down the volume of your alarm with a special treatment that we know helps kids with OCD called exposure and response prevention. Our job is to work as a team to help you 'boss back' OCD by facing these false alarms in small steps without doing your rituals."

Make this concept more interactive by asking the child how they might react if a kitten walked into the room, then ask how they might react if a tiger walked in the room or even make it playful by acting out the scene. Try providing other examples of helpful anxiety that are relevant to youth, such as studying when one is nervous about a test or jumping out of the way of an oncoming car. With children, we often talk about ERP as *bossing back* OCD. At the most basic level of explanation, bossing back is doing the opposite of what OCD wants you to do.

8.2.1.2 Goals of ERP

After building the rationale and orienting the family to how ERP works, introduce the goals of ERP. Exposure-based CBT aims to build tolerance for distress and to decrease anxious distress through repeated practice. One helpful way of explaining ERP is to compare it with learning a new skill that is relevant and interesting to the child (e.g., musical instrument, a sport, dance). For example, for a child who loves baseball, draw the comparison that when they first began playing, they likely could not throw a fastball or strike out their opponent. With persistence and practice, however, they learned new skills and became better at the sport "the more you practice, the better you get at the activity!" The same is true for ERP. Explain that confronting a feared situation will become easier over time as the child repeatedly practices being brave in that situation.

Similarly, the feeling of warming up after entering a cold swimming pool or the ocean is a helpful metaphor to explain a body's natural decrease in anxiety over time. Use Socratic questioning to illustrate on how the water feels really cold at first but if you stay in the water, it feels warmer over time. Prompt the child to reflect on the fact that the temperature does not actually change; instead, their body adjusts to being in the water, causing the water to feel warmer. Other ways to illustrate this point are by prompting the child to think about their fear the first time they rode a roller coaster or watched a scary movie and comparing the experience to how they might feel after doing the activity many times.

8.2.1.3 Normalizing Intrusive Thoughts

Intrusive thoughts are unwanted thoughts or images that enter an individual's consciousness. For children with OCD, however, some of these intrusive thoughts become salient and intensely distressing. Some children have a difficult time understanding these experiences and feel too embarrassed to verbalize the thoughts and associated distress. Psychoeducation regarding the nature of intrusive thoughts normalizes these experiences and sets the stage for doing ERP, during which children focus on these thoughts. Tompkins et al. (2020) suggest that labeling a thought as *bad* or *scary* makes us think it is important, which causes the mind to think about it more, thereby making the thoughts more frequent and/or distressing. When individuals with OCD try to push away the obsession, the thought only becomes stronger. There are several well-known prompts that demonstrate this concept. *Purple Elephant* is a version of this technique that includes the therapist prompting the child and family to imagine anything, except a purple elephant (Storch & Lewin, 2016). Use some of your engagement tools to be creative! Does your client enjoy playing a sport? Prompt them to think of anything in the world except their favorite athlete in a clown suit, for example. Processing this activity with the child and family highlights that pushing away thoughts tends to make them stronger and tougher to not think about. This technique can add to the child and family's understanding of how OCD, specifically intrusive thoughts, has become powerful.

8.2.1.4 Externalizing OCD

Externalizing OCD is an engaging strategy used with the child and family early in treatment. Personifying OCD as a separate entity removes self-blame both from the child and the caregiver, giving them an opportunity to unite together against a common enemy (Myrick & Green, 2012). Families often relate to this concept when comparing OCD to a bully who will not go away.

Externalizing OCD includes asking the child to name OCD and create an illustration of their OCD. If you or another family member is particularly skilled in drawing, you could ask the child to close their eyes and describe what OCD looks like and then draw the visual of it! Some children prefer to personify OCD with a familiar character, such as a villain from a movie or video game. Another idea is to use a photo or to print a coloring page of this character. For young children, choosing a tangible object, such as a stuffed animal, is often helpful to represent OCD.

8.2.2 Building a Fear Hierarchy

To optimally deliver ERP and create a hierarchy for OCD, it is crucial to understand the relation between obsessions and compulsions (Abramowitz et al., 2019; Conelea et al., 2012). Compulsions that look similar topographically (e.g., what the behavior looks like when observed) may serve different functions depending on the underlying obsession or fear. Function represents the *purpose* of the behavior and draws links between the action and associated antecedents and consequences.

Figure 8.1 depicts how the same ritual may be associated with a number of different obsessions. In this example, a handwashing ritual may *look* the same when observed topographically, but may reflect different functions, such as responding to a disgust feeling, trying to neutralize a harm obsession (e.g., getting sick, someone getting hurt), or achieving a feeling of symmetry. Understanding these connections will help a therapist select exposures appropriately.

The process of hypothesis testing and understanding the relation between obsessions and compulsions should start before initiating ERP and occur throughout treatment. Conelea et al. (2012) present a helpful framework for organizing and understanding function using a visual map to link obsessions with compulsions. A thorough functional assessment will prepare a therapist to make a hierarchy with the family. Next, general principles for building a hierarchy are described, followed by modifications to make this process more playful and engaging.

8.2.2.1 The Fear Thermometer

Prior to building a hierarchy, a scale measuring distress should be introduced to the child and family (e.g., 0–10 scale, stoplight, faces). The scale serves as a communication tool around a child's distress both within and outside of exposure. A common example is a *fear thermometer* with numbered anchors relative to an individual child's distress. One way to engage the child is to have them draw their own thermometer as an art project. They can create their own version by picking representations for different levels of distress, such as faces, colors, types of animals, or cartoon characters. Choose a range that meets the child's developmental level. Consider practicing using the scale with non-OCD situations (e.g., going to a new playground, riding a roller coaster) before using it for hierarchy items.

8.2.2.2 Creating and Climbing the Fear Ladder

A fear ladder (i.e., a fear hierarchy using a ladder metaphor) is an exposure treatment plan that lists out specific situations or feared stimuli that the client will gradually face without engaging in rituals or avoidance behaviors (Abramowitz et al., 2019). To introduce this concept to a child, you might say the following:

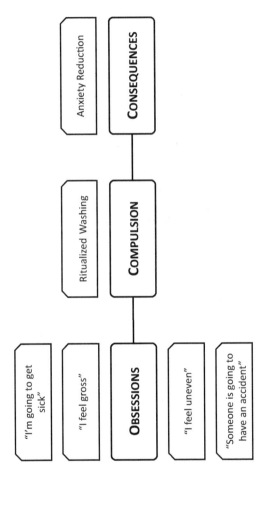

Fig. 8.1 Functional link between obsessions and compulsions

Example: Introducing the "Now we are going to focus on creating a plan together for how you are going to OCD. Today, we are making a fear ladder, which means we are going to talk about different situations that you might practice without doing any rituals or compulsions. I want you to use the fear thermometer to tell me how difficult something would be for you. Just like climbing a ladder, we don't start at the top or with the hardest practice first, we begin at the bottom of the ladder with something that feels like a small step."*boss back*

The next step is to identify specific situations that trigger the child's anxiety. Choose items that the child will practice in different contexts (e.g., office, home, community). Include situations, places, or things that are avoided or result in ritualizing on the hierarchy. When creating fear hierarchies for OCD, identify the obsession or fear the child is to focus on during the exposure, as well as any avoidances or ritualized behaviors the child should not engage in during or after the exposure. Ask the child and caregiver to rate items using the scale (e.g., fear thermometer) you introduced to the family. The goal is to identify items that represent low, middle, and high ranges of distress for a particular fear or target area. When trying to find ways to make an exposure easier or more difficult, consider changing the proximity of the stimulus, altering the amount of contact with the stimulus, combining more than one stimulus, having the caregiver present or not, or increasing or decreasing uncertainty around the task. It is important to note that sometimes building the hierarchy may be an exposure itself and a therapist needs to work towards the child sharing specific obsessions. Notably, caregiver perspective is especially important when creating hierarchies with younger children or children whose report is less reliable. Hierarchies for children should include specific items around reducing family accommodation as needed.

Hierarchies will constantly evolve throughout treatment and the initial hierarchy is meant to serve as a starting point for exposure work. To help facilitate engagement in hierarchy building, consider these options:

Create a *Sticky Note* Ladder

Write hierarchy items on sticky notes and ask the child to put them on the wall to create a sticky note ladder. The child can move around items as you build the hierarchy together. Figure 8.2 is an example of hierarchy items for a child who is fearful of bleach contamination and has compulsions of washing and counting.

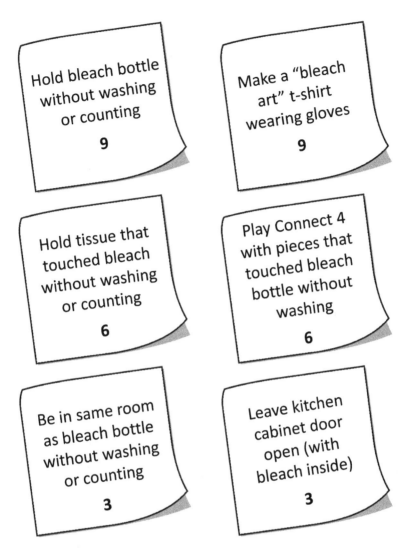

Fig. 8.2 Example of a *Sticky Note* Fear Hierarchy

Make a Bucket Game

Set up buckets on the other side of the room representing varying levels of difficulty (e.g., easy, medium, hard) or child's level of anxiety (e.g., a little, some, a lot). Write hierarchy items on pieces of paper. Ask the child to put cards into the bucket or even make it a basketball game by tossing the paper into the bucket.

Create Videogame Levels

Organize different hierarchy items into levels from easier to more difficult tasks. The child could design their own version or model the levels after their favorite game. For extra fun, create a hierarchy with a special or bonus challenge at the end of each level that they must complete before moving onto the next level.

8.2.3   Exposure and Response Prevention (ERP)

ERP is the main treatment ingredient in CBT packages for OCD treatment; therefore, it is imperative that ERP be part of your clinical intervention. This section will first focus on how to select an exposure with the family and general guidelines for delivering ERP. We will then discuss specific ways to use play to engage youth in exposure work.

8.2.3.1   Exposure Selection

The process of selecting an exposure should always be carried out collaboratively with the family. We have identified three steps for selecting engaging exposures for youth with OCD, detailed and summarized in Table 8.1.

The first step is to identify the current exposure goal and revisit the hierarchy. This goal is what you, the child, and/or their caregiver hope to achieve in completing an exposure during this session. Goals can be specific (e.g., eat more protein despite OCD food rules, wear a winter jacket the child believes is contaminated, tolerate uncertainty of what time mom will return from work) or broad (i.e., break food rules more generally, face contamination fears, tolerate uncertainty). Once you have identified the exposure goal, refer to the relevant hierarchy for exposure ideas for the session. Search for items in the hierarchy that relate to the exposure goal. In some cases, exposures listed in the hierarchy would achieve the identified goal in step one. In other cases, modifications to the exposure in the hierarchy would be necessary to achieve the goal. Aside from relevance to the identified goal, therapists

Table 8.1 Overview of how to select an exposure

Steps for exposure selection	Brief description
1. Identify current exposure goal	With family, identify the current exposure goal—whether specific or broad. Refer to fear hierarchy for exposure ideas related to the identified exposure goal
2. Integrate play (as appropriate)	Consider ways to integrate play into the exposure
3. Finalize exposure expectations	Conduct a *mini hierarchy* to titrate difficulty of exposure, clarify expectations, and finalize exposure before starting

should also consider selecting an exposure that is at the appropriate level of difficulty for the child, is engaging, and is one the child would be willing to attempt. Regarding exposure difficulty, it is better to pick an exposure on the easier side of the spectrum and later increase the difficulty than to start with an exposure that is too difficult and later attempt to reduce its difficulty. Think about exposure choice using the *Goldilocks principle*, meaning the goal is to find a task that is challenging yet doable (i.e., not too easy, but not too hard).

The second step is to brainstorm ways to integrate play into the exposure. As previously established, consider tailoring the exposure using activities (e.g., chess), franchises (e.g., Star Wars), and other things the child enjoys (e.g., cats). For further guidance on how to do so, refer to the section *Approaches to Integrating Play into Exposures*. In many cases, play can be integrated in some fashion. Once you have decided how to integrate play into the exposure, if applicable, finalize details of the exposure.

The last step is to conduct "mini" hierarchy building to clarify and finalize the exposure. "Mini" hierarchy building prior to the start of the exposure can be helpful to ensure the exposure task is clear, appropriately challenging, and engaging (e.g., playful enough to facilitate child's motivation). For example, a child with contamination fears may have "touch sink" as an item on their hierarchy. In presenting exposure options to the family and before agreeing upon an exposure, the therapist should try to be as specific as possible around the expected exposure task. In this example, further assessment might include specifying which sink the child would be touching (as child may perceive different sinks to have varied levels of contamination), whether the child will have direct or indirect contact (i.e., child touching the sink itself or an object that touched the sink), what part of the sink the child will touch directly or indirectly (e.g., faucet handle, side of the basin, drainage hole), what part(s) of their body will touch the contaminated item (e.g., elbow, one finger, two fingers, entire palm). Additionally, response prevention should be discussed and agreed upon prior to the exposure. For instance, this child may be asked to resist checking their hands to determine how contaminated they look; wiping, rinsing, or washing hands; or seeking reassurance from the caregiver.

8.2.3.2 Therapist Delivery of ERP

Prior to starting the exposure, clear instructions should be given about the expectations for the child, caregiver, and therapist. For younger children, coach caregivers on how to support the child during the exposure, such as how to respond if the child makes requests around ritualizing. Next, ask the child to approach the exposure stimulus. Once the exposure begins, try to help the child maintain contact with the exposure task. Examples include providing descriptive statements about the exposure itself (e.g., "Nice job being brave by breaking a rule with this game"), encouraging the child to decrease avoidance (e.g., "I want to focus on that incomplete feeling"), or increasing the difficulty of the exposure task itself (e.g., "Now touch it with your other hand, too"; Benito et al. 2020; Benito & Walther, 2015).

Given the goal of exposure is to create a new learning experience through building distress tolerance, attempt to avoid using strategies that purposefully reduce anxiety during exposure, such as using relaxation, providing accommodation, or distracting the child from the exposure. Additionally, there is no set length or rule for ending an exposure. While the inhibitory learning theory suggests that subjective reports of distress do not need to be reduced for exposure to end (Craske et al., 2014), an essential goal for OCD treatment is to ensure that children will continue to resist rituals related to the exposure after the session. If a child seems to be engaging in more approach behaviors and less avoidance, this is a good indicator that the exposure task is getting easier or they are tolerating their distress better. Natural reduction in fear (e.g., habituation) may occur within an exposure or through repeated practices though the habituation process is not necessary to end the exposure.

One engagement strategy that is especially helpful for younger children is for the therapist to play the role of OCD. You can either pretend to be OCD or use an object (e.g., puppet, stuffed animal) to represent OCD during the exposure. Playing OCD encourages the child to focus on the exposure task while also being silly and humorous. For instance, you could pretend to shrink in size as the child approaches the exposure task or "bosses back" OCD by doing the opposite of their rituals or saying things like "I don't have to listen to you."

8.2.3.3   Approaches to Integrating Play into ERP

This section details strategies for integrating play into exposures using games and creative arts. Examples for how to apply the approaches are provided. Some techniques lend themselves particularly well to certain core fears, while others have such varied applications that they span all core fears. Most, if not all, of these approaches can be used across several core fears. We strongly encourage you to be creative with application of these strategies.

Creating New Exposure Games

One way to integrate play into exposure is to create a new game. This gives you the ability to highly specialize a game towards a child's specific obsessions and associated triggers. The process of making a game with the child may be part of the exposure if constructing the game pieces is anxiety-provoking. The following are examples of different games that can be used in ERP.

Word Games Some children with OCD may avoid certain words or phrases associated with obsessional content. Constructing a word game is a fun way for kids to gradually approach this content by either first seeing the content, writing the content, or saying it aloud. These games can be particularly helpful for youth with illness worries, specific fears (e.g., ticks, severe weather, vomit), sexual obsessions, or morality concerns. A number of these games (e.g., Build a Flower, Word

Association) can also be used interactively during telehealth if you have a shared whiteboard.

Memory Game Build your own version of a memory game with "tiles" (e.g., paper cut into squares) featuring pairs of words related to the core fear you intend to target. The goal of this game is to have the child look at and think about content on the tiles. For example, for a child with obsessions about getting ill, create memory tiles with names of different illnesses (e.g., the flu, pneumonia, diarrhea). The exposure can simply consist of playing the game and thinking about the illnesses listed on the tiles. Alternatively, ways to increase difficulty might be to combine the game with other triggers (e.g., touching a germy surface before playing), having the child say the words aloud during the game, including pictures, or sharing facts or a story for each match made.

Go Feel Uncomfortable This game is based on Go Fish with cards involving avoided words or phrases. Make your own version of Go Fish "cards" with whatever materials you have on hand (e.g., paper cut into rectangles) featuring pairs of words or images related to the core fear you intend to target. Memory cards can also be used to play this game. For example, if a child worries about using "bad" words, make cards with the avoided content. The child then verbally asks, "Do you have a [avoided word]?" as part of the game. In this example, selection of words should be collaboratively decided with the child and caregiver. For an easier version, consider words that rhyme with or sound like the "bad" words. The exposure can consist of playing the game and thinking about if the child did something immoral by reading or saying the words written on the cards. Ensure the child resists any rituals, such as confessing.

Word Association Competition Compete to see who can think of the most words related to a word central to the core fear one would like to target. If your client has an unlucky color of red, take turns saying different words that are associated with that color (e.g., stop sign, cardinal, autumn leaves) to see who can come up with the most words. The goal would be for the child to engage in the game and resist any rituals. In this example, you could write the words with a red marker to make the task more challenging.

Build a Flower/Build a Snowman This game involves having a secret word or phrase that the other player must guess by giving letters. The secret word should be related to obsessional content that you are trying to target. If the child misses the letter, you draw one part of a flower or snowman until the child either guesses the word/phrase or the full picture is drawn. For example, for an illness related exposure, the therapist may make the secret word be "cancer" and the child guesses letters until they identify the word or lose when the flower or snowman is fully drawn.

Spin the *Exposure Wheel* This game is a fun way to introduce playfulness around choosing different aspects of an exposure by "spinning a wheel." To complete this game, identify different potential aspects of exposure and put them into a randomizer (e.g., a virtual wheel to spin, write them on slips of paper and place in a bowl). "Spin the wheel" to randomly choose aspects of exposure. For example, if a child is fearful of cartoons and fantastical media, collaboratively write down names of characters from cartoons and fantasy films on slips of paper and put them into a bowl. Take turns reading names on slips of paper and pulling up images of the characters. If a child habituates to the images, increase the exposure difficulty by watching videos of the characters instead. This particular approach also introduces more uncertainty, which may be another exposure target. To add even more uncertainty (as appropriate), the therapist could choose the characters without child input.

Secret Mission: Code Brave Design an adventure or special mission for the client that is relevant to their core fear. This game is especially helpful for children with morality concerns around breaking rules or doing something "wrong." For example, a Code Brave assignment might be to put an item in the grocery store back in the "wrong" spot without confessing. It is important to discuss these types of exposures with caregivers separately to provide the rationale and secure their agreement. Another Code Brave example is completing a scavenger hunt to search for feared stimuli or associated items. For instance, a child who is afraid of spiders might have scavenger hunt items including going to a spot they previously saw a spider, going to the basement, finding an outside spider web, or finding a real spider. Additionally, Code Brave can be used to target evenness/symmetry urges by moving personal items around or throwing away items to target hoarding.

Modifying Existing Games

Another way to use games is to make quick modifications to existing games to activate the child's core fear. Modifications can include changing or adding rules to gameplay or altering the physical pieces of the game (e.g., contaminating game pieces). Many of these approaches require owning board games although the specific board game is often flexible.

Change or Create New Rules Changing or creating new rules of board games may serve as an exposure for youth with rigidity, *not just right* (NJR) feelings, perfectionism, or morality concerns as part of their OCD. This approach often requires hierarchy building to identify what specific rule changes would activate or increase the anxiety you wish to target. For instance, an exposure task in a Monopoly game might include one or more of the following: the child moving pieces in the opposite direction, paying the *wrong* owner of space they land on, not collecting $200 when they pass go, or not going to jail when they get a *go to jail* card.

Contaminate Games Contaminate a preferred game or toy (e.g., board game, Legos, stuffed animals) with the goal of the child playing with the contaminated object. For example, a child who considers his younger sister to be highly contaminated given that she crawls on the floors of public places can play Scrabble with pieces touched by the child's younger sister before playing. During the Scrabble game, encourage the child to focus on the contaminated tiles and resist related rituals. Contaminating game pieces may be modified using sticky substances as well (e.g., small amounts of soda or honey).

Operation The game of Operation is useful to target health related fears or disgust. For example, each player describes an illness related to the body part where the item was removed. When the child removes the ankle bone, they share or read a story about bone cancer.

Pictionary Similar to word games, Pictionary is easily adapted across a wide range of core fears and helps a child approach feared content in a fun way. For example, if a child is fearful of bugs, a therapist and child can take turns drawing and guessing different items associated with insects. Pictionary is a game that is applicable for telehealth by using a shared whiteboard screen or holding up pieces of paper to the screen.

Simon Says Use Simon Says to encourage movement while activating a relevant core fear. For example, this game is helpful to target asymmetry or unevenness in body movements (e.g., tap your left hand but not the right). For children with sensory intolerance or NJR feelings with clothing, playing Simon Says while wearing clothes that do not feel right promotes distress tolerance while engaging in activities.

Creative Arts

Using art as a medium to complete exposures is very effective across a number of core fears. Below are some examples of ways to use integrate arts into ERP when treating pediatric OCD.

Baking/Cooking For contamination fears, bake and eat a preferred treat in the presence of a contaminant or with "contaminated" hands. For example, if a child is afraid of coming in contact with cleaners, a family may bake brownies with disinfectant wipes on the counter while resisting rituals. Cooking or baking using knives, if developmentally and clinically appropriate, can be an engaging exposure for youth who may avoid sharp objects due to self-harm obsessions. Changing proximity to the knife or altering the type of knife (e.g., plastic, butter, bread knife) are ways to make the exposure easier or harder. For perfectionism obsessions, purposefully altering a recipe, such as putting in too much or little of an ingredient, might be distressing for the child and can build tolerance for making small mistakes.

Artwork Using art across many different mediums is a creative and fun way to engage children in exposures. For children with NJR or incompleteness symptoms, consider asking the child to color outside of the lines, choose *incorrect* colors for objects (e.g., blue sun, red grass), and/or leave portions of the drawing incomplete without correcting. Art projects are useful for targeting avoidance related to sticky substances or disgust. Completing art projects using glue, finger painting, or shaving cream may target these feelings. Given these projects can become quite messy, be mindful of slowly approaching the task to ensure the exposure is manageable and not too difficult. Similar to using knives with baking, some children may avoid using scissors for fear of harming themselves or others. Art projects incorporating scissors can be utilized to help them approach the stimulus. To target hoarding, purposefully create a drawing or complete a coloring page to recycle. The child would *boss back* OCD by resisting the urge to save it or take it out of the recycling bin. To add some extra fun, consider making paper airplanes to fly into the recycling bin!

Media While not necessarily play, using media (e.g., video games, movie clips) can make exposures more engaging given these are typically preferred activities. For example, there are scenes from TV shows and movies appropriate for different ages that feature vomiting (e.g., Dora the Explorer, Arthur, Pitch Perfect 2, Cheaper by the Dozen). For intrusive images or thoughts, consider watching or reading the scene from Harry Potter and the Prisoner of Azkaban when Harry casts the Riddikulus spell to banish the Boggart. In the scene, the spell turns a Boggart, who feeds on fear, into something silly, taking away its power. Rather than avoiding scary thoughts, encourage children to use their own Riddikulus spell and imagination to change the distressing image/thought into something silly. One could sit with the funny version of the intrusive image or even draw a picture of it as an exposure.

Songs and Storytelling Another fun way to help youth approach feared content is for them to create a silly song or story. Change the information and level of detail of the story or song make it more or less difficult. For stories, use a *Roll-a-Story* format with dice to turn this activity into a game. Collaboratively identify and assign a character, setting, and problem that are related to obsessional content to each dice number (e.g., 1–6). The child then rolls the dice for each category to select prompts to be used in a story. For instance, a child with obsessions related to choking might roll the dice and be asked to produce a story involving a sibling (character), the bus (setting), and gagging (problem). Read the story as an exposure. Encourage details to create a vivid imaginal exposure as a way to increase the difficulty.

8.2.4   Family Involvement

Family involvement in pediatric OCD treatment is important and targeting family accommodation (e.g., family involvement in rituals, changes in routine in response to OCD) is associated with positive treatment responses (Anderson et al., 2015; Lewin et al., 2014). Since children spend the majority of their time outside of therapy, it is critical that families continue incorporating and reinforcing strategies or techniques learned in treatment (e.g., reducing accommodation, encouraging children to approach feared stimuli without ritualizing). The amount therapists use these strategies will depend on a child's presentation, motivation, and interactions within the family. Repeating play-based exposures completed during the therapy session at home is one helpful strategy to promote ERP at home. Encourage caregivers to participate in your session exposures to help build their confidence in completing similar exposures in the home environment.

Using positive reinforcement strategies is strongly encouraged, including verbal praise for brave behavior. Many children also benefit from a rewards system. Utilization of rewards to encourage children to complete between-session homework is an important way for caregivers to reinforce treatment strategies. Rewards can be tangible items (e.g., stickers, small toys) or privileges (e.g., staying up 30 minutes past bedtime, making a preferred treat, family movie night, having special time with a caregiver). As an example, create a *Bingo* chart filled with exposure practices that the child can earn a sticker or checkmark for completion. Once they have a bingo, the child can earn a reward. Most importantly, be creative and identify rewards that are reinforcing for the child.

Other helpful strategies for caregivers when doing ERP with children include modeling and scaffolding (Freeman & Garcia, 2008). One way children learn is by observing adults. Encourage parent modeling of brave behavior by demonstrating approach to uncomfortable situations and by calmly encouraging children to do the same. Other family members can model brave behavior by participating in exposures both in session and at home. Scaffolding supports a gradual approach to help the child face challenging situations, especially with unexpected triggers. To scaffold approaching an anxiety-provoking situation, a caregiver should first identify the child's emotion and empathize with their feelings. Second, brainstorm options to limit avoidance and help the child approach the situation in some way. Lastly, encourage the child to approach and praise them for brave behavior.

8.2.5 Relapse Prevention

Relapse prevention is typically incorporated towards the end of treatment and includes educating the family about the chronicity of OCD, possible reemergence of symptoms, and value of continued exposure practice. It is important for families to know that exposure does not end with treatment but should become part of a new lifestyle. Comparing OCD to a weed in a garden exemplifies how anxiety returns if you do not keep engaging in exposure. To help the child practice managing new or reemerging symptoms, ask them to pretend to be the therapist and help you with an OCD symptom. Children often find this to be a fun way to practice applying these skills to new situations.

Lastly, another part of relapse prevention is to focus on the child's progress and skill acquisition. Making a project, such as a video or book, promotes self-efficacy by reviewing ways in which a child has progressed and it documents skills the child has learned. This final project can be a helpful resource for families after treatment to review skills.

8.3 Conclusion

Cognitive behavioral therapy using ERP is a well-established and effective treatment for pediatric OCD. Integrating play and using playful approaches when delivering ERP for OCD can help promote treatment engagement and increase tolerability of exposures for youth. When using play in ERP, it is important to be mindful of the function of play with the primary goal to increase engagement and willingness rather than serving as a distraction. By being creative and playful with CBT for

OCD, children not only create new and helpful learning experiences but they can have a little fun too!

References

Abramowitz, J. S., Deacon, B. J., & Whiteside, S. P. H. (2019). *Exposure therapy for anxiety: Principles and practice* (2nd ed.). Guilford Publications.

Albert, U., Barbaro, F., Bramante, S., Rosso, G., De Ronchi, D., & Maina, G. (2019). Duration of untreated illness and response to SRI treatment in obsessive-compulsive disorder. *European Psychiatry, 58*, 19–26. https://doi.org/10.1016/j.eurpsy.2019.01.017

American Psychiatric Association. (2013). *Diagnostic and statistical manual of mental disorders* (5th ed.). Author.

Anderson, L. M., Freeman, J. B., Franklin, M. E., & Sapyta, J. J. (2015). Family-based treatment of pediatric obsessive-compulsive disorder. *Child and Adolescent Psychiatric Clinics of North America, 24*(3), 535–555. https://doi.org/10.1016/j.chc.2015.02.003

Benito, K. G., Machan, J., Freeman, J. B., Garcia, A. M., Walther, M., Frank, H., et al. (2021). Therapist behavior during exposure tasks predicts habituation and clinical outcome in three randomized controlled trials for pediatric OCD. *Behavior Therapy, 52*(3), 523–538. https://doi.org/10.1016/j.beth.2020.07.004

Benito, K. G., & Walther, M. (2015). Therapeutic process during exposure: Habituation model. *Journal of Obsessive-Compulsive and Related Disorders, 6*, 147–157. https://doi.org/10.1016/j.jocrd.2015.01.006

Conelea, C. A., Freeman, J. B., & Garcia, A. M. (2012). Integrating behavioral theory with OCD assessment using the Y-BOCS/CY-BOCS symptom checklist. *Journal of Obsessive-Compulsive and Related Disorders, 1*(2), 112–118. https://doi.org/10.1016/j.jocrd.2012.02.001

Craske, M. G., Kircanski, K., Zelikowsky, M., Mystkowski, J., Chowdhury, N., & Baker, A. (2008). Optimizing inhibitory learning during exposure therapy. *Behaviour Research and Therapy, 46*(1), 5–27. https://doi.org/10.1016/j.brat.2007.10.003

Craske, M. G., Treanor, M., Conway, C. C., Zbozinek, T., & Vervliet, B. (2014). Maximizing exposure therapy: An inhibitory learning approach. *Behaviour Research and Therapy, 58*, 10–23. https://doi.org/10.1016/j.brat.2014.04.006

Fineberg, N. A., Dell'Osso, B., Albert, U., Maina, G., Geller, D., Carmi, L., et al. (2019). Early intervention for obsessive compulsive disorder: An expert consensus statement. *European Neuropsychopharmacology, 29*, 549–565. https://doi.org/10.1016/j.euroneuro.2019.02.002

Foa, E. B., & Kozak, M. J. (1986). Emotional processing of fear: Exposure to corrective information. *Psychological Bulletin, 99*(1), 20–35. https://doi.org/10.1037/0033-2909.99.1.20

Franklin, M. E., Freeman, J. B., & March, J. S. (2019). *Treating OCD in children and adolescents: A cognitive-behavioral approach*. The Guilford Press.

Freeman, J., Benito, K., Herren, J., Kemp, J., Sung, J., Georgiadis, C., et al. (2018). Evidence base update of psychosocial treatments for pediatric obsessive-compulsive disorder: Evaluating, improving, and transporting what works. *Journal of Clinical Child & Adolescent Psychology, 47*(5), 669–698. https://doi.org/10.1080/15374416.2018.1496443

Freeman, J. B., & Garcia, A. M. (2008). *Family based treatment for young children with OCD: Therapist guide*. Oxford University Press.

Freeman, J., Sapyta, J., Garcia, A., Compton, S., Khanna, M., Flessner, C., et al. (2014). Family-based treatment of early childhood obsessive-compulsive disorder: The Pediatric Obsessive-Compulsive Disorder Treatment Study for young children (POTS Jr)—A randomized clinical trial. *JAMA Psychiatry, 71*(6), 689–698. https://doi.org/10.1001/jamapsychiatry.2014.170

Himle, M. B. (2015). Let truth be thy aim, not victory: Comment on theory-based exposure process. *Journal of Obsessive-Compulsive and Related Disorders, 6*, 183–190. https://doi.org/10.1016/j.jocrd.2015.03.001

International OCD Foundation. (2020). Retrieved December 7, 2020, from https://iocdf.org

Lewin, A. B., Park, J. M., Jones, A. M., Crawford, E. A., De Nadai, A. S., Menzel, J., et al. (2014). Family-based exposure and response prevention therapy for preschool-aged children with obsessive-compulsive disorder: A pilot randomized controlled trial. *Behaviour Research and Therapy, 56*, 30–38. https://doi.org/10.1016/j.brat.2014.02.001

Myrick, A. C., & Green, E. J. (2012). Incorporating play therapy into evidence-based treatment with children affected by obsessive compulsive disorder. *International Journal of Play Therapy, 21*(2), 74–86. https://doi.org/10.1037/a0027603

Storch, E. A., & Lewin, A. B. (2016). *Clinical handbook of obsessive-compulsive and related disorders*. Springer International Publishing.

Tompkins, M. A., Owen, D. J., Shiloff, N. H., & Tanner, L. R. (2020). *Cognitive behavior therapy for OCD in youth: A step-by-step guide*. American Psychological Association. https://doi.org/10.1037/0000167-000

Torp, N. C., Dahl, K., Skarphedinsson, G., Thomsen, P. H., Valderhaug, R., Weidle, B., et al. (2015). Effectiveness of cognitive behavior treatment for pediatric obsessive-compulsive disorder: Acute outcomes from the Nordic long-term OCD treatment study (NordLOTS). *Behaviour Research and Therapy, 64*, 15–23. https://doi.org/10.1016/j.brat.2014.11.005

Chapter 9
Superheroes and CBT for Youth

Sandra S. Pimentel and Ryan C. T. DeLapp

Keywords CBT · Superheroes · Child and adolescent psychotherapy

9.1 Introduction

> *You're much stronger than you think you are. Trust me.*
> —Superman

Child and adolescent cognitive behavioral clinicians strive to teach CBT principles, skills, and strategies in ways that are accessible, creative, and tailored to youth interests. For this, superheroes provide abundant material and opportunities. From comic books to cartoons, and television shows to blockbuster movies, superheroes are highly available models to many youth. Superhero content (for better or worse) is plentiful in the form of school supplies, clothing, costumes, stickers, and other goods. While noted for gender and racial representation (see McGrath, 2007), in addition to their increasing visibility across pop culture formats, modern superheroes are diverse and their narratives increasingly inclusive and relatable.

Comic books, often featuring superheroes, have long been used for promoting positive messages (e.g., Captain America and patriotism) and health education (Branscum & Sharma, 2009) as well as safety and resilience related to abuse (e.g., Spider-Man). Research also demonstrates that priming individuals with superhero social concepts or associated physical poses facilitate prosocial behaviors (Pena & Chen, 2017; Rosenberg et al., 2013). Beyond serving as models, superhero themes provide useful metaphors (Rubin, 2007); more directly, superhero stories can be

S. S. Pimentel (✉) · R. C. T. DeLapp
Department of Psychiatry and Behavioral Sciences, Montefiore Medical Center/Albert Einstein College of Medicine, New York, NY, USA

Anxiety and Mood Program Child Outpatient Psychiatry Division, Bronx, NY, USA
e-mail: spimente@montefiore.org; rdelapp@montefiore.org

R. D. Friedberg, E. V. Rozmid (eds.), *Creative CBT with Youth*,
https://doi.org/10.1007/978-3-030-99669-7_9

utilized for specific elements that may match a youth's experience, such as early parental loss or absence (Betzalel & Shechtman, 2017). Others have introduced incorporating superheroes into CBT with youth (Friedberg & McClure, 2015) as well as a more explicit "Superhero Therapy" as a format for delivering CBT and ACT-based strategies (Scarlet, 2017).

So, why superheroes? Superheroes provide clinicians infinite resources for teaching and executing CBT—their stories are engaging, imperfect, and generally encompass a series of trial-and-error efforts in problem-solving. Sure, some of their problems may involve stopping global destruction, but they have problems nonetheless! Every superhero has an origin story where learning and practice are emphasized, as superheroes often have superpowers, weapons, costumes, and/or props that they must learn how to use. Many also have sidekicks or a team of superheroes to help during their missions. This chapter provides transdiagnostic treatment recommendations drawing upon the superhero genre to enhance youth treatment engagement and cognitive behavioral skill building. We aim to demonstrate varied examples of and suggestions (as summarized in Table 9.1) for utilizing superhero metaphors, models, language, and associated accoutrements that can be used across youth ages, interests, and presenting concerns.

9.2 Case Conceptualization and Superhero Narrative

Cognitive behavioral case conceptualization drives treatment planning and intervention (Friedberg & McClure, 2015; Persons, 2012). A full conceptualization aims to develop a coherent framework for understanding a patient's presenting concerns via ongoing assessment and iterative "working hypotheses." In addition to a problem list, the biopsychosocial conceptualization includes origins of presenting concerns, predisposing and maintaining factors, protective factors and strengths; it incorporates family, culture, and context. While case conceptualization is beyond the scope of this chapter, clinicians often start CBT by providing a summary and synthesis of information gathered following comprehensive assessment. With this information, we tell the best understanding of the "story"—the diagnoses, yes, but more so how problems may have started and are interfering with functioning (e.g., going to school, making friends, sleeping, etc.), the interplay among thoughts, feelings, and behaviors (including avoidance or withdrawal), and the proposed plan for the course of treatment.

9.2.1 Origin Stories

Every patient has a story; every superhero has an origin story to which some youth can liken their own stories. Superheroes can be gods, humans transformed by accidents, tragedies, science experiments, or technologically advanced body suits;

Table 9.1 Superhero Adaptations and CBT Interventions

Superheroes adaptations		CBT intervention	Example
Superhero origin story	Using superhero background stories as metaphor for a patient's symptom etiology and to provide psychoeducation about CBT interventions	Psychoeducation & conceptualization Problem-solving Emotion recognition & expression Exposure & desensitization Behavioral activation Somatic management	For a child struggling with perfectionism, using the Avengers loss at the end of Avenger: Infinity Wars to discuss thoughts, feeling, and actions associated perceptions of failure
Superpowers	The concept of "superpowers" aligns with goal of skill acquisition and mastery	Problem-solving Emotion recognition & expression Exposure & desensitization Behavioral activation Somatic management	Therapist to patient: "What if I told you that you already have a couple of key superpowers for dealing with your panic attacks? Some skills that allow you to do battle with it"
Superhero missions	The concept of "superhero missions" aligns with challenges or obstacles patients must acquire and/or strengthen skills to complete	Problem-solving Exposure & desensitization Behavioral activation	Framing learning how to prepare to engage in exposures or resist avoidance and withdrawal urges
Training sessions	The concept of "training sessions" illustrates the importance of skill rehearsal	Problem-solving Emotion recognition & expression Exposure & desensitization Behavioral activation Somatic management	Framing repeated exposure practice as a "training sessions" to strength bravery superpower
Incredible Hulk's storyline	The Incredible Hulk provides a metaphor for several components of emotion regulation	Psychoeducation & conceptualization Problem-solving Emotion recognition & expression	Viewing Hulk transformation videos to provide psychoeducation about physiological arousal associated with anger
Superhero rating scales	Superhero themed scales can be used to help patients create emotional rating scales	Psychoeducation & conceptualization Emotion recognition & expression	Using images of brave superhero scenes to create a Bravery Rating scale
Next frame	An experiential exercise using comic strips	Problem-solving Cognitive coping	Using a scene from comic strip and prompting to use details from one frame to anticipate the thoughts, emotions, and actions of the superhero in the next frame of the comic strip

(continued)

Table 9.1 (continued)

Superheroes adaptations		CBT intervention	Example
Thought bubbles & villain thoughts	Using thought bubble illustration to support cognition awareness and the concept of "Villain Thoughts" to emphasize Automatic Negative Thoughts	Emotion recognition & expression Cognitive coping Desensitization & exposure Behavioral activation	"When I worry about what other people think. It's the Joker…it tricks me"
Power breaths & riding the wave	Framing somatic management strategies as superpowers that ultimately help with tolerating stressful situations	Somatic management Desensitization & exposure	Teen with panic disorder envisioned herself as a Super-Surfer with her "Super SurfBoard" to "ride the wave" of her intense physiological symptoms
Tools & props Superhero song Superhero poses	Using tools, props, and mimicking superhero actions to increase confidence in one's ability and motivation to engage in skill rehearsal	Problem-solving Emotion recognition & expression Exposure & desensitization Behavioral activation Somatic management	Anxious younger kid wears a "Brave Cape" or "Courage Cuffs" during in vivo exposures

they can also be mutants or royalty, of this universe or realm or even everyday folks among us. Superhero stories show early adversity and later resilience from that adversity. Further, grief, loss, anger, or social rejection offer entry points for the affective education that often occurs early in CBT. Skills can be framed as super-powers as illustrated below in a session with one teen patient:

T: *You mentioned you really liked Spider-Man?*
P: *Yea.*
T: *Can you tell me why he stands out to you from all the superheroes?*
P: *He lost his parents like me.*
T: *Right. And then he even lost his uncle too in a violent way.*
P: *He was bullied by kids at his school. And he lived in New York.*
T: *Like a lot of teenagers, you can see he dealt with a lot of social stuff too. The therapist in me likes that there's attention to his feelings of rejection and the grief he was working through. What can I say? Peter Parker was a science nerd, and I'm a psychology nerd.*
P: *(Laughs).*
T: *Spider-Man's story can actually be helpful for us in what we will work on. Understanding how his story led him to have certain feelings and expectations about the world and for himself. How he used something he was good at, science, and then had to learn a bunch of new stuff—from perfecting his costume to his web-shooter… In the movie, remember how rough it was for him in the beginning when he was learning?*

P: Yea, he got banged up.

T: Yea, and he set goals and kept at it. He found a way to help others and made connections. Like you, he had a really tough experience when he was younger and really struggled. Our job together is to figure out how with your story... you can use the strengths you have and maybe learn some new superpowers or skills that can help you achieve your goals.

P: Okay. But he got bit by a radioactive spider.

T: Good point. We can skip that part, deal?

In this dialogue, the clinician utilizes a natural interest of the teen patient by creating a shared understanding of his "origin story." The Spider-Man narrative offers language to discuss difficult experiences, such as sexual abuse, rejection, and loss, while normalizing that the emotions associated with such experiences are familiar. Additionally, Spider-Man's story features themes of perseverance and resilience that set the stage for discussing therapy's role within the teen's story—collaboratively working with the clinician to strengthen skills (e.g., framed as one's own superpowers) needed for his goal attainment.

[Authors' note: In the 1980s, Spider-Man powerfully revealed that he had been sexually abused as a child. Marvel Comics and the National Committee for the Prevention of Child Abuse joined forces as part of a mass education campaign for kids (and adults) on the effects of sexual abuse. In the comic supplement, Spider-Man disclosed his feelings of fear, helplessness, and shame and how he shared what happened to him with his trusted aunt and uncle, and the comic supplement itself provided additional guidance and strategies for youth (Gorner, 1985; https://www.chicagotribune.com/news/ct-xpm-1985-02-10-8501080651-story.html). This well-developed story line for arguably one of the most popular superheroes provides an impactful model for resilience.

As noted, superheroes are increasingly available and representative models, and this can aid in more meaningful inclusion for coping and mastery models. At the start of the Coping Cat workbook, an efficacious treatment for youth anxiety disorders (e.g.., Walkup et al., 2008), we learn the origin story of Coping Cat (Kendall & Hedtke, 2006). Born in September 1988, and starting off as a scaredy cat, the scene is set to understand how the workbook and treatment can help transform fear into coping. Soon after the movie "Black Panther" was released (and reinforcing the importance of representative models!), one young boy of color starting CBT for his anxiety exclaimed: "Oh I want to be the Coping Black Panther!" And so, that framed the treatment moving forward.

9.3   Superheroes and the Stories of Marginalized Groups

From X-Men's powerful fighter Storm, who was one of the first black female comic book characters to more modern America Chavez (see below) and Miles Morales, also known as "the Black Spider Man" and/or "the Puerto Rican Spider Man," diverse superhero models are available. Their origins as mutants who have been marginalized may be valuable models for youth from marginalized groups. For example, gender diverse, LGBTQ+, or neurodiverse youth may present with anxiety and mood difficulties connected to having been bullied or teased for being "different." They may encounter systems (e.g., schools, churches) that label them as such, and they may experience added challenges. The very origin of the X-Men series launched in 1963 during the Civil Rights movement reflected the times fraught with racism, bigotry, and disenfranchisement of Black Americans. X-men were mutants experiencing discrimination and anti-mutant sentiment, and they promoted tolerance—"Sworn to protect a world that hates and fears them." From these early days and characters such as Beast and Cyclops and through time with Storm and Nightcrawler to more modern mutant X-Men like Taki the "Wiz Kid" who has dyslexia, these characters have drawn youth (and adults) precisely because of their origin stories and their marginalization. One of the central messages of Professor X and the X-Men is embracing difference, challenging the notion of difference as meaning "broken" or "less than," and learning to harness the powers that come with these differences sometimes in the face of bigotry. How's that as a conceptual model for both acceptance and change skills in CBT?

9.4   Coping Is a Superpower

Coping skills *are* superpowers. There, we said it. Some we may already know and carry with us. Some we may even do regularly—like breathing!—and can learn to do in a particular way. Strengths-based conceptualization acknowledges what youth bring into the therapy room (or even the virtual Zoom room). Some skills youth must learn entirely, practice, tweak, and practice some more. As shown with this 14-year-old with panic disorder, the superpowers can be used to highlight strengths that they already possess:

T: Why do superheroes have superpowers?

P: To be able to fight the bad guys.

T: Right. Now like we talked about, anxiety isn't necessarily bad but when you have a full-blown panic attack, it feels pretty evil and dangerous for sure.

P: Definitely.

T: What if I told you that you already have a couple of key superpowers for dealing with your panic attacks? Some skills that allow you to do battle with it.

P: (Stares at therapist) I don't know.

T: One is something you already do without thinking…breathing.

P: Breathing? I feel like I can't even catch my breath sometimes.

T: I remember you saying that. It's a really scary feeling and a common one for people having a panic attack. Like we talked about, the threat switch got flipped and has set off the danger alarm. You have a superpower to help you reset. This is learning to breathe in a particular way. The regular breathing we don't often think about is like regular strength. This type of slower, and controlled breathing is like superpower strength, and it can be learned with practice.

P: Um, okay (skeptical)

T: I know, it seems simple but with practice when you are not having a panic attack, you can get better at it, and use it when that false alarm goes off.

The above example demonstrates an option for conceptualizing patient's presenting concerns and treatment interventions through the lens of superpowers. Of course, the therapist would have laid psychoeducational groundwork for understanding the panic cycle, including thoughts, physiological symptoms, and behaviors associated with triggering and maintaining panic attacks (e.g., Pincus et al., 2008, b). Furthermore, as in the above example, cognitive reappraisal strategies (discussed in more detail below) may be framed as superpowers as youth learn to identify their automatic thoughts and overestimation and catastrophic thinking errors. Like slowing down breathing, slowing down one's thinking and catching those catastrophic beliefs can be quite powerful!

The following sections will provide a few detailed examples of how the superhero genre can be intertwined into how some specific coping skills are introduced in therapy and how patients implement these skills. See Table 1 for a list of superhero adaptations for CBT interventions.

9.5 Problem-Solving

Superheroes face internal struggles as well as a host of external ones. Spider-Man and Batman fought crime in New York. Superheroes like Captain America, Captain Marvel, Wonder Woman, Superman, America Chavez as well as many others have a long history of fighting Nazis. The players in the "Save the World" edition of Fortnite become "heroes" tasked with, well, saving the world. Superheroes battle problems on all scales, from local to global, universal, and intergalactic problems. It's what they do. So, they can teach us a thing or two about problem-solving. Problem-solving skills training can be a transdiagnostic stand-alone treatment (e.g., D'Zurilla & Nezu, 2010) or be an important component of a broader CBT for youth across conditions, including anxiety (Kendall, 2006), depression (Becker-Weidman et al., 2010; Rohde et al., 2005), self-injurious thoughts and behaviors (Glenn et al., 2014), anti-social behavior (Kazdin, 2000) and in varied formats of delivery (e.g., cognitive behavioral group treatment for social anxiety Stand Up, Speak Out, Albano & DiBartolo, 2007).

Superheroes solve problems and they have missions. For some youth, clinicians can frame problem-solving skills in terms "superhero missions." Superheroes most notably put their problem-solving skills on display when they have "missions" and utilize their superpowers to navigate seemingly insurmountable obstacles. Problem-solving steps generally include some variation of the following: (1) Identity the problem, (2) Brainstorm options and alternatives, (3) Consider those options, (4) Make a plan, (5) Try it out, (6) Evaluate how it went, (7) Self-praise for effort. Superheroes, when faced with missions, follow the same general steps. Below are a few examples of utilizing the superhero mission theme to encourage growth in problem-solving skills.

9.5.1 Brainstorming

Youth with problem-solving skills deficits often fail to see and generate alternative solutions to the problems they are experiencing. As such, an essential skill in problem-solving is brainstorming. Superheroes have ideas. They are smart and clever. Often, they rely on the best science (real and imagined!). So, when teaching brainstorming, clinicians can enlist superheroes for a fun method of teaching this as a skill. For example, they might ask "Imagine you're on Wakanda? What would Black Panther say?"

"Imagine you're sitting in the X-Mansion. What would Professor X say? Storm? Wolverine?"

"Imagine you're in the Avengers Compound, what would Iron Man suggest? Thor? Black Widow? Nick Fury?" and/or "Imagine yourself around the Justice League table, what would Wonder Woman suggest? Superman? Batman?"
Observational Learning

Observational learning is a common source of skill acquisition for everyone—especially children (Bandura et al., 1966). Superhero stories are rich with illustrations of the problem-solving steps and thereby viewing superhero movie and/or cartoon clips or reading comic strips can be utilized as a great observational learning tool. Superheroes often are confronted with complicated emotions and competing agendas in pursuit of their missions, which provides an opportunity to prompt the patient to consider all of these factors while identifying a target problem, generating solutions, and evaluating the consequences.

Consider the dilemma Captain America faces when he is forced to confront and subdue his long-lost friend, Bucky. As depicted in the Captain America movies, Bucky was transformed into a brainwashed soldier called a Winter Soldier. For the sake of therapy, Bucky was an old friend who became a bad guy. Just this relationship dynamic alone can be relatable to young patients in that it sparks this question, "How do I treat a close friend who now does or says hurtful things?" Clinicians can simply summarize this backstory of the two friends and prompt patients to practice defining quite a complicated problem: completing the mission and trying to save his friend. Next, clinicians can show movie clips of their battle scenes and encourage patients to observe and evaluate the solutions Captain America implements to resolve both dilemmas. Lastly, clinicians can conclude this exercise by prompting patients to consider any parallels between Captain America's dilemma and their own lived experiences, thereby encouraging problem-solving skill acquisition and application.

9.5.2 Experiential Learning

Children may be reluctant to engage in talk-based therapy, especially early in the treatment process. Indeed, they rarely self-refer to treatment. A potential solution for establishing rapport, building trust, and introducing a framework for the course of treatment is to engage in an experiential problem-solving task. The clinician can introduce problem-solving skills by creating an activity that presents a dilemma the child must resolve. This does not require the clinician to have an in-depth knowledge of all dilemmas a particular hero has faced. Furthermore, in the early stages, it does not even require the therapist to discuss the presenting problems.

Consider the patient dialogue below of a 9-year-old girl with ADHD with emotional outbursts:

T: *Today, I was thinking we could talk about Shuri and how you said before that she was the true superhero in Black Panther.*
P: *Yea, she was. T'Challa would not have been able to do anything without her inventions.*
T: *I thought that was really interesting. Haven't heard that one before. So, I was wondering who's the better inventor - Shuri or Tony Stark?*
P: *Oooo. That's a hard one, but I think Shuri. She's got the smarts plus she knows how to use the Vibranium in her inventions.*
T: *So, what if Shuri and Tony Stark teamed up to build a spaceship?*
P: *That would be dope. I mean, I think Shuri is the better inventor though (laughs).*
T: *I have a game for us to play today. Let's say you are Shuri and I am Tony Stark. We have these Legos here and we are going to build a spaceship for the Avengers. But, here is the thing. We can't talk and we have to take turns building.*

From this point onward, the clinician can prompt the patient in identifying the problem (communication), generating and evaluating solutions (e.g., draw on a white board/blank paper, hand signals), solution implementation (e.g., building together using the selected strategies), and discussing what went well afterwards.

9.5.3 "Next Frame"

Another experiential exercise involves using comic strips for problem-solving skills training. As mentioned, comic books can be used to teach youth how to identify and name cognitions via thought bubbles and call outs. Clinicians and patients can draw, via comic book frames, the specific problem or challenge facing the youth. Each frame captures specific automatic thoughts, worries, assumptions, and/or frustrations that all comprise a problem the superhero must resolve, with multiple "next frames" lined up. As shown in Fig. 9.1, youth and clinicians can identify a stressful situation, consider multiple "Next frames" depending on the alternatives they select, and simulate different possible outcomes.

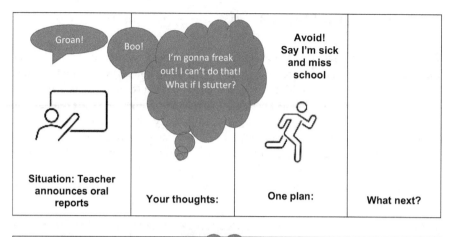

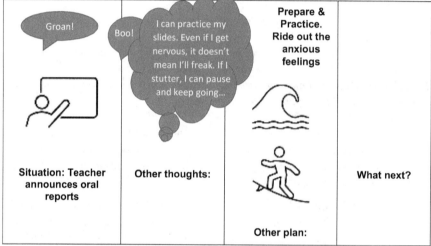

Fig. 9.1 Sample Next Frame

Following any of the aforementioned exercises, the clinician now has the option of personalizing the superhero's problem-solving to the child's presenting problems. The concept of generating a solution can be redefined as finding the most appropriate "superpowers" to manage the formidable foes (or the child's presenting concerns). In using a strengths-based approach, the clinician can first prompt the child to consider "superpowers" that are already possessed and evaluate their effectiveness. Similar to training sessions where superheroes are getting used to their powers (e.g., Scott Lang practicing shrinking in his Ant Man suite or Peter Parker practicing web-swinging through the city), clinicians can frame therapy as a means to strengthen these superpowers. Also, the problem-solving framework creates space to emphasize the importance of identifying a variety of coping responses—many heroes require more than one power.

9.6   Emotion Recognition and Expression

A common goal within most cognitive behavioral interventions is to support growth in a child's emotion regulation skills, as such skills are transdiagnostically applicable (Uhl et al., 2019). A core element of emotion regulation is the ability to mindfully observe and identify emotional states at varying intensities (also known as affect labeling). And the importance of affect labeling is accentuated by its ability to promote regulation of autonomic and behavioral responses to perceived negative affect (Torre & Lieberman, 2018).

9.6.1   Introducing Affect Labeling

An essential ingredient to building such emotional awareness is applying the thought-feeling-behavior model to various emotional states. Superhero stories provide dilemmas that are accessible to children and assist children as they observe and describe components of the thought-feeling-behavior model.

T: Do you believe the thought-feeling-behavior model can be used to describe a person's response to any situation? I mean any situation?

P: I guess

T: You like Spider-Man, right?

P: Uh huh

T: How do you think Peter Parker felt when he first learned about his Spidey senses? What emotions did he have?

P: I guess scared. But maybe a little excited too because he was able to climb on the wall and stuff.

T: Why do you think he was scared and excited to be climbing walls?

P: I mean…who doesn't want to be able to climb walls, jump really high, and swing from building to building. It's just cool. But, I guess it would be weird to all of a sudden be able to do this.

T: Look at that. You just used the thought-feeling-behavior model. Feelings…scared and excited. Behavior…Climbing on walls. Thoughts… "This is weird and cool." Now, if you can do this with Peter Parker, I know you can do this for your own situations throughout the week.

If youth have limited emotional vocabulary, clinicians can provide a list of emotion types and use thoughts and actions displayed in superhero comics, cartoons, and movie clips to improve affect labeling skills.

9.6.2   The Incredible Hulk and Emotion Recognition

The Incredible Hulk's super strength powers directly parallel the emotion regulation construct. As the story goes, Dr. Bruce Banner, a smart and well-accomplished scientist, gains super strength by way of experimental malfunction that must be well-managed, or he risks uncontrolled destruction when provoked. He is a representation of the range of emotion regulation and dysregulation. The distinction between Dr. Banner and the Incredible Hulk represents a great visual model for psychoeducation about the emotion of anger.

Consider an 8-year-old male who is presenting with explosive angry outbursts in response to task difficulty (e.g., homework, losing in video games) and transitioning from preferred to non-preferred activities (e.g., transitioning from screen time to bedtime). The child and parents present to treatment with limited awareness of triggers or early signs of worsening mood—often explaining, "He goes from 0 to 60 with little warning." Conceptually, there could be a myriad of other factors influencing the angry outbursts (e.g., family–child relationship, reinforcement schedules, biological predispositions); however, after functional assessment, the evident deficits in emotional recognition and expression represent an early treatment target that can also increase the child's treatment buy-in.

Specifically, Dr. Banner's seemingly instantaneous transformation into the Incredible Hulk provides a clear visual of various targets for improving emotion regulation because on closer examination, there are clues that can help. Therefore, his transformation into the Hulk exemplifies the youth's seemingly instantaneous outbursts and associated interventions—psychoeducation about changes in the autonomic nervous system arousal, behavioral patterns that vary by emotional intensity, consequences of behavioral patterns at higher intensity, and learning to connect one's emotions to their values. Dr. Banner's story also provides an opportunity to educate about the thought-feeling-behavior model within the context of anger without requiring the child to acknowledge or describe the severity of their own emotional outbursts.

A particularly therapeutically rich scene comes from the 2003 movie production of Hulk where Bruce Banner is engaged in a physical altercation with Major Glenn Talbot (Lee et al., 2003). During the scuffle, Major Talbot is depicted penning Banner to the floor and Banner communicates, "You are making me angry." Talbot's non-compliance with Banner's effort to emotionally communicate his anger results in Banner's transformation to the Hulk and the subsequent destruction of property and physical aggression.

In processing this scene with a patient, there are several potential treatment relevant topics. The most obvious observation is the physiological changes depicted in Dr. Bruce's transformation into the Hulk that resemble the arousal of the sympathetic nervous system (e.g., changes in skin color, muscle tension, tachycardia, increased breathing). Also, the scene depicts an example of how Dr. Banner has had to develop strategies for early self-awareness of his changing emotional intensity (i.e., "You are making me angry")—an example that is particularly germane to the aforementioned case describing a "0 to 60" emotional escalation. This element of the scene provides an opportunity to prompt the child to consider what Banner might have noticed to signify that his transformation to the Hulk felt imminent—awareness that this situation has previously triggered him, changes in physiology, or awareness of aggression urges.

Next, Major Talbot's unresponsiveness to Banner's expression of "You are making me angry" depicts how emotional reactivity can partly result from under-developed emotional communication skills or environments not responding to one's efforts to communicate emotional distress and assert needs. To this end, this problem-solving example can be used to prompt kids to identify alternative forms of emotional communication and assertiveness skills—preferably reframing Dr. Banner's "You are making me angry" to "I am starting to feel angry right now and I would like for you to give me some space to calm down." Also, this example highlights the importance of providing psychoeducation and coaching caregivers and adults within the child's environment (e.g., teachers). They can improve the child's efforts to engage in effective communication, especially during the early phases of treatment when the child's communication results in seemingly ineffective, accusatory approaches, such as "You are making me angry." Clinicians can support parents and other caregivers with instruction about how to provide validating responses that successively reinforce growth in healthy emotional expression and regulation (Meyer et al., 2014). Lastly, the resultant property destruction and physical aggression in the clip present an opportunity to discuss the consequences of unmanaged anger.

9.6.3   Superhero Rating Scales

Superheroes can provide good examples for creating emotion rating scales. Consider identifying scenes from comics, television shows, or movies where superheroes display the targeted emotion and create a scale anchored by different displays of this emotional intensity. Superhero narratives are rich with displays of the range of affect including, fear, sadness, anger, bravery, hope, excitement, and triumph. Dr. Banner and the Incredible Hulk are, once again, a great illustration of the spectrum of calm to uncontrolled emotion. The creation of a "Hulk Meter" (as shown in Fig. 9.2) displaying the shades of Banner's physical transformation into the Hulk can become a tool for patients (especially younger children) to communicate their emotional intensity to parents and other adults in their lives (e.g., teachers). Of note, the "transformation" portion of scale represents an opportunity for clinicians to encourage patients and their families to identify early signs of "transformation" (e.g., physiological arousal, patterns of negative statements). Similarly, a "Brave Meter" featuring superheroes and their acts of bravery along a continuum of low to high bravery can be utilized to help children communicate how much bravery they perceive an exposure task might require and/or serve as a metric of progress—"I have achieved a Captain America level of bravery today."

Fig. 9.2 Sample Hulk
Meter. Clinician and
patient can collaborate to
select images to anchor the
scale

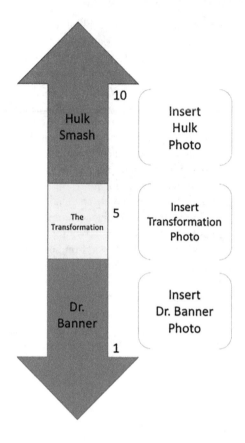

9.7 Cognitive Coping Skills

Cognitive coping skills as superpowers apply transdiagnostically. Early phases of
CBT for youth involve learning to self-monitor their thoughts, feelings, and actions
on worksheets, self-monitoring forms, or daily diaries. An integral focus of CBT is
supporting youth in better understanding how their thought patterns are associated
with presenting concerns. The recognition of cognitive distortions, or negative
thought patterns that often unrealistically and/or rigidly construe perceived experiences, is an important component of cognitive therapies. It is imperative that youth
initially possess a framework to mindfully observe and describe their cognitive
experiences. Below are a few options for supporting such self-awareness:

9.7.1 Thought Bubbles

Clinicians teach youth to pay attention to their thoughts or cognitive distortions
(e.g., thinking errors or "traps") that may be associated with their uncomfortable
feelings (see, for example, Coping Cat, Kendall & Hedtke, 2006). As such, comic

books and graphic novels are a useful format for teaching youth to pay attention to their "thought bubbles." Quite straightforwardly, comic books with superheroes can be used to teach youth the process of cognitive interventions: that is, how to identify thoughts in various situations, acknowledge certain thoughts and connect them to certain feelings, and validate those feelings (e.g., "If the character is feeling like nobody likes them, it makes sense they are sad and want to skip class"). This may require either clinicians to have their own collection of comic books or invite youth to bring in and share their favorites.

The clinician and patient often review the CBT-comic books together, stopping on certain frames to connect a character's thoughts with emotional cues and other aspects of the story. Specifically, clinicians can read a superhero comic in-session, prompt youth to observe the thought bubbles throughout the story, and generate dialogue about how each character's momentary thoughts are influencing the youth's reactions within the story. Next, clinicians can create comic strips where the child chooses the superhero's dilemma and then provide empty thought bubbles for the child to complete. The ultimate goal of the thought bubbles is to inspire youth's curiosity about their own thought bubbles.

9.7.2 Villain Thoughts

Children often closely identify with the superhero protagonist and are intrigued by the hero's ability to resist, thwart, and overpower the efforts of the crafty villain. The superhero provides an opportunity to support youth in casting themselves as the superhero while externalizing their negative thought patterns as a villain.

Youth can learn to use "thought bubbles" to express what they are thinking in situations and to spot the Villain thoughts. Clinicians can inquire, "As you're thinking about your math test, what's in your thought bubble?" Automatic thoughts can be fast! Youth can develop a new relationship to their thinking by using the thought bubbles to *slow down* those automatic thoughts and take a closer look. By externalizing their thinking process, youth become primed for the cognitive reappraisal process.

An occasional concern about cognitive therapies is their ability to be accessible across the age span. Incorporating superhero, and in particular, superhero comic book callouts that say power phrases like "Pow!," "Splat!," "Boom!," "Zap!" can be quite engaging for younger patients. Moreover, these power phrases can be used to stop automatic negative thoughts (ANTs) in their tracks and battle them in a developmentally appropriate way. One 6-year-old learned to "SPOT and STOMP!" the monster ANTS with—you guessed it—his Super-Spotter and Super-Stomper! He designed, drew, and colored them in comic book frames (picture ski goggles with lasers and large red platform boots) and practiced, with significant specific labeled praise for reinforcement, how he would enter his room when he got scared of monsters in his room.

Box 9.1 Example of Superhero Language in Cognitive Work
Perfectionism is my Kryptonite. It freezes me.
My mind reading is like a messed up telepathy power.
"Shoulds" are like Fortnite Husks in my brain
When I'm depressed it's like all my thoughts are evil shape-shifters

Given that unmanaged ANTs can perpetuate unwanted, unproductive behaviors for youth, CBT-based interventions often prioritize strengthening a child's ability to evaluate the factual nature of their thinking to promote more flexible, realistic thought patterns; a skill also known as cognitive restructuring. Cognitive distortions are a collection of commonly experienced ANT patterns and they make us vulnerable. Also known as "thinking traps," sometimes youth get "stuck" in these thought patterns and cognitive restructuring can help to get them unstuck—if they can learn to see them coming! All-or-none thinking keeps youth from seeing nuances and the possibilities in the middle. Catastrophizing assumes the worst possible outcomes. Overestimation errors miscalculate and predict the increased likelihood of bad events happening with often the added whammy of underestimating our ability to handle outcomes. Jumping to conclusions leads us to skip over and miss information. For anxious or depressed youth, fortune telling typically doesn't predict a joyful future. Helping youth identify these vulnerabilities in their thinking can be an important first step in catching, challenging, and changing these thought habits. Superheroes have strengths and vulnerabilities. Adapting superhero language, youth can be encouraged to spot the vulnerabilities in their own thinking. Please see text box for samples (Box 9.1).

Learning how to recognize these vulnerabilities and patterns allows us to see them, examine them more closely, and come up with a plan. Cognitive coping skills include teaching youth how to use dispute handles or Socratic questioning in service of cognitive restructuring. They can learn to challenge their maladaptive thinking, ask clarifying questions, and test the assumptions in their thoughts. The dialogue with a teen diagnosed with Social Anxiety and OCD presented below illustrates the process:

P: I really screwed up. All my friends hate me.

T: What happened?

P: I was talking way too much about the movie. I was excited but being a terrible friend. I think I annoyed them. And then I apologized a few times for being annoying and they were like "STOP it's fine"

T: Wow, "terrible friend" sounds harsh. Did your friends know you were excited to see it?

P: Um yeah, of course.

T: Let's take a closer look at those thoughts? What do we know about your thinking traps?

P: Feeling like I have to be perfect is my Kryptonite.

T: *How can knowing that help you here?*

P: *I feel like I have to be a perfect friend and that sets me up to feel bad. And I think I'm not then I apologize over and over again.*

T: *Right. And what about the mind reading?*

P: *It's super negative messed up telepathy.*

T: *Now, I have no idea if you were talking too much or what that even means, and I have no idea if some of your friends got annoyed, but what I do know is that a messed up telepathy power is not a source that can be trusted!*

P: *Yea.*

T: *How would you react to a friend who is excited about something?*

P: *I'd want to hear about it.*

T: *Do you ever get annoyed with your friends?*

P: *Sometimes.*

T: *Me too. It's normal. Do you know that ALL of them got annoyed? There's that all-or-none thinking.*

P: *No, I guess not. But they got annoyed when I kept apologizing.*

T: *They all did?*

P: *Well one of them.*

T: *Can you spot the effects of the Kryptonite?*

P: *It turned my excitement over something into worry, then I obsessed, then I apologized a lot, and then I kept thinking about it over and over.*

T: *That's some powerful Kryptonite. Even the most powerful Superman has a vulnerability that he has to watch out for. How can knowing this help you?*

In this example, the therapist works with the youth, first, to recognize and name their cognitive distortions, and second, how they can begin to challenge them to create alternative scripts and more effective coping. Notice, the goal is not positive thinking per se—sometimes we annoy our friends!—it is understanding how to make our thinking more realistic and helpful. Superhero language can aid in this skill building.

9.7.3 Coping Self-talk

Coping self-talk can be framed as a superpower. While therapists can use superhero language to spot thinking traps, they also can work with youth to incorporate this language and associated metaphors into developing more effective self-coaching. Please see Box 9.2 (Authors' note: This teen taught their therapist about America Chavez comic books, a more modern character who had been unknown to the therapist. They noted that they were drawn to America Chavez as a superhero because she is a "Latina, lesbian, tough girl" and her origin story includes having two mothers from an alternate universe. The teen patient also described appreciating that the superhero attended college at Sotomayor University, another meaningful reference for them in a nod to the Supreme Court Justice who had been born in a familiar

Box 9.2 Examples of Superhero Language in Coping Self-talk
I'm fortune-telling again. I have to remind myself that I do not have the power to time travel to the future. I'm more powerful when I remind myself to stay in the present
Flexible thinking is like Vibranium
Like America Chavez, I can punch through the dimensions in my thinking into other possible realities. Instead of jumping to conclusions, I can use my ability to jump dimensions to think about what else is possible

neighborhood—the Bronx!. This teen became increasingly and meaningfully excited to (1) teach the curious therapist about the character and plot advancements, and (2) review the America Chavez comic books with an eye toward therapy themes and skills. Therapists are off the hook for feeling as if they have to know all the characters or shows!).

In addition to this type of representativeness, and as previously noted, therapists further can utilize superheroes as models for adaptive thinking. Wonder Woman and Captain America are famously optimistic and hopeful; they are also determined and pragmatic. Despite, and likely because of great adversity, superheroes adapted how they think and approach the world. When faced with superhero problems (e.g., saving the world, stopping crime, helping humanity and the like), they do not succeed by surrendering to their vulnerabilities, insecurities, or anxieties. They succeed in (1) reflecting, (2) engaging in more flexible thinking, (3) problem-solving, (4) developing a plan, and (5) finding and using social support.

9.7.4   Strengths Check

In addition to their super-strengths, superheroes possess many favorable everyday strengths and qualities that help them with their struggles. Sure they can teleport and crush things, and they are smart, funny, hopeful, curious, sassy, determined, etc. These strengths are as important for enacting those superpowers. After all, as we learned with Spider-Man, "with great power comes great responsibility." And, further, that sense of responsibility gives more power. Across diagnoses, youth may present with negative self-perceptions. From a strengths-based CBT perspective, clinicians can work with youth to identify and affirm their basic strengths. Youth are tasked with recalling or selecting as many strengths as apply from a pre-existing list (see Fig. 9.3) and then clinicians can discuss how treatment will support patients in enhancing their strengths during their "superhero missions."

This is a STRENGTHS CHECK

Funny	Like dancing	Cheerful
Kind	Thoughtful	Good hug giver
Like Drawing	Scientist	Listen to music
Curious	Compassionate	Friendly
Sassy	Like reading	Creative
Like to play sports	Sense of humor	Like videogames
Helper	Like animals	Like poetry
Care about the environment	Musical	Tell fun jokes
Responsible	Care about others	Clever
Fun	Dependable	Like stickers
Energetic	Quiet	Like cooking
Easy-going	Focused	Cheerful
Friendly	Giving	Smart

Fig. 9.3 Strengths Check

9.7.5 Self-validating Thoughts

Many superhero narratives depict a real struggle, and at times, a temporary defeat at the hands of the villain. Therapists can seek out any examples of temporary set-backs, losses, rejections, defeats, and failures. Furthermore, these examples can be used to metaphorically validate the difficulty of managing "villainous" thoughts (or cognitive distortions). For example, after Thanos obtained the last infinity stone, there was a collective dismay and sense of failure experienced by the Avengers at the end of *Avengers: Infinity War* (Russo et al., 2018), as their powers appeared insufficient relative to Thanos' newly obtained strength. Sadness, anger, shock, and a sense of failure are all illustrated as the Avengers witness their comrades instantaneously vanishing. Clinicians can prompt patients to observe and describe the cognitive reactions to their perceived or actual momentary defeats or setbacks (e.g., not passing a test, not receiving a party invitation, or having an awkward peer interaction) and generate a sense of self-compassion and self-validation. Below is a therapeutic dialogue with a 10-year-old boy with social anxiety:

T: So, how was school today? Were you able to practice any of your brave goals [of raising your hand to ask or answer a question]?

P: No. I really wanted to but my Villain thoughts were telling me, "They will laugh at you" and that if I asked the teacher to repeat what she said, "They will think I'm not paying attention."

T: Ooh sounds like the Villain thoughts were pretty powerful. I know that you have talked a lot about wanting to feel more brave in school. What made the Villain thoughts seem so strong?

P: I don't know. They just made a lot of sense to me at the time. With all my nervous issues, they tell me what I want to hear. "Don't do it."

P: It's tough to not know what others will do or think. I know others who have similar Villain thoughts. But, just a quick reminder. Why do we call these thoughts your Villain thoughts?

P: I know. I know. Because they trick me sometimes.

T: Yes, they can be tricky and their trickiness can be frustrating and hard to deal with. Does Batman win every small battle with the Joker?

P: No.

T: But he does eventually learn how to beat him in the end—sometimes even using what he learned from the battles lost to help him to triumph in the end. We keep at it. And remember—sounds like you did a good job at labeling the Villain thoughts this time. So how can we use this attempt for next time you try to practice?

As demonstrated in the dialogue above, acceptance-based strategies can be essential for overcoming nonlinear treatment progress and maintaining treatment motivation. Often, there are both internal and external motivators creating pressure for children and adolescents to change their ways; with these pressures engender guilt, resentment, frustration, and hopelessness as ANTs continue at times as relentless foes. It is important to help patients develop empathy and compassion as they learn to manage ANTs and develop a concept for incorporating their setbacks into the bigger triumphant narrative.

9.8 Behavioral Interventions

Superheroes are tasked with learning how to "strategically" access and unleash their superpowers in response to dilemmas or adversity. But, even superheroes are fallible with acting on emotionally rooted impulses that ultimately interfere with strategic execution of their mission. Similarly, youth patients are often engaged in therapy because they, too, are struggling to manage emotional impulses. The superhero genre offers an opportunity to normalize these experiences via depictions of similar struggles. Furthermore, superhero examples provide opportunities to discuss the emotion-action urge relationship, highlight how certain action tendencies can interfere with superhero missions, and prompt a conversation about interventions that could help the superhero better achieve their goals.

9.8.1 Exposures

For anxious avoidance, consider the Incredible Hulk's refusal to emerge to battle after succumbing to Thanos in defeat in the 2019 movie production *Avengers: End Game* (Russo et al., 2019). Regardless of Dr. Banner's coaxing and frustrating pleas for the Incredible Hulk to be brave and unleash his super strength to help with the mission, the Hulk refused and stayed hidden. The Hulk! This example provides an opportunity to normalize that even superheroes can struggle with anxiety. In this case, importantly, the Hulk illustrates how perceived setbacks and failures can cause one to lose confidence in their superpower. Exposure therapy is an intervention that encourages repeated engagement with feared stimuli until one develops less emotional reactivity or, more importantly, develops new expectations about their emotional tolerance and/or the likelihood of negative outcomes (Peterman et al., 2019).

Clinicians can introduce the concept of exposure therapy as a series of training sessions that help everyone (superheroes and children) acquire new confidence or regain lost confidence in their superpowers. Exposure therapy comes in different forms— *imaginal exposure* is used to encourage cognitive and emotional processing of feared thoughts, images, or imagined scenarios (Kearney, 2005*), in vivo *exposure* is used to reduce avoidance of situations that include feared stimuli (Kearney, 2005), *interoceptive exposure* used to promote tolerance of feared somatic sensations (Boettcher et al., 2016), or *prolonged exposure* to promote tolerance of feared emotional, physiological, and cognitive reactions to feared traumatic memory (Rossouw et al., 2018). Regardless of the exposure format, the superpower metaphor is far-reaching where superpowers are targeted specifically (e.g., strengthening powers to participate in class, tolerate the forces of dizzy sensations, stay in line when feeling panic) or more generally (e.g., superpower of bravery). Once the patient's target superpower is identified, a hierarchy of "exposure training sessions" can be created to strengthen their superpower to improve preparedness for their "superhero missions." The concept of "superhero missions" can be applied to designing exposures, consistent with Albano & DiBartolo, 2007, "Mission is Possible" tasks in their group CBT for socially anxious adolescents.

If anxious youth are struggling to engage in exposure training sessions, clinicians may benefit from utilizing a superhero-friendly technique that dates back to the 1960s. Emotive imagery is a systematic desensitization technique where imagery triggering positive or neutral emotions are used to neutralize the fear response as individuals engage with a feared stimulus (Lazarus & Abramovitz, 1962). In this approach, an imaginal exposure narrative is created where the patient's superheroes of choice are interwoven into the narrative in a way that fosters competing emotional states (e.g., curiosity, excitement) that support the patient's participation and tolerance of the exposure. In a case example presented by Lazarus and Abramovitz (1962), a child with school refusal engaged in an imaginal exposure where he was assigned by Batman and Robin to participate in a surveillance mission at his school where he monitored the whereabouts of his feared teacher. Such imagery appeared to trigger positive emotions in the boy and encouraged his engagement in the exercise. While the active ingredient of change in helping youth develop competing, non-fear-based associations with the initially fearful stimuli is exposure therapy (and not desensitization strategies, such as emotive imagery; Knowles & Olatunji, 2019), it is possible that strategies like superhero themed emotive imagery can support youth in developing an initial confidence of being able to tolerate exposure exercises. Once this foundation is formed, subsequent exposure exercises, rooted in inhibitory learning theory principles (Knowles & Olatunji, 2019; McGuire & Storch, 2019), can be designed to reduce reliance on desensitization strategies and deepen the effectiveness of exposure exercises. See the "Enhancing Superpowers" section below for more adaptations and desensitization strategies for enhancing motivation for exposure therapy.

9.8.2 Behavioral Activation

The superhero genre can be used to address depression-induced withdrawal or avoidance. Behavioral activation, or the intentional scheduling of and engagement in activities that promote enjoyment, a sense of mastery, and value, is an effective stand-alone (McCauley et al., 2016) and a component within a cognitive behavioral (Chorpita & Weisz, 2009) intervention for depression. This skill encourages growth in the superpower of resisting the force of withdrawal urges and daring to adhere to daily routines and typically enjoyable, valued activities despite the force's discouragement. Similar to exposure therapy, it can be helpful to engage youth during in-session behavioral activation training sessions to help the patient practice this "superpower." Consider the example of a 16-year-old nonbinary teen experiencing a depressive episode presented below.

P: I don't even know why I am here. This is pointless. I don't have anything to say to you.

T: Can you tell me how you are feeling?

P: You know how I am feeling. I am depressed and talking about it with you is not going to help.

T: You know. I get it. Sometimes when we feel depressed. We don't want to talk. We don't want to do anything really. And yet you still came.

P: [interrupts] My mom made me.

T: Well I mentioned to you before that our meetings don't only have to be about having in-depth conversations about your depression. Sometimes, there is *power* in doing activities - even if in silence. How about this? We can go for a walk around the building together and then check back in.

P: I guess that's fine.

[After the walk]

T: So, how was that for you?

P: I mean it's not like depression's gone or anything, but I do feel a bit better.

T: That's interesting. Any idea how something like taking a walk could have an effect (even if it's small) on your mood?

The above scenario illustrates how in-session behavioral activation can be utilized for in vivo mood activation, especially when children and adolescents appear unwilling or unable to engage in more cognitively demanding conversations about their depression. More superhero themed activities could include watching movie clips with exciting scenes, scene reenactments, or engaging youth in superhero themed hypotheticals (e.g., who's a better inventor—Shuri or Tony Stark, Do you think the Civil Rights Movement would have been different if Black Americans had access to Vibranium?)

If using behavioral activation in this way, patients may express doubts as to whether engaging in pleasurable activities when experiencing negative affect (e.g., sadness or irritability) will in fact lead to mood improvements. Lean into this doubt; encourage them to use the activity like a behavioral experiment where they generate a prediction for the impact the activity will have on their mood and then compare their prediction with their actual experience. In the above scenario, a slight perceived benefit or even the fact her mood did not get worse can be viewed as evidence that this intervention is effective—even if seemingly minutely so. Clinicians can help youth contrast the consequences of chronic avoidance or withdrawal (e.g., remaining in bed all day, avoiding text messages, canceling plans) against using behavioral activation to resist these urges (e.g., by starting the morning routine, answering at least two texts/day, planning to attend an event for at least 30 min) to understand the long-term benefits of consistently applying this intervention. By establishing realistic expectations for behavioral activation, youth learn that consistency is key in reducing the severity of their depressed mood, recurrence of stressors, and ruminative thoughts (McCauley et al., 2016; Ritschel et al., 2011).

The ultimate goal (regardless if using in vivo activation or not) is to inspire motivation for patients and their families to express a commitment to routinely practice behavioral activation in response to depressed moods and to proactively continue prioritizing pleasurable and mastery-inducing activities in their daily schedules as a means of reducing the vulnerability towards depressed moods (also known as ABC PLEASE skills in DBT-A; Rathus & Miller, 2014*). Aside from supporting the activity scheduling process (e.g., identifying superhero themed activities and social interactions), the superhero genre can be used to sustain motivation towards ongoing practice of behavioral activation. Clinicians can contrast the patient's anticipated outcomes associated with chronic withdrawal/avoidance (e.g., staying in bed all day, avoiding texts/calls from friends, neglecting school assignments) with using the behavioral activation superpower (e.g., keeping a regular sleep schedule, answering at least a few texts from friends, starting some assignments)—particularly linking this superpower with better preparation for the patient's daily missions.

During the COVID19 pandemic and beyond, these superpowers may be particularly relevant for youth and young adults, who may be especially vulnerable to the associated mental health impacts of social isolation and feelings of loneliness (e.g., Bu et al., 2020; Loades et al., 2020). As the global pandemic has reminded us of our interconnectedness, so too does the superhero narrative remind us of our interconnectedness. From Earth to other planets and galaxies, superhero stories challenges are prefaced on this interdependence. In this context, therapists further can assist youth patients to contextualize any mental health sequelae and strategize accordingly.

9.9 Somatic Management

Learning strategies to regulate and tolerate adverse somatic experiences is a transdiagnostically relevant skill set—especially when a primary goal is improving emotion regulation (Loevaas et al., 2019). There is no shortage of somatic management strategies to introduce in treatment (e.g., paced breathing, progressive muscle relaxation, meditation, yoga); however, the challenge can be creating a convincing rationale that inspires youth patients to try and then actually employ these strategies. Once again, the superhero genre offers options for identifying how these strategies enhance the efforts of the child's favorite superheroes to complete their missions.

9.9.1 Power Breaths and Superhero Breathing

Breathing is powerful. Breathing is often an essential somatic management strategy that CBT clinicians teach their patients. These include variations on diaphragmatic breathing, belly breathing, and controlled breathing where youth learn and practice the mechanics of inhaling through the nose for a count, drawing breath to fill their bellies, and slowly exhaling through the mouth. It can feel like we are losing our power or even have no power when our bodies are anxious, riled up, or jumpy. That's where teaching Power Breaths comes in!

Superhero breathing combines teaching these breathing strategies with superhero poses. Youth can extend their arms out at the start, then when drawing their inhale, pull their arms in with elbows pulling to their torso, and the exhale is where the superhero magic happens—they can shoot their arms out and up in the air like a superhero flying and breathing out of their mouths.

9.9.2 *"Riding the Wave"*

Per our clinical observations, a common barrier to the perceived effectiveness of somatic management strategies is when youth have unrealistic expectations that engaging in these strategies will result in instantaneous relief. Such expectations can backfire—generating beliefs that "I am not doing it right" or "I knew this stuff doesn't work." The Silver-Surfer who uses his surfboard-like craft to surf through the elements can be utilized to more accurately conceptualize the benefits of somatic management strategies. The activation of the sympathetic nervous system (or our "Fight, Flight, or Freeze" response) is associated with the onset of various affective states (e.g., anxiety, fear, anger; Kreibig, 2010) and often includes uncomfortable physical sensations that somatic management strategies seek to relieve. While this system's effects may be felt instantly, the "Peace and Relax" response of our parasympathetic nervous system can be a gradual process. Rather than instant stress relievers, somatic management skills can be construed as superpowers that help patients to "surf or ride the wave" of their uncomfortable somatic arousal and emotional states. One teen with panic disorder who enjoyed surfing envisioned herself as a Super-Surfer with her "Super Surf-Board" to "ride the wave" of her intense physiological symptoms.

9.10 Enhancing Superpowers: Supplemental Interventions for Enhancing CBT Intervention

Superheroes rarely act alone. Though they often get recognized for their awestriking superpowers, they always have a team of supporters. Young patients are no different. CBT superpower skill sets can be extremely useful in addressing the cognitive, emotional, and behavioral components of emotion dysregulation. Youth may continue to struggle with low motivation to attempt new skills, experience difficulty engaging with a primarily talk-focused intervention, or feel alone in their efforts to resolve problem areas. The following recommendations provide options for how to utilize the superhero theme to enhance patient motivation for and follow through with skill practice.

9.10.1 *Using Superheroes to Seek Social Support*

Superhero missions operate better with a team. As part of basic problem-solving skills, clinicians teach and encourage youth to identify their team by asking for help. Social support in the form of capable adults and peer relationships is a key and consistent element in youth resilience (Masten, 2014). In teaching problem-solving, clinicians can teach effective help-seeking: whom to ask and how to ask. Again, superheroes can provide a model. More recent movies emphasize the message of teamwork to solve the biggest problems. Individuals may have their strengths, but when they seek help and join forces with others, they become more formidable. What is better than a group of Super Friends? Recall the Wonder Twins, the famed superhero sibling duo, who would join hands and declare: "Wonder Twin powers, activate!" in order to activate their superpowers. Sometimes, superheroes have side-kicks like Batman has Robin. They may pair up for alliances or they may form a Fantastic Four. Or, like Thor, they seek counsel from their parents. Sometimes, they already exist as a powerful team of warrior women like the Amazons or special forces team of Wakandan women like the Dora Milaje (Special shout out to portrayals of powerful women). When superheroes tackle universal problems, they assemble a team.

Therefore, as part of superhero resiliency training and problem-solving, youth can learn to assemble their own teams and grow their social capital. Why might it be helpful to form this team? Who is on their team? Who can they talk to when they are feeling down? Who supports them? Who can they talk to if they are having a hard time with reading or math? Who can they reach out to when they need a laugh? With whom can they play a video game or card game? Who can they ask about soccer strategy? Who can they contact to supercharge their coping powers? See Fig. 9.4 as a sample worksheet to support youth in assembling their support networks.

As noted, youth rarely self-refer to therapy. Seeking treatment can be a (super) powerful way for a child and family to grow their team. Showing vulnerability and sharing difficult experiences may be challenging but they are also acts of bravery. Clinicians can normalize help-seeking in the superheroes that seek help all the time. For example, Chris Evans, the actor who plays Captain America, has openly talked about going to therapy and for his anxieties and "noisy brain."

9.10.2 Behavior Plans

Therapists can work with caregivers and youth to set up at-home behavior plan targets as superhero missions. These superhero missions can be utilized for youth academic tasks, social problem-solving, and shaping compliance behaviors. Clinicians can work with parents and youth to set up at-home behavior plan targets as superhero missions that, for example, encourage chores (Operation House Clean!), increase responsibilities (Operation Dog Walk), or ensure at-home exposure practice (Operation Brave Talk). Just about anything can be converted into a Superhero Mission.

One young boy diagnosed with ADHD-Combined Type, with hyperactivity and organizational skills deficits needed help organizing his school materials. He seemed consistently "on the go"! For him, The Flash provided a guide for Operation Slow Down and Operation School Stuff. The Flash's greatest strength was his speed; his speed was also his greatest vulnerability. The therapist, patient, and caregiver color coded school folders by subject, and the patient received "Flash points" for

Who is on your team?

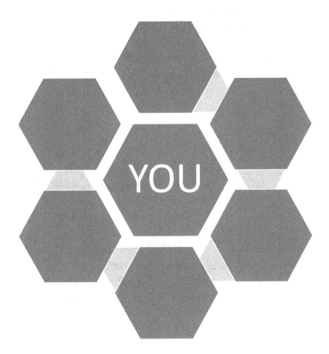

Some questions to help:

Who are some trusted adults?

Who can you talk to when you need support?

Who can you reach out to for school-related questions?

Who can play games or sports with?

Who makes you laugh or smile?

Fig. 9.4 Assemble Your Super Team

accurately placing school assignments in the proper designated folder. He earned "Flash points" for organizing his backpack and using the identified folder bin on the desk in his room. He could also earn points for appropriately managing with restlessness (e.g., quiet fidget toy, asking the teacher for a "shake break" to shake out his body jumpiness, etc.). Instead of receiving frequent attention for his disorganization and hyperactivity, he learned how to embody The Flash by receiving reinforcement for adaptive behaviors.

With respect to behavior plans and charts themselves, especially for younger children, the internet provides a multitude of options for colorful superhero themed forms, both generic and specific heroes, that can be personalized, downloaded, and printed. Parents and youth can work together to create and design charts based on youth's preferred characters and collaboratively decide where in the home these will be displayed. Further, superhero materials simply can be used as reinforcers and rewards (e.g., superhero themed stickers, prizes, Spidey-bucks, etc.). Parents can learn to incorporate superhero type language into their specific labeled praise: "You helping to clean up without asking was a superpower move. So proud of you!"

9.10.3 Superhero Tools and Props

With younger kids especially, CBT therapists can incorporate props to creatively teach skills throughout the course of treatment, capitalizing on imagination, play, and fun. Imagine your own favorite superheroes. What are they wearing? What are they carrying? What are their weapons or tools of choice? How do they unleash their might powers?

Many superheroes wear costumes. They may wear capes, masks, or cuffs or technologically superior suits made of Vibranium. They may carry a lasso, hammer or protective shield. Therapists can join imaginary forces with their youth patients in creating therapy props that aid in skill building and practice. Prop building typically requires only minimal arts-and-crafts supplies, and therapists can enlist parents in their creation as well. Anxious younger kids can wear a "Brave Cape" or "Courage Cuffs" to encourage in vivo exposures as they embark on their superhero mission of battling their worries. With construction paper or cardboard and colorful markers, therapists and patients can create a SuperShield to fight off those scary monster thoughts.

A strategy often taught to youth receiving exposure and response prevention (ERP) treatment for obsessive compulsive disorder is externalizing and naming their OCD (e.g., Franklin et al., 2019). At times, OCD can throw some pretty villainous thoughts and youth can frame and name these as supervillain-type characters: Germeo, Doomsayer, and a recent favorite, Sir Boss-A-Lot. Youth can draw out these characters so they can recognize OCD's tricks, and further, gather their own superhero "gear" to do battle with them. Sir-Boss-A-Lot was no match for the Bossy Blaster. Therapists and youth can borrow Thor's powerful hammer (e.g., made out of a foam noodle) to crush Germeo or Wonder Woman's Lasso of Truth (e.g., made out of braided yarn with glitter) when challenging Doomsayer's tall tales.

During the COVID19 pandemic, some youth have expressed anxiety about wearing masks, for example, due to sensory discomfort or breathing difficulty. One strategy that has assisted some youth is likening masks to superhero masks or superhero shields that help to protect them from the virus. As an added superhero bonus, these masks also help to protect others, as we know superheroes do. Connecting public health promoting behaviors to altruistic and greater good may increase motivation and compliance (e.g., Brooks et al., 2020). Having younger kids pick out masks with their favorite superhero characters printed on them may be a simple motivation booster. Then, as other superheroes do, they can practice using their mask shields for increasing amounts of time or during varying activities. Pairing wearing a superhero mask with watching a preferred superhero cartoon or playing a preferred videogame can pack a behavioral super-punch! Generally, therapy props can be utilized for a multitude of skills and behaviors that therapists and parents can shape over time. Capes can also be "SuperHelper Cape" as part of behavior plans to increase chore compliance. One young SuperHelper wisely enlisted the robotic room vacuum as her side kick!

Superhero, or otherwise, therapy props can be utilized to promote initial engagement in in vivo exposures. One younger child with selective mutism summoned the strength of his Super Sparkle Speaking Stick before his first speaking exposures, including holding it out of sight when unmuting his microphone to speak to his kindergarten teacher for the first time during virtual learning. His fear ladder included repeated speaking exposures across settings with the Super Sparkle Speaking Stick and then, being mindful of safety behaviors (see Rachman et al., 2008) without it. He learned that the Super Speaking Power was within him all along!

In another example, one youth presented with PTSD symptoms and a phobia of dogs after witnessing a dog attack a family member at a local park. Her anxiety further generalized from that park to all parks, and she began to avoid socializing with peers for fear they would want to go to the park to play. Importantly, she also presented with a love of Wonder Woman and was immediately drawn to a talking Wonder Woman figure in the therapist's office. Pressing a button at its base resulted in various empowering and inspirational sayings, including, "You are a warrior" and "You are a one-woman army." The patient worked with the therapist on an illustrated trauma narrative with Wonder Woman making an appearance in her comic book style drawings. When preparing for her first out-of-office exposure to the park up the street with the therapist and her mother, she asked if she could bring the Wonder Woman figure with her because "She reminds me I can do it even if I'm scared." They even joked that they were, in fact, a four-women army. The patient carried Wonder Woman to that park, and then another, and then the park where she witnessed the dog attack, and then when she first started petting dogs. The patient gained increasing confidence and was able to practice without needing to carry the (physical) Wonder Woman with her.

9.10.4   Finding your Superhero Song

The 80's-kid clinicians among us may recall the television series, "The Greatest American Hero," with its introductory theme song and chorus, *"Believe it or not, I'm walking on air, I never thought I could feel so free"* (sing it with us!). Take a moment to recall the original Superman theme song by famed composer and conductor John Williams in all its orchestral glory. Superheroes have anthems and superhero shows and movies have soundtracks and scores. For some youth who may connect through music, clinicians can help them to find their Superhero Song. What is a song that pumps them up and reminds them of their powers? What is a song they can listen to before an exposure? What is a song that gets them dancing and behaviorally activated? What is a song that grounds them if they are restless? Superhero songs can then be added to a playlist or bookmarked on their smartphones, laptops, or tablets to cue up when needed.

9.10.5 Superhero Poses

As noted earlier, physically engaging in superhero type poses can prime for prosocial behaviors (Pena & Chen, 2017; Rosenberg et al., 2013). Working with younger patients involves more engaging, lively, and interactive intervention elements; as Dr. Phil Kendall, one of the pioneers in adapting CBT for youth and developer of Coping Cat, famously emphasizes child therapists have to get out of the chair and "get on the ground" to meet youth where they are. Similar to emotive imagery exercises or superhero breathing exercises noted above, superhero poses can be incorporated to supercharge, if you will, skills learning and practice. Fly like Superman when you exhale! Some youth with social anxiety may have deficits in their social skills including poor eye contact, slouching, speaking in low volume or other nonverbal and verbal avoidance-related behaviors, and may benefit from social skills training (e.g., Mesa et al., 2015). Reference to superhero poses embodying improved posture, head up, and more direct eye contact may be helpful for some youth. The young Coping Black Panther referenced earlier would ready himself for problem-solving and exposures by assuming the Wakanda Forever stance. One child with separation anxiety engaged their "Confident Coping Pose" while another her "Sassy Stance" to face their anxiety exposure challenges. Picture Wonder Woman, Captain Marvel, and Storm (with a dash of Beyonce and Lizzo).

9.11   Conclusions

Superheroes provide ample material for infusing creativity in the delivery of CBT for youth and families. Whether as metaphor, model, or message for resilience and coping, they can join clinicians, youth, and families as they assemble the therapy team. Superheroes come in many recognizable forms, and they include everyday heroes among us. A goal in incorporating superheroes into youth CBT is to connect their story with that of a meaningful hero to them, and in essence to becoming aware of their own superpowers. We will conclude where we began with a quote from Superman (and one of the most well-known actors to play him, Christopher Reeve): "I think a hero is an ordinary individual who finds strength to persevere and endure in spite of overwhelming obstacles."

References

Albano, A. M., & DiBartolo, P. M. (2007). *Cognitive-behavioral therapy for social phobia in adolescents, stand up, speak out, therapist guide*. Oxford University Press.

Bandura, A., Grusec, J. E., & Menlove, F. L. (1966). Observational learning as a function of symbolization and incentive set. *Child Development, 37*, 499–506.

Becker-Weidman, E. G., Jacobs, R. H., Reinecke, M. A., Silva, S. G., & March, J. S. (2010). Social problem-solving among adolescents treated for depression. *Behaviour Research and Therapy, 48*(1), 11–18.

Betzalel, N., & Shechtman, Z. (2017). The impact of bibliotherapy superheroes on youth who experience parental absence. *School Psychology International, 38*(5), 473–490.

Boettcher, H., Brake, C. A., & Barlow, D. H. (2016). Origins and outlook of interoceptive exposure. *Journal of Behavior Therapy and Experimental Psychiatry, 53*, 41–51.

Branscum, P., & Sharma, M. (2009). Comic books: An untapped medium for health promotion. *American Journal of Health Studies, 24*(4), 430–439.

Brooks, S. K., Webster, R. K., Smith, L. E., Woodland, L., Wessely, S., Greenberg, N., & Rubin, G. J. (2020). The psychological impact of quarantine and how to reduce it: rapid review of the evidence. *The Lancet, 395*, 912–920.

Bu, F., Steptoe, A., Fancourt, D. (2020). Loneliness during lockdown: trajectories and predictors during the COVID-19 pandemic in 35,712 adults in the UK. *medRxiv*.

Chorpita, B. F., & Weisz, J. R. (2009). *Modular approach to therapy for children with anxiety, depression, trauma, or conduct problems (MATCH-ADTC)*.

D'Zurilla, T. J., & Nezu, A. M. (2010). Problem-solving therapy. In K. S. Dobson (Ed.), *Handbook of cognitive-behavioral therapies* (pp. 197–225). Guilford Press.

Franklin, M., Freeman, J., & March, J. (2019). *Treating OCD in children and adolescents: A cognitive-behavioral approach*. The Guilford Press.

Friedberg, R. D., & McClure, J. M. (2015). *Clinical practice of cognitive therapy with children and adolescents: The nuts and bolts* (2nd ed.). The Guilford Press.

Glenn, C. R., Franklin, J. C., & Nock, M. K. (2014). Evidence-based psychosocial treatments for self-injurious thoughts and behaviors in youth. *Journal of Clinical Child and Adolescent Psychology, 44*(1), 1–29.

Gorner, P. (1985, February). Spider-man unfolds web of child abuse. *Chicago Tribune*.

Kazdin, A. E. (2000). Treatments for aggressive and antisocial children. *Child and Adolescent Psychiatric Clinics of North America, 9*, 841–858.

Kendall, P. C. (2006). *Cognitive-behavioral therapy for anxious children: Therapist manual*. Workbook Publishing Inc..

Kendall, P. C., & Hedtke, K. A. (2006). *The coping cat workbook*. Workbook Publishing Inc..

Knowles, K. A., & Olatunji, B. O. (2019). Enhancing inhibitory learning: The utility of variability in exposure. *Cognitive and Behavioral Practice, 26*(1), 186–200.

Kreibig, S. D. (2010). Autonomic nervous system activity in emotion: A review. *Biological Psychology, 84*(3), 394–421.

Lazarus, A. A., & Abramovitz, A. (1962). The use of "emotive imagery" in the treatment of children's phobias. *Journal of Mental Science, 108*(453), 191–195.

Lee, A. (Director), & Arad, A., Franco, L., Hurd, G., & Schamus, J. (Producers). (2003). Hulk [Motion picture]. Universal Pictures.

Loades, M. E., Chatburn, E., Higson-Sweeney, N., et al. (2020). Rapid systematic review: The impact of social isolation and loneliness on the mental health of children and adolescents in the context of COVID-19. *Journal of the American Academy of Child and Adolescent Psychiatry, 59*(11), 1218–1239.e3. https://doi.org/10.1016/j.jaac.2020.05.009. Epub ahead of print.

Loevaas, M. E. S., Sund, A. M., Lydersen, S., Neumer, S. P., Martinsen, K., Holen, S., … Reinfjell, T. (2019). Does the transdiagnostic EMOTION intervention improve emotion regulation skills in children? *Journal of Child and Family Studies, 28*(3), 805–813.

Masten, A. S. (2014). *Ordinary magic, resilience in development*. The Guilford Press.

McCauley, E., Gudmundsen, G., Schloredt, K., Martell, C., Rhew, I., Hubley, S., & Dimidjian, S. (2016). The adolescent behavioral activation program: Adapting behavioral activation as a treatment for depression in adolescence. *Journal of Clinical Child & Adolescent Psychology, 45*(3), 291–304.

McGrath, K. (2007). Gender, race, and latina identity: an examination of marvel comics' amazing fantasy and araña. *Atlantic Journal of Communication, 15*, 268–283.

McGuire, J. F., & Storch, E. A. (2019). An inhibitory learning approach to cognitive-behavioral therapy for children and adolescents. *Cognitive and Behavioral Practice, 26*(1), 214–224.

Mesa, F., Le, T., & Beidel, D. C. (2015). Social skill-based treatment for social anxiety disorder in adolescents. In K. Ranta, A. M. La Greca, & L. J. G.-L. Marttunen (Eds.), *Social anxiety and phobia in adolescents* (pp. 289–299). Springer International Publishing.

Meyer, S., Raikes, H. A., Virmani, E. A., Waters, S., & Thompson, R. A. (2014). Parent emotion representations and the socialization of emotion regulation in the family. *International Journal of Behavioral Development, 38*(2), 164–173.

Pena, J., & Chen, M. (2017). With great power comes great responsibility: Superhero primes and expansive poses influence prosocial behavior after a motion-controlled game task. *Computers in Human Behavior, 76*, 378–385.

Persons, J. B. (2012). *The case formulation approach to cognitive-behavior therapy*. Oxford University Press.

Peterman, J. S., Carper, M. M., & Kendall, P. C. (2019). Testing the habituation-based model of exposures for child and adolescent anxiety. *Journal of Clinical Child & Adolescent Psychology, 48*(sup1), S34–S44.

Pincus, D. B., Ehrenreich, J. T., & Mattis, S. (2008). *Mastery of anxiety and panic for adolescents riding the wave, therapist guide (treatments that work)*. Oxford University Press.

Pincus, D. B., Ehrenreich, J. T., & Speigel, D. A. (2008). *Riding the wave workbook (treatments that work)*. Oxford University Press.

Rachman, S., Radomsky, A. S., & Shafran, R. (2008). Safety behaviour: A reconsideration. *Behaviour Research and Therapy, 46*(2), 163–173.

Ritschel, L. A., Ramirez, C. L., Jones, M., & Craighead, W. E. (2011). Behavioral activation for depressed teens: A pilot study. *Cognitive and Behavioral Practice, 18*(2), 281–299.

Rohde, P., Feeny, N. C., & Robins, M. (2005). Characteristics and components of the TADS CBT approach. *Cognitive Behavioral Practice, 12*(2), 186–197.

Rosenberg, R. S., Baughman, S. L., & Bailenson, J. N. (2013). Virtual superheroes: Using superpowers in virtual reality to encourage prosocial behavior. *PLoS One, 8*(1), e55003. Retrieved from https://journals.plos.org/plosone/article?id=10.1371/journal.pone.0055003#s5.

Rossouw, J., Yadin, E., Alexander, D., & Seedat, S. (2018). Prolonged exposure therapy and supportive counselling for post-traumatic stress disorder in adolescents: task-shifting randomised controlled trial. *The British Journal of Psychiatry, 213*(4), 587–594.

Rubin, L. C. (Ed.). (2007). *Using superheroes and villains in counseling and play therapy: A guide for mental health professionals*. Routledge.

Russo, A.; Russo, J. (Directors), & Feige, K. (Producer). (2018). *Avengers: Infinity war* [Motion Picture]. Walt Disney Studios; Motion Pictures.

Russo, A.; Russo, J. (Directors), & Feige, K. (Producer). (2019). *Avengers: End game* [Motion Picture]. Walt Disney Studios; Motion Pictures.

Scarlet, J. (2017). *Superhero Therapy, Mindfulness skills to help teens and young adults deal with anxiety, depression, and trauma*. New Harbinger Publications.

Torre, J. B., & Lieberman, M. D. (2018). Putting feelings into words: Affect labeling as implicit emotion regulation. *Emotion Review, 10*(2), 116–124.

Uhl, K., Halpern, L. F., Tam, C., Fox, J. K., & Ryan, J. L. (2019). Relations of emotion regulation, negative and positive affect to anxiety and depression in middle childhood. *Journal of Child and Family Studies, 28*(11), 2988–2999.

Walkup, J., et al. (2008). Cognitive behavioral therapy, sertraline, or a combination in childhood anxiety. *New England Journal of Medicine, 359*, 2753–2766.

Chapter 10
Using Superheroes with Children who have Chronic Illnesses

Laura Nabors and Olutosin Sanyaolu

Keywords Children · Superheroes · Imagery · Play · Anxiety · Chronic illnesses

10.1 Introduction

Children with chronic illnesses or chronic medical conditions may experience significant anxiety (Pinquart & Shen, 2011). Coping strategies featuring distraction, such as positive imagery, often facilitate child adjustment reducing worry about coping with medical procedures (Nabors et al., 2019a, b). Use of positive imagery and play techniques may serve as a safety valve, allowing children to express and release feelings of anxiety (Bolig, 2018; Gordon & Paisley, 2018). Play is a child's method of communication and offers a means of connecting with adults while discussing anxiety-provoking experiences from a position of power and may offer solace to the child (Bolig, 2018; Crenshaw & Kelly, 2018). Moreover, fantasy play is an important part of the child's play repertoire, playing a key role in children's abilities to assimilate experiences and developing mastery and understanding of events in their lives (Rubin & Livesay, 2006). In this chapter, our focus is to discuss use of superheroes in fantasy play, particularly for children with chronic illnesses who are coping with anxiety or pain related to their medical conditions.

Children may select play experiences relative to their experience in their situation, and thus use of superheroes may be ideal in situations where a child needs support or needs to feel empowered when he or she is coping with stress (Rubin & Livesay, 2006). And, superheroes overcome problems, in ways that are not available to children (Rubin & Livesay, 2006). As such, superheroes to defeat pain and support children through medical fears, are a supportive play technique for young

L. Nabors (✉) · O. Sanyaolu
Health Promotion and Education Program, School of Human Services, University of Cincinnati, Cincinnati, OH, USA
e-mail: naborsla@ucmail.uc.edu; sanyaooa@mail.uc.edu

© The Author(s), under exclusive license to Springer Nature
Switzerland AG 2022
R. D. Friedberg, E. V. Rozmid (eds.), *Creative CBT with Youth*,
https://doi.org/10.1007/978-3-030-99669-7_10

children facing medical procedures and pain related to chronic medical conditions. Fradkin et al. (2017) mentioned that the notion of empowered superheroes to help children in stressful situations, providing them with courage and hope to cope with stressors, has been discussed since the 1940s. Introducing a superhero, that the child identifies as a friend and protector, also may be a way for the adult to build a relationship with a child (Rollins, 2018) and encourage a coping focus, emphasizing active coping, which may help the child manage anxiety and pain related to medical procedures. Developing a superhero story, and then making a book depicting the superhero's deeds, allows the child to capitalize on the healing powers of art therapy. This process helps the child tell his or her story and cope with and perhaps gain a sense of control over anxiety-provoking or traumatic experiences (Eaton et al., 2007; Freeman, 1991; Mellenthin, 2018a, b). Involving storytelling and art while discussing superheroes to fight illnesses, and enlightening children about the use of imagery and metaphor, may enable this technique to be used with older children with chronic medical conditions (e.g., Freeman, 1991). To integrate this technique into clinical practice, it is recommended that the therapist/counselor assess the child's needs. Next, the therapist selects a play-based intervention that "matches" the child's needs for growth and learning new skills. In turn, engaging in play builds rapport and encourages indirect expression of feelings, further solidifying the therapeutic relationship (Seymour, 2016). Involving parents, as observers, and then as play partners, helps them learn to use play techniques to advance child coping and adaptation, improving the "therapeutic reach" of techniques (Seymour, 2016).

10.2 Theoretical and Empirical Foundations

Superhero play and story relies in part of the value of metaphor in therapy. The superhero is a symbol of power for good outcomes, and as the child becomes the superhero, he or she engages in mastery play and can master coping with feelings and issues that the child might not be able to engage in without the superhero's strength and help. The superhero may provide feelings of safety in the child's mind with the superhero scene. These scenes contain some of the overwhelming nature, stress, and fear related to traumatic events, and the child often plays through feelings, expresses feelings, and reviews stressful, traumatic events that have occurred (Crenshaw & Kelly, 2018). Medical trauma results when a child feels stress, fear, and a lack of power (Gordon & Paisley, 2018). This trauma may be stored in "emotional memory" and play with the superhero (figure or imaginary play) allows the child to work through trauma, with mastery, in a safe environment to tell his or her story (Gordon & Paisley, 2018).

Superhero stories follow a similar archetype. The hero overcomes a threatening outside force. The "power or powers" of the superhero are used for good, to restore goodness and ensure that everything turns out well (Gross, 2018). In addition, the story may be a form of metaphor, that engages the child with his or her audience, in our case, the therapist or parent, to bring people to the child's "lived experience"

(Kestly, 2018, p. 118). Within the story the adult can add an optimistic, positive theme with the child overcoming problems, instilling a positive coping framework and encouraging a problem-solving attitude for the child (Kress et al., 2019). If therapists see disasters such as floods, fire, etc. in children's play or stories while engaging the superhero "metaphor," it may be a time to support the child and project positive coping to bolster the child's ego strength (Crenshaw & Kelly, 2018). The therapist also may create new endings. For example, if the child is "locked" in a traumatic event, thinking it will never end in his or her perceptions, then the therapist reviews or replays the event within the superhero context and can interject that the traumatic event has passed and the child is now in a new situation that is safe. The therapist also may "create" different events through play that allow the child to review feelings related to traumatic events that occurred, which the child has been unable to discuss (Crenshaw & Kelly, 2018).

As play unfolds, the therapist or adult encourages emotional expression and discusses how the child is like the superhero, a problem-solver who actively copes with difficult situations finding ways to be successful. For instance, the therapist begins by helping the child select or create his or her superhero to be the main character. Then, during play, the superhero models positive coping behaviors and expressing feelings to encourage the child to act in the same manner. The superhero discusses how it is difficult to problem-solve and act differently, and that it may take several attempts to problem-solve to a "successful" solution to a difficult situation. Additionally, the superhero models coping techniques, such as deep breathing and muscle relaxation that "increases" the superhero's power deal with painful situations. A young child may say, "This is just like me." And, agreeing with this, often strengthens a child's self-concept. Alternately, a child might mention, "This is what I need to do" and the therapist may reply, "Yes, and you can do it, because you are a superhero in your own life story!" Through play exploration and telling the superhero's story, both from the child's point of view and weaving in success plans (thereby enhancing problem-solving), the superhero story allows the child to reach a "congruence" between feelings, thoughts, and plans for future action, which helps reduce discomfort and feelings of dissonance for the child (Crenshaw & Kelly, 2018; Kress et al., 2019). The therapist or adult "teaches" coping skills and the superhero story sets a "safe stage" for modeling positive coping skills, capitalizing on vicarious learning for the child.

10.3   Clinical Applications

Pretend play and art materials such as small dolls or figures, puppets, stuffed animals, cars, and LEGOs® are commonly used to build a play city (village, town, or perhaps a hospital) and a doll or figure can be designated as the superhero (Kress et al., 2019). As play continues, the story of the superhero and how he helps usually unfolds. Our team often uses Playmobil© hospital toys to recreate a hospital experience (Nabors et al., 2013). The superhero frequently comes to save the day, explaining the child's feelings to health professionals and parents. The therapist works with the child, while parents observe, to teach breathing, muscle relaxation, and imagery to facilitate pain coping and a relaxation response for dealing with fears. Here are some "sample" techniques. The superhero talks about the child's wishes for "fun," as the hospital is at times a lonely and isolating place. A play telephone is used and the child "calls" the superhero to express what he or she is feeling to convey thoughts and needs. Or, the child uses his or her eyes as a camera and draws a picture of his/her room and tells the therapist how the superhero feels staying in this room. The therapist then talks about the feelings of loneliness and provides ideas for keeping busy, such as drawing in a sketchbook or writing down a game to play with parents when they return for a visit. The therapist may connect with Child Life Specialists, if this service is available, so they can connect with the child during times when parents and family are not visiting.

Another tool is for the therapist to help the child "create your own superhero self" through drawing or art projects. To do this, the child constructs him or herself as a superhero. This superhero masters feelings of insecurity and fear related to medical procedures and pain related to chronic illness. During repeated play or storytelling with the superhero, the child develops a representation which will be internalized to improve ego strength, thereby strengthening self-concept (Crenshaw & Kelly, 2018). Developing superhero stories, with the superhero self as the main character, is a method for assisting the child in telling his or her story. The child then internalizes a representation of a self that masters fear, expresses feelings, and is a problem-solver taking positive actions to cope with medical illness. It is important through the play and story to allow the child to express the pain and suffering he or she has experienced. This allows the child to express the journey that he or she is traveling in the safety of the superhero environment (Crenshaw & Kelly, 2018; Gordon & Paisley, 2018). During stories or play, the therapist asks the child about his or her thoughts and feelings. To help the child process memories, the therapist focuses on the senses by asking the child what he or she smelled, heard, saw, and felt during an event (Gordon & Paisley, 2018). It may be helpful to add, that although pain occurred with the doctor or nurse, "Doctors and nurses are here to keep you safe and help you get well." It is important to understand that younger children commonly engage in "magical thinking," thinking he or she caused health issues through misbehavior (Nabors & Liddle, 2017). Consequently, through superhero play, the therapist corrects misconceptions and describes medical conditions and their waxing and waning course in language that the child understands. Similarly, modifying or correcting magical thinking in relation to things that promote wellness is important. For example, eating apples may not cure cancer although it can improve nutrition and be one thing that contributes to improved health.

Stauffer (2021) used superhero stories, created through drawing, to help children overcome "stuckness" in therapy. Children created their own superhero, thinking of the superhero's, "...strengths, characteristics, abilities, clothing, tools, vehicle, home environment, and mission..." (Stauffer, 2021, p. 21). Clients drew pictures of the superhero's life over several sessions and processed the superhero's story. The story and drawings were kept in special place (i.e., a box or folder) to be accessed during subsequent sessions. The therapist noted that after the superhero story unfolded, children showed a "renewed sense of purpose and energy" (Stauffer, 2021, p. 21), and the child actually absorbed or "took on" some aspects of the superhero's personality and coping abilities. Playing through the superhero's story in drawings allowed children opportunities to, "…connect with others, feel capable, display courage, and feel as if they count" (Stauffer, 2021, p. 21). These activities apparently improved children's self-concept and sense of empowerment (noted by Rubin & Livesay, 2006). It is noteworthy that children in Stauffer's (2021) study did not have primary diagnoses of medical conditions although they experienced trauma. These authors believe, however, that therapists using superhero stories will see positive outcomes, as children work through worries, concerns, and pain related to their medical conditions in an "empowered" way as the superhero aids in mastery of feelings related to difficult life experiences. Superhero stories are useful when children are unable to directly verbalize their feelings or are "stuck" in telling their story or expressing emotions.

10.3.1   Medical Trauma and Anxiety

Locatelli (2020) stated that medical trauma can lead to emotional and behavioral problems. In a case study, she used play with a preschooler who was exhibiting emotional and behavioral problems, secondary to medical trauma (Locatelli, 2020). The child experienced significant anxiety and pain related to blood transfusions, and the child used action figures to express feelings related to medical experiences. At times, feelings of anger were directed toward the therapist. Eventually, the figures were used to heal herself and the therapist, showing positive resolution and mastery. We recommend that superhero or action figures are available during the play session. This permits the child to reenact traumatic experiences in play situations where he or she experiences mastery while expressing feelings. These ideas harken back in time to suggestions for mastery play posited by Virginia Axline (1981). During play, children provide figures of everyday people with magical powers and these figures become superheroes, with healing superpowers (Nabors et al., 2013). In play work with children at a local Ronald McDonald House, small Playmobil figures depicting parents, doctors, and nurses became superheroes, using other small toys (e.g., a flower or a radio) to heal other figures who represented someone who was ill, usually with an illness similar to the child (Nabors et al., 2013). Providing an accepting environment (Axline, 1981), where superhero figures embody healing superpowers, sets the stage for a child who has experienced medical trauma. After playing through the trauma and expressing feelings, the child may exhibit improvements in behavioral and emotional functioning (Locatelli, 2020).

Children coping with chronic illnesses often experience anxiety and worry related to medical procedures. Simultaneously, many do not have coping skills for dealing with anxiety. Superhero play affords "teachable moments" when the therapist provides ideas for coping. Nabors et al. (2019b) worked with children who were preparing for or recovering from medical procedures related to their illnesses at the Ronald McDonald House. .This team taught children anxiety management skills (e.g., breathing, imagery, relaxation) and developed a coping menu with children's personalized tools for anxiety management (Nabors et al., 2019b). One common coping technique on the coping menu included a superhero that helped the child fight pain or worry related to his or her chronic illness. The superhero may be well-known, such as "Superman" or "Aqua man." At times, however, the superhero was a unique character. One girl owned a stuffed pillow of an emoji, who was her hero. This pillow came with her to "needle" appointments (e.g., venipunctures and blood draws). The pillow sang, whistled, and played the role of an imaginary friend, saying encouraging words so that she could cope with pain. When she stayed overnight in the hospital, the emoji pillow, whom she described as "my friend 'Peri' who is my hero" slept by her on the bed so she had someone to give "hugs" and someone to, "watch out for me." Thus, Peri helped allay fears and worries and was a source of comfort.

For other children, superheroes were there to protect children and help them cope with stress and difficult feelings (e.g., fear related to medical procedures; Nabors et al., 2019b). Often, superheroes had a fight song or phrase that infused the child with courage. One child carried a stuffed animal that spun a protective shield with its tail. This shield was a force field, enabling the child to gain strength and deal with medical procedures. One fight song by another child went something like this, "My hero will save the day. It will all be O.K. I can make it with her by my side." Shepherd and Kuczynski (2009) employed emotive imagery through the voice of a cartoon character with a 10 year boy who suffered from nighttime fears of ghosts and zombies. He was afraid of sleeping in his own room. The child used his favorite cartoon character, the "Tasmanian Devil," to imprison the zombies and ghosts. The boy practiced imprisoning the zombies and ghosts (i.e., seeing and hearing all the scenes, using emotive imagery) during a therapy session. This intervention was partially successful after practicing it in session. The boy used the imagery at home, and then reported being free of fears in the next session. Encouraging children to apply imagery with successful endings, such as imagining being strong to cope with medical procedures, facilitates coping in medical settings. Another idea is for the child to provide him- or herself with a superhero name and tell a positive story about overcoming anxiety or an obstacle related to medical fears. To illustrate, explicit imagination of a child being a superhero who rises above fears and obstacles, such as fear of pain related to needle sticks by taking superhero breaths to relax, has the potential to reduce anxiety among children (Muris et al., 2011).

10.3.2 Learning Coping Skills

Superheroes also teach the coping skills. For pain, the superhero models proper breathing techniques. Therapists teach positive imagery, with the superhero imagining being at a birthday party or trip to the beach—imagining all the sights, sounds, and smells of each place. Similarly, therapists teach or model relaxation, giving themselves a superhero name, and then demonstrating making a fist like a rock and then dangling fingers like spaghetti strings to model relaxing muscles. Alternately, the superhero makes his or her body strong like a "rock" and then relaxes into a "sponge" to be able to float in the sea—this is another form of whole body muscle relaxation (Nabors et al., 2019b). Another teaching technique is to use either an action figure or be a superhero and show the child how a superhero says what he or she thinks and feels to nurses and doctors, so the child benefits from learning how to communicate with the medical team.

Mellenthin (2018a, b) presented the "Superhero in the Mirror" technique. Mellenthin (2018a) reported that this technique assists children to "...realize their inner strengths and sense of empowerment, in a playful, fun activity" (p. 70), which allows children to learn about the "superhero powers inside of them" (p. 70). She recommended use of dramatic play materials, such as a cape, wand, mask, shield, or sword. The child is instructed to look into a mirror (without the "dress-up" play materials) and describe who and what he or she sees. Next, the child dresses in different costumes using different props (e.g., cape, wand, magic tiara) and identifies different superhero powers (Mellenthin, 2018b). The child talks about what it would be like to be a superhero with special powers and discusses who he or she would rescue or help and how this would occur (Mellenthin, 2018a, b). The therapist explores what it would feel like to be a superhero with superpowers. Then, the child is asked to imagine being the superhero and to describe how the superhero would cope with the current situation that is stressful or traumatic (Mellenthin, 2018a). The child practices being the superhero and problem-solves his or her present challenges. Homework is assigned which includes practicing becoming a superhero. The child looks into a mirror, states a problem, which superhero he or she is, and reviews how the superhero tackles or solves the problem. This technique is practiced daily or every few days (Mellenthin, 2018b, p. 29). Therapists may want to send home a mask, or another prop, as a reminder for the child to practice this technique. Inviting parents to observe a session, or reviewing this technique with them, helps parents to learn the technique to facilitate their child's practice. The child, as a superhero in the mirror, practices positive self-talk and praises coping efforts. Role-modeling of relaxation techniques, like breathing and muscle relaxation, also can be tasks for the "superhero in the mirror."

Children with chronic illnesses, who are bedridden, may not be able to stand in front of a mirror or try on clothes, so we have modified the technique for use with this population. If children cannot use a mirror or try on clothes, then they could draw a superhero and a mirror and then discuss special powers the superhero has to help others cope through "trouble spots." For another example, they can learn breathing (smell the flower and blow out the birthday candle), while drawing a picture of the superhero using his or her relaxation powers. The therapist also may use prompts to guide the child in practicing positive imagery, discussing the story of a superhero who flies a child to his or her "happy place." Additionally, the superhero comforts the child and identifies, with the counselor's help (using a stage whisper to coach the child), negative thinking that can be changed to more positive self-talk and coping statements. Making a poster, picture, superhero mask, or story to have a product reviewing what was practiced during the therapy session, provides a tangible "reminder" of the work that occurred during a session. The child then explains the product and the story behind developing it to parents, reviewing what he or she learned. This also provides the child with additional practice using positive and mastery coping with the superhero story.

10.3.3   Coping with Pain

Superheroes are imaginary role models for practicing relaxation or other pain management strategies. Fradkin et al. (2017) mentioned that if the child does not have a positive role model in a situation, then the superhero fulfills this role, instilling "...confidence, resilience, and courage" (p. 137). Stories are used to introduce cognitive-behavioral anxiety management and pain management techniques. Through storytelling, within the superhero framework, coping occurs through a play-based medium. Delivering treatment through play and allowing the child to challenge worries with the help of a superhero and story capitalizes on the fact that children naturally overcome fears through play (Clark & Garland, 2018). Nabors et al. (2019b) used superheroes as one technique to encourage coping in children with chronic illnesses, residing at a local Ronald McDonald House, waiting for medical appointments or surgery. Children were instructed to, "Pick a hero to help you get rid of your worry. Make up a movie to play in your head. In the movie let your hero make your worry go away! Play this movie in your head when you have worry that is getting too big. Talk back to your worries to defeat them." This challenge strategy helps the child "fight back" against repetitive thoughts about hospital procedures. Practicing using other anxiety management strategies, as superpowers of their superhero provides children with opportunities to review coping strategies. One such strategy is relaxation (using deep breathing—smell the rose and blow out the candle. "Remember when you breathe in, fill up on air and make a beach ball with your tummy"), relaxation ("be a rock, then let your body be a sponge"; while the therapist modeled whole body muscle tensing followed by relaxation of all muscles), and distraction ("Let's think of something fun, like your birthday party, to chase away worry thoughts.") (Nabors et al., 2019b). The superhero's successes could also be recorded through drawing and art by the therapist and child to have a storybook to read to review coping strategies when the therapist was no longer present.

Parents commonly mention that a child's "fighting spirit" helps him or her cope with exacerbations of or medical procedures related to the child's medical condition (Nabors et al., 2018). Superhero play allows the child to share this spirit with his or parents. The superhero battles pain or anxiety related to a chronic illness, and at the same time, through the joint narrative, the therapist teaches the child anxiety management and pain management strategies. Similar strategies relieve anxiety and pain. These include positive imagery (of the superhero battling pain and making anxiety shrink), teaching deep breathing, distraction (have fun drawing a picture of the hero), and relaxation, (make a superhero fist and then relax it). Our instructions for deep breathing involve practice with the superhero, "Let's practice some breathing. Here's how it works. Smell the rose, and then blow out the candle. Now, rest for a count of 10. Let's take another breath where we smell the rose and blow out the candle and then rest." We recommend allowing the child to select the number of breaths, but typically, at least three calming breaths are recommended.

10.3.4 Storytelling

A joint storytelling technique is helpful in promoting coping within families (Trees & Koenig Kellas, 2009). Sharing positive stories, with the parent and child taking turns telling stories with "coping narratives" increases bonding and encourages the child to think positively about mastering stressful situations. Parents facilitate child emotional expression and encourage use of positive imagery during painful medical procedures. The superhero story is uplifting for parents as well, as they often need to think positively as they face the stress of their child's illness (Nabors et al., 2018). For instance, the child tells his or her parent/therapist a superhero story, and then, in order to ensure positive therapeutic support, the parent/therapist interjects comments about problem-solving and coping in anxiety-provoking situations while encouraging emotional expression. One anxiety-provoking situation for children includes communicating with doctors and nurses. Within the superhero story and play, the therapist helps the child "practice" through the "voice of the superhero" communicating feelings and ideas about procedures to doctors and nurses. Children often use the story in a repetitive fashion as a "stress reliever." For example, one young girl, undergoing cancer treatments, developed a "magical unicorn" as her superhero. When she was in pain or bored at the hospital, she thought of the magical unicorn jumping a fence to her happy place—a garden with rainbows and lots of pink grass for her unicorn to eat. She rode on her unicorns back to this garden, picked flowers, ran and played when she needed to relieve stress. Boys may tend to pick superheroes who take "action" such as "Thor" with his magical hammer to fight back and get well when there is a problem related to the medical condition. Another boy had "The Flash" say encouraging statements, such as "You can do it," a mantra to help the boy successfully cope with venipunctures for blood draws. If the therapist is flexible, allowing the child to lead the way, and using a humanistic approach, the child will often use the superhero to help him or her with things about the chronic medical condition that are stressful or anxiety-provoking.

The child may also tell his or her story through drawing the storyline of a superhero's battle with pain or journey through a medical procedure. The child makes his or her story like a cartoon or develops a book to tell the story of the superhero. The story may unfold over several sessions or be a short story completed in one visit. Drawing is a powerful tool for emotional expression and healing (Malchiodi, 2013; Stauffer, 2021). The child decides whether the therapist or the child keeps the story when it is completed. Similar to joint storytelling, the therapist inserts pages into the book, where the superhero problem-solves about things like communicating with the medical staff and parents. In the story, the superhero asks the medical team to show the procedures to the child. Or, alternately, if the child needs to be distracted during a medical procedure, such as a needle stick, the child reviews his or her story during the needle stick and practice taking deep breaths and relaxing with the superhero or thinking of positive places to visit with the superhero. Many times, parents are coaches, reviewing the story which will support the child in thinking positively, as he or she copes with medical procedures and visits.

10.4 Case Example

Garrett was a seven-year-old boy attending the second grade at a rural elementary school.[1] He was, at times, unable to complete his class work due to migraine headaches. He felt pressure in his nose and pain in his eyes before a migraine was in "full force" and he had to lie down at the nurse's office. Often, he needed to go home and rest, and it could be 2 or 3 days before he returned to school. Garrett had been suffering from migraines for 2 years. His mother and father thought that the migraines were related to stress as Garrett was having some difficulty keeping up in school.

After obtaining parent permission, the counselor spoke with Garrett's teacher and completed a classroom observation. His teacher noted that his performance was below average in reading speed and comprehension. However, his spelling and math skills were good. Garrett did a "very nice job" recalling facts in social studies, and only had difficulty in this subject when reading comprehension was involved. The counselor's observation in the classroom was consistent with the teacher's report, in that the therapist observed Garrett fidgeting and looking into the distance during reading periods, and avoiding raising his hand or stating that he did not want to read aloud if the teacher requested that Garrett read aloud in the classroom. Garrett also tended to talk to others and avoid assignments where students read and then answered questions about the reading material. During one of the observations the counselor noticed that Garrett became pale and quiet as the students read a story aloud. After a few moments Garrett said, "My eyes are sore and hurt, and it hurts in my head over my eyes." The teacher then dismissed Garrett to go and visit with the nurse. Garrett went to the nurse's office and laid on a cot in the office. The nurse called his mother and he went home.

Garrett's mother, when providing historical information, reported that his migraines occurred two to three times a month. Typically, they began at school, but could also start at home. Usually, migraines began when Garrett was completing homework. Garrett had his eyesight tested and had been to see his pediatrician, who

---

[1] This character (Garrett) is based in part, on Dr. Nabors' work with several clients and, in part, fictional. The name is a pseudoname and is not related to any person who worked with Dr. Nabors. The grade in school is also fictional, developed for this case presentation.

was in the process of determining if referral to the pediatric headache clinic was warranted. His mother reported that children's pain medication helped "a bit," but did not fully alleviate his headaches. Laying down and sleeping were the "best" remedies to help Garrett find relief.

When Garrett returned to school, the counselor asked to meet with him. She asked Garrett how often he had headaches. Garrett said he was not sure, but they were "bad" and "hurt very much." Garrett said "They (headaches) come and I can't do anything about them." Garrett said he slept to feel better, and he added, "When I sleep, I don't get to play with my friends or on my Tablet." Garrett said he hoped the headaches "Get well soon."

Garrett spontaneously spoke about his school progress. Garrett said he felt very worried that he was not understanding reading assignments. He reported when he could not understand a reading passage his eyes hurt and there was a band around his head. He said he was very nervous that he was not doing well in school, like his older sister. He reported that his father, and his mother, always were happy with his sister, because she did well at school. He then mentioned, "They are sad about me, because I can't read good, and because I have to come home from school a lot." Garrett confessed that he started to worry and feel bad every time "I see a book, because I know I can't read good."

After completing her observations and interviews, the counselor proposed several ideas to help Garrett. First, she referred his parents for an evaluation of academic achievement with the evaluation team at Garrett's school. Until the evaluation was completed, she recommended that Garrett's teacher allow him to complete math problems or write a story when he felt that a reading assignment was becoming too difficult for him to complete. The counselor referred Garrett for an evaluation at a pediatric headache clinic at the local children's hospital. The counselor also asked Garrett's parents if she could work with Garrett on some relaxation techniques to help him feel better when he began to feel worried about his school work. She discussed using relaxation and positive imagery as two anxiety management techniques to use with Garrett. Because Garrett was feeling powerless and unable to control migraines, the counselor planned to introduce these techniques using a superhero, who would be able to overcome tension in his forehead and eye area.

Garrett was friendly and established rapport quickly. During the second session, the counselor discussed ways to reduce tension and "fight" his worries. The counselor provided psychoeducation about the mind-body connection. "When people feel worried, they may tighten their forehead and eye muscles, resulting in a headache." The counselor said that she had some ideas to lessen tension and cope with worry so that Garrett could relax and feel less tension. The counselor stated that her lessons and the relaxing exercises might not stop headaches, but maybe could make them better. She described how muscle tension in the head can have a role in headache pain. She also discussed how pain messages then can travel to the brain and we feel hurt. The counselor helped Garrett relax so his head was not as tight or painful. She taught Garrett ways to fight back against the thought that he would always get a headache if he had "hard" reading work to finish for school.

Garrett's counselor asked Garrett to select his favorite superhero to help him. Garrett selected the "Incredible Hulk" and said the "Hulk is my favorite - he's a nice doctor and he turns into a big hero to fight the bad guys." The counselor and Garrett discussed how his headache Hulk could help him fight the idea that he would immediately get a headache if the reading was too difficult for him. Garrett said, "Well, the Hulk can smash the headache." The counselor expanded on this notion, stating, "The Hulk could also smash your thoughts that say you have to get a headache." Garrett responded, "Well, maybe, then it wouldn't even start," and he smiled brightly. He then drew a picture of the Hulk smashing his thoughts saying "My headache is coming, his thoughts were in a train moving toward him." Drawing a story about this and discussing how his superhero could save him was helpful for Garrett.

Next, the counselor pretended she was "Wonder Woman," her superhero, and as Wonder Woman, she demonstrated a gentle massage on her forehead to increase relaxation. The counselor used her index finder and made small circular motions on her forehead (above her eyes) and at the sides of her eyes. Garrett, as the "Hulk" practiced this as well. They also practiced squinting their eyes and then relaxing them and keeping them closed to release tension in the eye area. Garrett said, "The Hulk really likes this X-ray eye squint, and it will help X-ray out the pain." The counselor praised Garrett's efforts at practicing and they recorded his strategies: (a) smashing thoughts that a headache always comes, (b) massage, and (c) X-ray eye squints on an Incredible Hulk strategy poster that Garrett kept at his desk at school. The counselor made a copy of this poster and provided it to Garrett's mother so that they could discuss the strategies and practice them at home.

The therapist continued to meet with Garrett and his superhero, whom he affectionately named "The Hulkster" as he discussed his worries about school and pleasing his parents. In the persona of the Hulk, Garrett developed a "play" routine where the Hulk told his parents and the teacher about his concerns. Over the next few weeks, the counselor was pleased to learn that Garrett told his parents and teacher about his worries. The evaluation at the headache clinic was helpful as Garrett was provided with medication to use in cases of severe headache (e.g., when he must lie down because of pain). The educational evaluation indicated issues in the area of reading comprehension; programming was developed to assist Garrett in remediating his reading deficits. At the end of the school year, Garrett had about one headache a month, and proudly said, "I don't have to go home every time my head hurts." His parents were pleased with Garrett's progress. Both his parents and the teacher reported that his superhero strategies of relaxation and positive thinking—in terms of being able to stop pain—were helpful additions to cope with eye strain and negative thoughts about head pain.

10.4.1 Case Synthesis

The case of Garrett is an example of using superheroes in treatment. It highlights use of explanation, so the child understands the rationale for therapeutic techniques applied by the superhero. These authors find that children understand and benefit from explanations of the purpose of the actions of their superhero. Garrett gained agency by selecting a superhero that he could identify with and "liked." While the therapist would not have chosen "Hulkster," Garrett found meaning for this superhero which led to increased efficacy in mastery as he "won" against the headaches. When a child has a somatic concern, it is advisable to rule out medical causes and make referrals to pediatricians and connect with them to ensure that medical treatment is not indicated. Furthermore, the child had a key role in developing and implementing the positive imagery, ensuring that it "worked" and was acceptable to him. Thus, personalizing positive imagery potentially improves its meaning for the child, increasing chances for the child to practice and/or apply the intervention. Practicing using the intervention during sessions (or at home, with parents) provides opportunities for the child to learn, improving chances that the child will apply the intervention when it is needed. In this case, Garrettt showed immediate progress, which is gratifying and reinforcing. However, if Garrett had needed to learn other techniques, the superhero as trainer, teacher, and alter ego was already in place, and the therapist could easily work on other intervention techniques mentioned in this chapter to increase the child's "tools" for coping with headaches.

10.5 Conclusion

As shown in examples and ideas for intervention, we believe that the superhero story is uplifting for the child and parent (Nabors et al., 2018). Moreover, this metaphor allows the child to express anxiety and stress related to medical procedures (Freeman, 1991). Using a joint storytelling or narrative approach provides a medium for the therapist to teach coping skills to the child (Trees & Koenig Kellas, 2009). For example, we teach problem-solving skills in stories and provide examples of ways to communicate feelings and needs to doctors, nurses, and other health professionals. The superhero is important for children's play as affording opportunities for mastery of stress and anxiety in a "safe space" (Rubin & Livesay, 2006). Moreover, it is a child-centered technique; child-centered approaches are empowering and healing for children (Axline, 1981). It is our hope that this chapter has provided some ideas for clinicians and health professionals to build upon, as they use superhero stories, play, and drawing in their work to support children coping with stress, pain, and worry related to their chronic medical conditions and possible medical procedures associated with these conditions.

References

Axline, V. M. (1981). *Play therapy*. Ballantine Books.

Bolig, R. (2018). Play in children's health-care settings. In J. A. Rollins, R. Bolig, & C. C. Mahan (Eds.), *Meeting children's psychosocial needs across the health-care continuum* (2nd ed., pp. 79–118). Pro-Ed, an International Publisher. Retrieved from www.proedinc.com

Clark, S. L., & Garland, E. J. (2018). Integrating play and cognitive-behavioral interventions to treat childhood worries and generalized anxiety disorder. In A. A. Drewes & C. E. Schaefer (Eds.), *Play-based interventions for childhood anxieties, fears and phobias* (pp. 107–123). The Guilford Press.

Crenshaw, D. A., & Kelly, J. E. (2018). Play therapy in assisting children with medical challenges. In L. C. Rubin (Ed.), *Handbook of medical play therapy and child life: Interventions in clinical and medical settings* (pp. 57–68). Routledge.

Eaton, L. G., Doherty, K. L., & Widrick, R. M. (2007). A review of research and methods used to establish art therapy as an effective treatment method for traumatized children. *The Arts in Psychotherapy, 34*(3), 256–262. https://doi.org/10.1016/j.aip.2007.03.001

Fradkin, C., Weschenfelder, G. V., & Yunes, M. A. M. (2017). The pre-cloak superhero: A tool for superhero play and intervention. *Pastoral Care in Education, 35*(2), 137–144. https://doi.org/1 0.1080/02643944.2017.1306874

Freeman, M. (1991). Therapeutic use of story-telling for older children who are critically ill. *Children's Health Care, 20*(4), 208–215. https://doi.org/10.1207/s15326888chc2004_3

Gordon, J., & Paisley, S. (2018). Trauma-focused medical play. In L. C. Rubin (Ed.), *Handbook of medical play therapy and child life: Interventions in clinical and medical settings* (pp. 154–173). Routledge.

Gross, S. (2018). The power of optimism. In T. Marks-Tarlow, M. F. Solomon, & D. J. Siegel (Eds.) *Play and creativity in psychotherapy* (pp. 359–375). Terry Marks-Tarlow, Marion F. Solomon and Mind your brain, Inc./W.W. Norton and Company.

Kestly, T. (2018). A cross-cultural and cross-disciplinary perspective of play. In T. Marks-Tarlow, M. F. Solomon, & D. J. Siegel (Eds.) *Play and creativity in psychotherapy* (pp. 110–127). Terry Marks-Tarlow, Marion F. Solomon and Mind your brain, Inc./W. W. Norton and Company.

Kress, V. E., Paylo, M. J., & Stargell, N. A. (2019). The use of play and creative arts in counseling. In V. E. Kress, M. J. Paylo, & N. A. Stargell (Eds.), *Counseling children and adolescents* (pp. 228–252). Pearson Education, Inc.

Locatelli, M. G. (2020). Play therapy treatment of pediatric medical trauma: A retrospective case study of a preschool child. *International Journal of Play Therapy, 29*(1), 33–42. https://doi.org/10.1037/pla0000109

Malchiodi, C. A. (2013). *Art therapy and healthcare*. The Guilford Press.

Mellenthin, C. (2018a). Play-based treatment for school-related fears and phobias of children. In A. A. Drewes & C. E. Schaefer (Eds.), *Play-based interventions for childhood anxieties, fears and phobias* (pp. 60–77). The Guilford Press.

Mellenthin, C. (2018b). *Play therapy: Engaging & powerful techniques for the treatment of childhood disorders*. PESI Publishing and Media, PESI, Inc.

Muris, P., Huijding, J., Mayer, B., van As, W., & van Alem, S. (2011). Reduction of verbally learned fear in children: A comparison between positive information, imagery, and a control condition. *Journal of Behavior Therapy and Experimental Psychiatry, 42*(2), 139–144. https://doi.org/10.1016/j.jbtep.2010.11.006

Nabors, L., Bartz, J., Kichler, J., Sievers, R., Elkins, R., & Pangallo, J. (2013). Play as a mechanism of working through medical trauma for children with medical illnesses and their siblings. *Issues in Comprehensive Pediatric Nursing, 36*(3), 212–224. https://doi.org/10.3109/0146086 2.2013.812692

Nabors, L., Cunningham, J. F., Lang, M., Wood, K., Southwick, S., & Stough, C. O. (2018). Family coping during hospitalization of children with chronic illnesses. *Journal of Child and Family Studies, 27*(5), 1482–1491. https://doi.org/10.1007/s10826-017-0986-z

Nabors, L., & Liddle, M. (2017). Perceptions of hospitalization by children with chronic illnesses and siblings. *Journal of Child and Family Studies, 26*(6), 1681–1691. https://doi.org/10.1007/s10826-017-0688-6

Nabors, L., Liddle, M., Graves, M. L., Kamphaus, A., & Elkins, J. L. (2019a). A family affair: Supporting children with chronic illnesses. *Child: Care, Health and Development, 45*, 227–233. https://doi.org/10.1111/cch.12635

Nabors, L., Stough, C. O., Combs, A., & Elkins, J. (2019b). Implementing the coping positively with my worries manual: A pilot study. *Journal of Child and Family Studies, 28*, 2708–2717. https://doi.org/10.1007/s10826-019-01451-3

Pinquart, M., & Shen, Y. (2011). Anxiety in children and adolescents with chronic physical illnesses: A meta-analysis. *Acta Paediatrica, 100*, 1069–1076. https://doi.org/10.1111/j.1651-2227.2011.02223.x

Rollins, J. A. (2018). The arts in children's health-care settings. In J. A. Rollins, R. Bolig, & C. C. Mahan (Eds.), *Meeting children's psychosocial needs across the health-care continuum* (2nd ed., pp. 119–165). Pro-Ed, an International Publisher. Retrieved from www.proedinc.com

Rubin, L., & Livesay, H. (2006). Look, up in the sky! Using superheroes in play therapy. *International Journal of Play Therapy, 15*(1), 117–133. https://doi.org/10.1037/h0088911

Seymour, J. W. (2016). An introduction to the field of play therapy. In K. J. O'Connor, C. E. Schaefer, & L. D. Braverman (Eds.), *Handbook of play therapy* (2nd ed., pp. 3–15). Wiley.

Shepherd, L., & Kuczynski, A. (2009). The use of emotive imagery and behavioral techniques for a 10-year-old boy's nocturnal fear of ghosts and zombies. *Clinical Case Studies, 8*(2), 99–112. https://doi.org/10.1177/1534650108329664

Stauffer, S. D. (2021). Overcoming trauma stuckness in play therapy: A superhero intervention to the rescue. *International Journal of Play Therapy, 30*(1), 14–27. https://doi.org/10.1037/pla0000149

Trees, A. R., & Koenig Kellas, J. (2009). Telling tales: Enacting family relationships in joint storytelling about difficult family experiences. *Western Journal of Communication, 73*(1), 91–111. https://doi.org/10.1080/10570310802635021

Chapter 11
The Force Awakens: Mindfulness-Based Cognitive Therapy Using Star Wars

Drea Letamendi

Keywords Mindfulness · Common elements · Youth · Adolescents · Pop culture · Storytelling · Parasocial relationships

11.1 Introduction

"The Force" is an invisible energy. You cannot see it or touch it, but if you focus your attention on the sensations within and around you, you can connect to its presence. The Force refers to a metaphysical and ubiquitous power in the Star Wars universe, a galaxy far, far away. It is an obscure energy source that "exists between all things" but requires balance, insight, and intention to harness. According to Star Wars mythos, only those who are intuitively connected to the mystical energy—called Force-users, Force Adepts, or Force-sensitives—are able to convert the energy of the Force into extraordinary abilities. These practitioners can harness their skills for good, as seen in characters such as Luke Skywalker, Yoda, or Rey. Or, if they choose so, they can let their negative emotions guide their manipulation of the energy, or be consumed with them, as seen in Sith characters like Darth Maul or Emperor Palpatine. Though it stems from fantasy, the concept of The Force—and its themes and characters in the stories of Star Wars—holds a pathway to learning about the therapeutic practice of mindfulness.

This chapter will cover teachable moments found in Star Wars related to self-awareness, self-compassion, and centering the self in response to maladaptive

D. Letamendi (✉)
Counseling and Psychological Services, Student and Campus Resilience, UCLA, Los Angeles, CA, USA
e-mail: aletamendi@orl.ucla.edu

© The Author(s), under exclusive license to Springer Nature Switzerland AG 2022
R. D. Friedberg, E. V. Rozmid (eds.), *Creative CBT with Youth*, https://doi.org/10.1007/978-3-030-99669-7_11

191

patterns common among youth with anxiety, traumatic stress, and mood disorders. Characters such as Kylo Ren and Rey from the Star Wars sequel trilogy introduce us to realistic, relatable, and sometimes upsetting psychological features such as negative thinking patterns and dysregulated internal states. Strategies covered will review how youth can notice thoughts and manage their reactions to negative patterns to disengage from self-criticism rumination and dysphoric moods. This chapter will also review how youth can harness the compelling and restorative influences of the "parasocial" relationship—the strong, personal connections one has with a fictional character and their story. The chapter will incorporate useful meditative-like strategies for using mindfulness with teens, in order to help gain relief from negative psychiatric symptoms as well as support growth, identity building, and establishing a unique purpose in the universe.

11.2   Mindfulness Becoming Mainstream

Mindfulness refers to the state we are in when we are paying attention to our present-moment experiences with openness and intention. More broadly, mindfulness is "living in the now." When we bring awareness to the experience we are in, simply being with our emotions and thoughts, and observing ourselves without judgment, we can experience immediate relief, calmness, and insight. There are benefits to "just being." Research-supported effects of mindfulness for adults include improved control over anxiety, improved sleep, decreased intrusive thoughts, lower stress, better attention, enhanced memory, improved enjoyment, and greater personal satisfaction (Creswell, 2017; Hoge et al., 2017; Tang & Bruya, 2017; Schmidtman et al., 2017;Noonan, 2014). Younger generations are more likely to seek mindfulness to help manage the distractions of modern technology (cell phones, social media, email, etc.; Gray, 2017).

Over the past three decades, mindfulness has become one of the most recognized terms in the field of clinical psychological science. Moreover, in the last 10 years, the general public has become knowledgeable about the basics of mindfulness as a well-being practice. Schools, universities, and tech companies have implemented mindfulness-based wellness centers to enhance quality of life and prevent stress-related health conditions such as burnout.

Mindfulness is also appreciated in our cultural entertainment landscape. Mindfulness themes can be spotted in Taylor Swift's song lyrics ("Shake it Off"), Disney's emotionally driven films such as *Inside Out* (2015) and *Soul* (2020), Oscar-nominated drama *Sound of Metal* (2019), and the anime series *Avatar: The Last Airbender* (2005–2008). Additionally, *Star Wars: The Jedi Mind* (2020) is a self-care book that takes quotations and lessons from Star Wars and pairs them with practices such a breathing, posture, and meditation. The 2020 film *The Mindfulness Movement* featured household figures such as musicians, news anchors, and spiritual leaders speak to the benefits of mindfulness. And, in January of 2021, the self-help calming app *Headspace* joined forces with the streaming service *Netflix* and released a series of 20-min episodes of mindful practices, officially injecting mindfulness into the massive pop culture bubble.

11.3 Mindfulness-Based Cognitive Therapy

When used as a therapeutic technique, mindfulness is a conscious effort to make oneself aware of one's present internal emotional and cognitive states without forming *attachment* to them. The therapeutic tool includes observing, describing, and participating in our own reality, nonjudgmentally, and with effectiveness (Robins et al., 2004). Effectiveness refers to the skills we build to examine thoughts and feelings intentionally and with curiosity, without interpreting them as facts or fuel to act upon. The most fundamental difference between mindfulness-based interventions and traditional CBT is the inclusion of *acceptance* perspectives and strategies into CBT's direct change framework (Fielding, 2009). That is, a growing number of new wave cognitive behavioral therapists use mindfulness training coupled with traditional CBT techniques to help clients recognize and accept their negative cognitions simply as *streams of thinking rather than absolute truths.* Clients are encouraged to allow those streams to naturally flow through their mind. Their thought patterns, therefore, do not represent rigid architecture that dictates their decisions and behavior (Segal, 2017; Kaipainen et al., 2017).

In clinical settings, mindfulness training aims to develop individuals' competence in certain social and emotional faculties—fostering self-awareness and regulation of cognitions and emotions as well as developing and cultivating kindness toward the self and others. The macro goal of mindfulness can include decreased suffering, increased happiness, and increased in self-control.

Mindfulness practice has been found to reduce anxiety found in generalized anxiety disorder, social anxiety disorder, panic disorder, test anxiety, illness anxiety, and depressive disorder with anxious distress (Creswell, 2017; Hoge et al., 2017; Dundas et al., 2016; Kim et al., 2016; Surawy et al., 2015). Mindfulness-Based Cognitive Therapy (MBCT) emerged as a solution for practitioners in areas of the field who do not agree that individuals must discard or shift all of their negative thinking in order to achieve contentment or relief from their anxiety, depression, or traumatic stress. Several versions of clinically based mindfulness training including mindfulness-based stress reduction (MBSR; Kabat-Zinn, 1990) and MBCT (Teasdale et al., 2000) have received "high" *quality of research and dissemination* scores as designated by the U.S. Department of Health and Human Services (USDHHS) National Registry of Evidence-Based Programs and Practices (Substance Abuse and Mental Health Services Administration, 2013).

Mindfulness-Based Cognitive Therapy for Children (MBCT-C) can produce immediate improvements in measures of executive function, metacognition, attention, and behavioral regulation compared to controls (Black, 2015). Mindfulness training also shows improvements in depressive symptoms, anxiety symptoms, rumination, externalizing problems, and prosocial skills among youth 6–18 years old, and the approaches are feasible and acceptable for diverse groups of youth (Black, 2015). While mindfulness-based training programs may differ by types of meditation practices, treatment duration, and number of practice sessions, this chapter refers to the common elements of these approaches (sometimes referred to as common practices or key ingredients), which represent identifying the specific, shared techniques and practices that make up evidence-based protocols for specific problem areas among youth and adolescents (Chorpita et al., 2005, 2007; Fielding, 2009), rather than focusing on a particular manual.

11.4 A Rey of Hope: Case Conceptualization

Introduced in *Star Wars: The Force Awakens* (2015), Rey is a clever scavenger from the desert world of Jakku. Self-sufficient and inventive, she spent most of her childhood and young adulthood alone, discovering ways to survive in the harsh and windy climate of the remote, desolate planet. Rey is Force-sensitive—meaning that she is attuned to the flow of the mysterious, binding energy of the Force—but in her early years is unaware of this extraordinary power. Though she has few memories of her early childhood, Rey carries one formative flashback of her parents leaving her on Jakku when she was very young, just a few years old. In some versions of her memory, she is screaming for her parents not to leave her, watching them fly away on a ship as the junk boss Unkar Plutt restrains her by the arm. Rey believes, at times, that she was abandoned on the desolate planet, or even traded, no different than a piece of junk or a scrap part.

As part of a comprehensive clinical assessment, in addition to noting difficulties and challenges, it is essential to enumerate a client's strengths and protective (or resilience) factors. Generally, psychological resilience is our ability to mentally and emotionally cope with hardships. As Rey demonstrates, resilience includes accessing our mental capacities, engaging our personal assets, and using external resources in order to protect ourselves from the hazardous effects of life's stressors. As we will see, living resiliently—accepting reality, shifting perspectives, facing difficult situations with openness—is similar to living mindfully.

In *Star Wars: The Force Awakens*, Rey exemplifies key resilience skills, which can easily be remembered as the "7 C's." The first six include **competenc**e (for instance, building a repulsorlift speeder out of scraps in order to haul materials during foraging, and learning various alien dialects); **creativity** (fashioning the lenses from the stormtrooper helmet into a pair of usable protective goggles); **confidence** (carrying strong internal conviction, a sense of integrity, persistence, and self-recognition when she has done well for the day); **character** (handling situations with a solid set of morals and values, such as rescuing BB-8, a spirited astromech droid, from being sold for parts by a greedy scavenger, Teedo); **coping** (tolerating the absence of her parents through managing her emotions, creating scratch marks on the side of the walker to mark the passage of time as a reminder of her progress and countdown until her family returned); and **control** (empowering herself by building traps, computers, and learning how to use a quarter staff to protect herself from others). In speaking of resilience, Rey embodies a remarkable ability to create routine, predictability, and even gratifying moments out of the randomness and harshness of the backwater planet. The 7th "C" of resilience is **connection,** an ability that Rey learns to foster throughout her relationship building with Han Solo, Luke Skywalker, and, later, Ben Solo.

> People keep telling me they know me. I'm afraid *no* one does.—Rey

Rey's enigmatic background has become one of the most discussed topics within the Star

Wars fandom during the sequels era. Even Rey is fixated on the questions of her origins—carrying troubled thoughts of her background, suffering nightmares, flashbacks, and intense visions of her past, and having difficulty remembering and understanding some aspects of events. Due to her non-traditional origins on her adopted planet, Rey has been described as an analogue for the experiences of foster youth, biracial individuals, and U.S. immigrants (Letamendi & Ratcliffe, 2017; @Blerdgirljedi, @rhymable_, @Porscheirielle, @JennaBellaJ, @Mjrjt, and @theroyalmilktea, 2020). Her self-awareness, self-concept, and sense of sociocultural identity are not underdeveloped or overly fragile, but Rey often feels she is navigating a world in which she is constantly the *other*.

One of the first goals of the mindfulness-based therapist is to develop a working model of what particular internal experiences (thoughts, feelings, and bodily sensations) the client finds unacceptable or challenging. Rey's separation from her parents is internally coded as abandonment, betrayal, and rejection. Rey not only wonders who she is in relation to family of origin, but she silently struggles to understand whether she has any value. How is she any different than the scraps and parts she sees littered along the landscape of the forgotten planet of Jakku? According to the Children's Bureau, abrupt removal and separation of a child from their original family/home can be distressing and confusing for them, sometimes leading to long-term social and emotional effects. Rey's early years resemble the challenging experiences—she is not placed in a supportive, enriching, and loving home after she is separated from her parents, which creates a vulnerability for further trauma. The emotions that may trouble Rey include loneliness, emptiness, confusion, feeling damaged, feeling unliked, and feeling unforgiven. An enumeration of difficult internal experiences like this one provides the clinician with a road map of potential targets for mindfulness and acceptance strategies while also setting up the potential for problem solving, addressing barriers, and anticipating setbacks.

11.5 Early Successes: Mindfulness in Daily Living

For the most part, Rey lives in quietude. Relying on her own intuitiveness and occasionally learning from the traders and off-worlders in Niima Outpost, Rey is a product of her environment as well as her inborn abilities of persistence, determination, and patience. She adopted multiple languages as she managed the harsh social and geographical climate of Jakku. She crafts and designs tools and shelter out of the scraps and wreckage leftover from Imperial-Class Star Destroyers. Rey is resilient not simply because she has the innate capacity to tolerate adversity; she is resilient because the social and ecological elements of her world taught her to be so. In MBCT, "mindfulness in daily living" is the practice of bringing moment-to-moment awareness into all aspects of one's daily life (Kabat-Zinn, 1996). Specifically, as part of our daily habits, this includes choosing one activity and intentionally bringing our awareness to that singular activity. We can do this when walking, eating, or engaging in other daily or routine tasks. When our attention wanders and we are drawn toward past experiences or future concerns, we can gently guide our mind back to our breath, to the present moment, and the activity we are engaged in. MBCT also refers to the "3-Minute Breathing Space," a brief exercise focusing full attention on the movement and sensations of each in-breath and out-breath as it occurs. Breathing exercises can be performed before and during a mindful activity to weave formal meditation practice into daily life (Segal et al., 2002). Early in treatment, homework assignments can include sessions dedicated to mindfulness in daily living—bringing awareness to both pleasant activities (walking, eating, showering), and unpleasant activities (chores, cleaning, exercise) during the week and recording the awareness of corresponding somatic, emotional, and cognitive reactivity.

Rey shows us multiple examples of mindfulness in daily living during the film *Star Wars: The Force Awakens*. We shadow her throughout a day of work as she is gathering scraps, traveling to the outpost with her wares, retrieving rations, cooking, and eating her daily meal. In one powerful scene, she sits quietly on a mound of sand, revealing that her home is in fact the carcass of an old AT-AT. She examines and puts on a scavenged X-wing helmet, taking in the moment. One might assume that Rey is wrapped in fantasy, but it is more intuitive to understand she is experiencing her internal states consciously, experiencing her reality as it is, and connecting to the universe authentically. She allows herself to contemplate her life in relation to the ghosts of the warships and vehicles she has made her home. She relates her existence beyond the desert village and its menagerie of beings and creatures that live there now and those that came before her.

11.6 Mindfulness and the Force: Behavioral Practices of Meditation

How does stillness, quietude, and curiosity provide Rey emotional growth? As earlier stated, mindfulness has noticeable benefits: It increases our ability to recognize emotional states within ourselves, dials up our self-compassion, and strengthens our ability to self-regulate—meaning, we're more likely to not only tolerate heavy emotions but actually learn how to manage and lessen their intensity. In following the emotionally complex characters such as Rey and Kylo Ren in the Star Wars sequels, we can draw some helpful parallels between mindfulness training and *harnessing the Force*. For instance, Force-users are taught to attend to the present moment with the aim to sense an energy within and around them, while calmly acknowledging and accepting one's feelings, thoughts, and bodily sensations. In order to develop the skill of mindfulness, there is a correspondingly explicit emphasis on the importance of practice. Like with mindfulness, Force-practitioners know they must learn to respond wisely to what's happening to them, rather than reacting blindly and lashing out. A distinction between the Sith and Jedi: As part of their practices, Sith emphasize that negative emotions must be explored and that their energy cannot be avoided. They are taught to notice negative feelings such as anger, jealousy, and hatred, and to not *judge* those experiences as unwanted or useless. In fact, Sith *value* negative emotions. They allow those emotions to inform their actions. And when taken to an extreme, this approach can be destructive. Characters who lean too far into the Dark Side such as Emperor Palpatine can serve as an example of tipping the balance.

Thus, the general practices of both Jedi and Sith—acting with awareness, observing/noticing oneself, articulating and labeling emotions, non-judging, non-reactivity, metacognition, and acceptance/letting go—are, in fact, conceptual and functional elements of mindfulness that support mental health growth such as trauma recovery, anxiety management, and stress reduction. Finding examples of these exercises and mapping them to the client's lived experience can help the client better conceptualize their own patterns and even increase their motivation to change them.

An important outcome of mindfulness is the improvement of self-awareness, which is our capacity for introspection. Self-awareness is essential in helping us understand how our emotions and thoughts guide us, drive our decisions, and help us form ideas about the world. On the hidden island of Ahch-To, where Rey discovers Jedi Master Luke Skywalker has been living in isolation for years, we can see how Rey's practice of meditation leads to further knowledge about the self. Though he was reluctant at first, Luke begins to teach Rey about the Force, and employs mindfulness principles when he asks Rey to use stillness as a form of self-learning, to draw her focus and attention inward, to use intentionality and observation so that she can increase insight.

> The Force is not a power you have. It's not about lifting rocks. It's the energy between all things, a tension, a balance, that binds the universe together.—Luke Skywalker.

In many ways, Luke's early teachings represent a therapeutic approach. He is scholarly as well as experiential: He knows he must teach theory but also allow Rey to learn through practice. He describes the Force as an energy "between all things." It is a balance. It is inside of us. It binds us. Luke is also stern in his warnings about what the Force is and what it isn't. "It is not a power you have," he contends, assuring Rey that that the energy she can harness has no owner; it moves freely within and among the beings of the universe. The Force, for once, becomes crystal clear. It is not about genetics (or *midi-chlorians*). Or IQ. Or something you have to be born with. Quite simply, it's our ability to notice. And the most powerful statement Luke makes is that the Force "does not belong to the Jedi" and thus, the Force does not belong to *anyone*, even those who have the power to harness it. Luke's messages are powerful, in the same way that we are empowered knowing our thoughts, feelings, and impulses are simply material that flows within us and do not define us.

Formal practice behaviors of these concepts can include the following: In a *sitting meditation*, the youth engages in intentional mindful awareness while seated with crossed legs on a cushion on the floor or in a straight chair. In a *body scan*, the youth lies on their back on the floor or couch with their eyes closed while gently drawing their attention to different regions of the body in a sequential manner. In using *posture*, the youth can align their head, neck, and body, with the intention to prepare their positioning for other meditative exercises such as a sitting meditation. Finally, movement meditations may be employed, such as *mindful walking*, which comprises attending to sensations in the body, particularly the shifts of weight and balance as well as noticing the ground beneath the feet during a slow-paced walk. Nearly all mindfulness approaches suggest locating (and finding in advance) a consistent place of meditative practice, and administering repeated, routine sessions for continued growth. Rey, for instance, often finds a stable and level ground overlooking the horizon as her place of meditation.

One key aspect should be clear: mindfulness is not necessarily about staying "immobile." Sensory exposure activities might aggravate symptoms in youth with a history of bodily trauma (assault, medical trauma, physical and sexual abuse). Paying close, sustained attention to their internal experience is sometimes not tolerable, especially if it invites contact with traumatic thoughts, images, memories, or even re-traumatic physical sensations. As such, youth who have suffered trauma may respond with feelings of anger, humiliation, hatred, self-loathing, and other negative feelings that can interrupt primary goals of the practice. For trauma survivors, complete silence or complete darkness is sometimes not possible or indicated. In teaching mindfulness activities, for instance, healing practitioners may want to minimize the potential dangers of meditative states to trauma survivors who may experience their body's stillness as triggering or re-traumatizing. Combining mindfulness and movement (breathing, yoga, sound, music, etc.), can sometimes be more helpful than traditional meditation for these reasons.

11.7 Confronting Discomfort—The Dark Side of the Force

Though she is remarkably receptive and willing to gain new skills, Rey struggles to stay present when facing negative emotions. Her most prominent difficulty from the clinical perspective is her fear and avoidance of intense and upsetting internal states. With practice, Rey must learn the ability to know what's happening in her body but not get carried away by what she learns. On the sacred island of Ahch-To, Rey opens up to Luke about the changes she is noticing when meditating—and her fear associated with these changes.

Something inside me has always been there. And now it's awake. And I'm afraid.—Rey

In a teachable moment, in order to help Rey grow more tolerant of her distress, Luke encourages her to engage the fundamental principles of mindful awareness, to reach out "with your feelings." With determination, Rey guides herself to sit in meditative stillness, and allows her mind to be drawn directly to her internal state, knowing it may lead to dark places. Here, Luke gently invites Rey to stay aware of her own experience, even if it ushers in anger, and, subsequently, fear. As she stills her body and mind, visions begin to overtake Rey. Dark imagery and sounds call to her, and we witness a shocking, penetrating rise of ominous energy burst into her mind. When she slips out of the meditative vision, Rey and Luke react to this moment, both a little shaken. "You went straight to the dark," he tells her, somewhat fearfully. "It offered you something you needed…You didn't resist."

Stemming from the notion that universal processes are at work in all humans is "the natural conclusion that there is an equality shared between the experiences of therapist and client" (Fielding, 2009, p. 28). The mindfulness-based therapist works from this perspective to reduce the power differential, and both practitioner and client can interpret difficulties as practice, and a normal part of the process. Each moment is a learning experience. Notably, the therapist should be vigilant for signs that the client is experiencing difficulties related to past adversities and traumas, and in turn, sensitively guide the client to relate skillfully rather than retreating away entirely or being blown away by intense experience. Though Luke is shocked by the intensity and immediacy of Rey's distress, he employs noticing and naming as part of the exercise, e.g., "The feeling of anger is arising in you."

Later, in a moment of solitude, Rey practices mindfulness methods with more autonomy when she feels drawn to a cavern located below the black sea rocks of Ahch-To. Convinced that there might be answers within the cave, Rey descends into the blackness, allowing her mind to wander and flow. In the dream-like, glistening chamber, Rey approaches a reflective wall. She sees multiple images of herself, mirrored back to her over a hundred times. "Let me see them," she commands, toward the splintered reflection, "my parents." She's filled with familiar feelings: Fear, confusion, uncertainty, being lost. Suddenly, two shadowy, indistinct, distant images begin approaching her on the other side of the blurry glass. They slowly concretize, and form into ghostly human bodies. Then, unexpectedly, the blurry images merge. Rey is staring at the simple and clear reflection of herself. She gapes at her own face. Rey never felt so alone.

The Ahch-To cave is an analogue of *expanding awareness*. Here, Rey is directly facing her fear, named as her ultimate worry that she may never know where she comes from or who she truly is. Rey asks herself what she must endure to find herself, to better *know* herself. She must endure the emotions of loneliness, isolation, scatteredness. She must be willing to observe her reality along with the sensations it brings her. The cave is not gentle or withholding. She sees herself fragmented, split into pieces. Not a whole person. Rey is simultaneously nothing and everything.

Dear child, The belonging you seek is not behind you…It is ahead.—Maz Kanata

To her surprise, Rey doesn't find the answer she is seeking within the cave. But, the Ahch-To cave tells her that where she comes from is not the actual answer she seeks. Though she feels disappointment, this moment conveys Rey's growing self-awareness and cognitive flexibility. She accepts the fear, the unknowing, and the realization that the person she is to become is defined within. Rey begins to let go of who she thinks she's supposed to be and embraces who she is now.

11.8   Kylo Ren and the Dark Side Struggle

Introduced in *Star Wars: The Force Awakens*, Kylo Ren is a young, Force-sensitive warrior who lands a commanding role in the galactic military dictatorship known as the First Order. Wrapped in long, black robes and concealed by a battered combat helmet, Ren has the potential to be a formidable villain. His unconventional, 3-bladed red lightsaber is much like his personality: rugged, fiery, fragmented, and unfinished. Indisputably, Ren is perceived by others as unpredictable and reckless. He is often consumed with anger. His emotional outbursts and frenzied tantrums reveal the flood of hate coursing through his body. And yet, given the full narrative of his journey, Ren is unconvincing as a true villain—he's unable to present himself as confident or unwavering. Ren struggles to form an all-embracing self-identify; he cannot fully access the evil stirring inside him because some semblance of Jedi faith remains at his core. Ren battles with an internal conflict that creates doubts and weaknesses within him, and as such, we're unable to see him as the figure he so desperately wants to be, Darth Vader.

Ren has reason to confuse his emotions as facts. Born as Ben Solo, Ren was hand-picked and recruited by the mysterious master of the dark side of the Force, Supreme Leader Snoke. Son to Leia Organa and Han Solo, Ben carried a unique ancestral makeup that Snoke wanted to possess—he assumed Ben had inherited something sinister from his grandfather, Darth Vader. As an adolescent, Ben began to struggle with mixed emotions and confusing urges, and Leia sensed that Snoke was threateningly close to narrowing in on him to harness that spark of darkness for his own advantage. As Leia explained, Snoke was interested in Ben because "He knew our child would be strong with the Force. That he was born with equal potential for good or evil."

Knowing full well of his Skywalker bloodline, Snoke brings Ren way out to the Rarlech system to train him as a dark warrior, hoping to groom him into a combatant as strong as Darth Vader. During a formative exercise, Snoke uses the Force to suspend Ren over the edge of a deep cliff. With his Force abilities still underdeveloped, Ren, terrified, is unable to resist Snoke's grasp. Snoke admonishes Ren, explaining that Ren *should* be afraid because he isn't in control of himself. Ren feels powerless, and Snoke knows this is how to bond him: connect helplessness to anger. Snoke proceeds to coach Ren by telling him to use his powerlessness to "turn to anger." As part of this exercise, Snoke releases Ren from his Force grip, advising him to convert his fear into anger, and then turn his anger into power. Ren follows obediently and manages to sustain his body over the cliff.

11.9   Reactivity to the Internal Experience

Kylo Ren offers a study of emotional attachments. Like Rey, Ren sometimes experiences himself as different and isolated from the world around him. He doubts that others feels what he does—the intensity of his conflicting emotions, the constant pull between the light and dark side, the deeply felt urges to lash out against the universe. What is clear is that Ren displays and handles emotions differently than the extremes of Jedi Masters or Sith Lords. Luke Skywalker, for instance, would have coached Ren to subdue and inhibit his negative emotions of rage, jealousy, and fear. Entertaining those feelings, according to the Jedi, would lead to bad decision-making, unhealthy attachments, and malicious behavior. The Sith philosophy, in contrast, encourages warriors to engage their uncomfortable feelings and convert them to mental and physical strength. As Palpatine had once instructed Anakin Skywalker, "I can feel your anger…it makes you stronger, gives you focus." Both extremes, however, place an inflated amount of value and power in emotional states.

Kylo Ren's "darkness" might be explained by the therapist as psychological pain or psychache. It was said that as a youth he suffered nightmares, upsetting visions, and terrifying voices from his past. In the Star Wars universe, the Dark Side of the Force is not unlike a negative energy or spirit that we can be made aware of. All of us, at some level, encounter feelings similar to the ones causing Ren struggle and difficulty. We can normalize his self-doubt, self-hatred, and mistrust of others. When we are hurt, we also feel the impulse to strike others; we, too, want to lash out, to scream with rage. The conflict between the light and dark side lives in us, manifesting simultaneously in the self-protective urge to destroy one another and the hope that people unconditionally care about us nonetheless.

> I want to be free of this pain.—Kylo Ren

Some youth treat emotions as if they are facts about the world—the stronger the emotion, the stronger their belief that the emotion is based on fact, e.g., "If I feel rageful, the world must be trying to destroy me"; "If I am scared, others are unsafe and mustn't be trusted." However, if we assume our emotions represent facts, we may use them to justify maladaptive actions (Linehan, 2015*). Youth who struggle with unbalanced mood states, fluctuations, or very intense emotions may experience moments of feeling "stuck" in their despair. Searching for a way to get "unstuck" or reconcile the turmoil, some feel they have one option: choose a side. So, stop trying to be better, stop trying to find "good" within themselves. Stop searching for ways to be happy. Stop trying to climb out. Sink deeper within the vast emptiness. This also means stop fighting urges. Let malicious *thoughts* permeate the mind. Allow them to exist freely. The distinction between acceptance and consumption is key. Noticing the how, what, where, and when of harmful emotions builds wisdom and even tenacity. But *immersing* oneself in distressed states and surrendering to their influence can slow down progress. Mindfulness offers the strategies with which to increase awareness of harmful mental processes (e.g., negative automatic thought, rumination, harsh judgments, etc.) while also growing aware of maladaptive reacting.

During his struggle, Ren holds conviction that he can grow more powerful if he were able to harness the darkness within, but instead he feels overwhelmed, disorganized, and conflicted by the tension. Here, we see how he is impacted by secondary emotions, or, in mindfulness terms, reactivity. Primary emotions simply refer to the initial feeling we experience in a situation. Secondary reactions, in contrast, are the reactions we have in response to initial emotions.

Mindfulness-based treatments emphasize the notion that secondary reactions result from a lack of awareness and acceptance, avoidance, or suppression of the primary experience. Ren's primary emotions are in the realm of sadness, despair, hopelessness—after all, he lacks a sense of belonging or achievement, as evidenced by his narrative of rejections from his father, Han Solo, and his mentor, Snoke. Feeling "weak" when noticing his emotions may lead to reactions such as anger and hostility. For Ren, he dodges his primary feelings of sadness and jumps right into the secondary emotions—he becomes impulsive, rageful, and destructive. Unable to contain the intensity of these feelings, he lashes out behaviorally. Then, because "there is good in him," as General Leia reminds us, Ren faces additional feelings of regret, guilt, and shame. These "lapses" between the light and dark are a tumultuous imbalance, such that Ren cycles back and forth between anger and shame. To his disappointment, Ren is unable to "successfully" convert his anger to dark power because he's not yet reconciled or even understood the sadness within him. Ren may hate Ben Solo, but he's nowhere close to loving Kylo Ren.

11.10 Holistic Practice: Luminous Beings We Are

Mindfulness-based practice always considers the whole client within a holistic system. That is, mindfulness embraces the mind and body as intertwined and connected, never separate. In addition, similar to the teachings of the Force, a client learns that the whole self is not separate from the greater relational and systemic whole. Thus, moment-to-moment observations are understood *in relation to* and *as part of* the universal human experience. This includes the sense of belonging and connectedness to one's neighborhood, community, society, and, yes, even the universe, in the largest sense. In clinical practice, such awareness is further aimed at helping clients to engage in more effective responses to each and every moment, consciousness, and sensation, even if they include stressful interactions.

> For my ally is the Force, and a powerful ally it is. Life creates it, makes it grow. Its energy surrounds us and binds us. Luminous beings we are. Not this crude matter.—Yoda

When Ren's mind wanders into his early learnings as a student of Jedi Master Luke Skywalker, he becomes emotionally dysregulated. Perhaps a sense of uncertainty grows when Ren recalls the Jedi lessons of patience and serenity or thinks about the tenets of treating all life forms with respect and dignity. As a Padawan, he was asked to serve as a guardian rather than destroyer, and there is a mismatch with how he sees himself now. Unable to manage the tension within, he turns toward to his grandfather for clarity. "Forgive me," Ren says to the charred, melted, deformed helmet worn by Darth Vader. "I feel it again. The call to the light." He asks the spirit of Darth Vader to show him the power of the darkness again. Alone with a heap of burnt metal, Ren searches for purpose, for a way to cauterize the turmoil within him rather than understand the relationship of these experiences as a whole.

One goal for mindfulness-based work is the search for *intrinsic wholeness*, which involves helping the client to dismantle beliefs that they are damaged or broken because of their past experiences or because they struggle with emotional pain. This involves promoting the awareness of self that is larger and more valued than the fragmented pieces: the pain of disappointment, past traumas, or psychological problems. As clients grow aware of their wholeness, they learn to be *containers* of their experience and not synonymous with their experiences; they are more than the sum of their parts. For instance, Ren can conceptualize his tensions and struggles as direct responses to the abuse he experienced, as natural reactions stemming from unwanted experiences. When he feels ready to inhabit his body with full ownership, he understands that no matter how many scars he has incurred, his original wholeness is still intact.

Formal practice behaviors of these concepts can include the following: During a *body scan,* youth attend to specific body sensations that arise such as tension, numbness, or pain. During a *sitting meditation*, youth can allow feelings of disappointment, sadness, anger, or grief to arise within them. Using the metaphor of *quicksand* ("the more you struggle, the more you suffer"), youth can practice the skill of naming emotional difficulties and letting go. By using storytelling and *upstream narrative*, youth can acknowledge that despite the turmoil associated with psychache, life can have joyful and satisfying moments that take place "upstream" or between currents. The upstream concept widens the lens on a problem by asking youth to consider imagining important landmarks in their journey that may be out of view in this moment. To advance their work, youth can be taught to adopt a "both—and" paradigm by looking for the synthesis between opposites, appreciating that their reality is complex, multi-layered, and integrated. Finally, when thoughts of anger, hate, and hostility arise during meditation practice, they can practice *affirmations* or *self-statements* of love and compassion. Adding and repeating specific positive words and phrases of loving feelings will eventually broaden their repertoire of responses to negativity.

It is likely that the pressures of light and dark have created much confusion in Ren's concept of his personhood, future, and purpose. His identity dualism, the self-fragmenting of his two personas, serves as a self-protective defense. But it cannot last. The fallacy of the Light vs. Dark side lies in the notion that we can fundamentally be characterized by "one side." We fail by believing in the myth that we must be "good" one hundred percent of the time, by not allowing ourselves mistakes or lapses in judgment. Realistically, we are both. We must grant ourselves the permission to experience and even honor conflicts within us, to find self-acceptance in the mixture between "light" and "dark," and the self-compassion to forgive ourselves when we lose control, to give ourselves a truer vision of our remarkable, magnificent place in this universe.

11.11   Parasocial Relationships—Finding Connection Not So Far, Far Away

A parasocial relationship (sometimes called a parasocial interaction or PSI) is a kind of relationship experienced by an audience in their mediated encounters with television, film, comics, and other forms of entertainment. Though they are one sided, parasocial relationships are very real personal connections one experiences with fictional characters. Common among all age groups, these emotionally charged relationships between a viewer and a media character typically involve three elements: (1) attachment and friendship (security, comfort, and trust); (2) personification (human-like needs and qualities such as hunger, sleep, and play); and (3) social realism (Richards & Calvert, 2017). Just as a friendship evolves through spending time together, parasocial relationships evolve by watching characters on our favorite TV shows, and relating to their personal lives, idiosyncrasies, and experiences.

As it turns out, social surrogates can represent safe social connections insofar as they can provide the psychological experience of a connection with few emotional threats compared to the real counterpart. Fictional friends are consistently available, reliable, and predictable, for the most part. Fictional loss, however, can be impactful. For instance, following the airing of the last episode of the television show *Friends*, researchers found that adult viewers anticipated experiencing the same negative reactions to parasocial breakups as they experience when their real social relationships dissolve (Eyal & Cohen, 2006).

The stories in entertainment media have provided us with a way to process, cope, connect or be transported from the world around us. It may not be surprising that the majority of us have turned to entertainment media during the COVID-19 pandemic to comfort our anxieties, manage our fears, and affirm our hopes. According to a *Fandom* report from October 2020, 74% of pop culture fans say they're spending more time with entertainment media compared to the months before the pandemic. Nearly half of viewers agree that they've permanently changed the way they engage with entertainment given their pandemic viewing habits. And many of us turned to familiar stories and characters we to help us cope; during the pandemic, nostalgic entertainment has provided fans a chance to connect with families and a way to share what we love with others in an otherwise solitary time (Paul, 2020).

Those of us experience grief and loss amidst the pandemic are struggling to find normal routines, stability, and peace during this tumultuous time. The predictability of fictional stories—the fact that they have a beginning, middle, and end—help us find clarity and concreteness during times of uncertainty. Stories might be particularly healing, because they provide a safe and healthy outlet that allows us to begin approaching our own emotions surrounding grief and loss. Many of our clients turn to stories to see others just like them overcome adversity and hardship; observing important traits such as empathy, compassion, and fallibility and seeking these traits within themselves.

Formal practices of these concepts can augment or accompany traditional mindfulness-based exercises. Youth can be taught to embrace the connections they have with characters from comics, sci-fi, and fantasy by identifying traits and abilities they relate to or admire. One exercise may include exploring their favorite character's "Wiki page," a unique online profile which houses their personality, abilities, and values, followed by guiding the client to create their own Wiki page with the similar elements of their own identity. Each Wiki page includes a character summary, quotation, background, trivia, origins, and picture. While youth build their own Wiki, they may begin to consider the traits and abilities that define them, or that matter most to them. Therapists will note that for some, building a "background section" may be adverse or negative, and that youth may cite both negative and positive experiences as "turning points" or core components of their identities. Finally, nailing just one biographical quotation can be formative as a practice, and can evolve over the course of therapy. A suggested prompt to generate a client's Wiki quotation might be "What is something *you've said* or something *said to you* that best represents who you are?"

11.12   Conclusion

To summarize, our meaningful, undeniably powerful connections to stories can be a particularly healing component of our mindfulness journey. Our moment-to-moment empathy for Rey in her quest for belonging can be exercised throughout the entirety of the Star Wars sequel saga. Similarly, our ability to find compassion for Ben Solo can stem from our own identification of discomfort and tension within our emotional selves. For many of us, witnessing characters face and overcome a fictional crisis can help us to process difficult or painful feelings like anguish and sorrow; and to uplift our spirits and encourage us to stay resilient, strong, and hopeful about our own futures.

References

@Blerdgirljedi, @rhymable_, @Porscheirielle, @JennaBellaJ, @Mjrjt, & @theroyalmilktea (Hosts). (2020, July 17). Rey *is* the biracial experience [Audio podcast episode]. In *Sistas with Sabers*.

Black, D. S. (2015). Mindfulness training for children and adolescents: A state of the science review. In K. W. Brown, J. D. Creswell, & R. M. Ryan (Eds.), *Handbook of mindfulness: Theory, research and practice* (pp. 283–310). Guilford Press.

Chorpita, B., Becker, K., & Daleiden, E. (2007). Understanding the common elements of evidence-based practice: Misconceptions and clinical examples. *Journal of the American Academy of Child and Adolescent Psychiatry, 46*(5), 647–652.

Chorpita, B. F., Daleiden, E. L., & Wiesz, J. R. (2005). Identifying and selecting the common elements of evidence based interventions: A distillation and matching model. *Mental Health Services Research, 7*(1), 5–20.

Creswell, J. D. (2017). Mindful interventions. *Annual Review of Psychology, 6i*(18), 18–26.

Dundas, I., Thorsheim, T., Hjeltnes, A., & Binder, P. E. (2016). Mindfulness-based stress reduction for academic evaluation anxiety: A naturalistic longitudinal study. *Journal of College Student Psychotherapy, 30*(2), 114–131.

Eyal, K., & Cohen, J. (2006). When good *friends* say goodbye: A parasocial breakup study. *Journal of Broadcasting and Entertainment Media, 50*(3), 502–523.

Fielding, L. (2009). A clinicians' guide to integrating mindfulness into evidence-based practice: A common elements approach. Theses and Dissertations. 31. Retrieved from https://digitalcommons.pepperdine.edu/etd/31.

Gray, K. (2017, June 1). *Here's why millennials are so dedicated to practicing mindfulness.* Brit + Co. Retrieved from https://www.brit.co.

Hoge, E. A., Guidos, B. M., Mete, M., Bui, E., Pollack, M. H., Simon, N. M., & Dutton, M. A. (2017). Effects of mindfulness meditation on occupational functioning and health care utilization in individuals with anxiety. *Journal of Psychosomatic Research, 95*, 7–11.

Kabat-Zinn, J. (1990). *Full catastrophe living: Using the wisdom of your body and mind to face stress, pain, and illness.* Delacourt.

Kabat-Zinn, J. (1996). Mindfulness meditation: What it is, what it isn't, and its role in health care and medicine. In Y. Haruki, Y. Ishii, & M. Suzuki (Eds.), *Comparative and psychological study on meditation.* MBSR Training Materials.

Kaipainen, K., Valkkynen, P., & Kilkku, N. (2017). Applicability of acceptance and commitment therapy-based mobile app in depression nursing. *Translational Behavioral Medicine, 7*(2), 242–253.

Kim, M. K., Lee, K. S., Kim, B., Choi, T. K., & Lee, S. H. (2016). Impact of mindfulness-based cognitive therapy on intolerance of uncertainty in patients with panic disorder. *Psychiatry Investigation, 13*(2), 196–202.

Letamendi, A., & Ratcliffe, A. (Hosts). (2017, Nov 8). A Rey of hope (No. 1) [Audio podcast episode]. In *Lattes with Leia.*

Noonan, S. (2014). Veterinary wellness: Mindfulness-based stress reduction. *Canadian Veterinary Journal, 55*, 134–135.

Paul, M. (2020, October 7). *The state of fandom.* Fandom. Retrieved from https://www.fandom.com/articles/state-of-fandom-2020

Richards, M. N., & Calvert, S. L. (2017). Measuring young U.S. children's parasocial relationships: Toward the creation of a child self-report survey. *Journal of Children and Media, 11*(2), 229–240.

Robins, C. J., Schmidt, H., III, & Linehan, M. M. (2004). Dialectical behavior therapy: Synthesizing radical acceptance with skillful means. In S. C. Hayes, V. M. Follette, & M. M. Linehan (Eds.), *Mindfulness and acceptance: Expanding the cognitive behavioral tradition* (pp. 1–29). Guilford Press.

Schmidtman, E. A., Hurley, R. A., & Taber, K. H. (2017). Secular mindfulness-based interventions: Efficacy and neurobiology. *Journal of Neuropsychiatry and Clinical Neurosciences, 29*(2), A6–A83.

Segal, Z. (2017, January 10). *Mindfulness based cognitive therapy as maintenance treatment for unipolar depression.* UpToDate. Retrieved from http://www.uptodate.com

Segal, Z. W., Williams, J. M. G., & Teasdale, J. D. (2002). *Mindfulness-based cognitive therapy for depression: A new approach to preventing relapse*. Guilford Press.

Substance Abuse and Mental Health Services Administration. (2013). National registry of evidence-based programs and practices. Retrieved from http://www.samhsa.gov

Surawy, C., McManus, F., Muse, K., & Williams, J. M. (2015). Mindfulness-based cognitive therapy (MBCT) for health anxiety (hypochondriasis): Rationale, implementation and case illustration. *Mindfulness, 6*(2), 382–392.

Tang, Y. Y., & Bruya, B. (2017, May 9). Mechanisms of mind-body interaction and optimal performance. *Frontiers in Psychology, 8,* 647.

Teasdale, J. D., Segal, Z. V., Williams, J. M. G., Ridgeway, V. A., Soulsby, J. M., & Lau, M. A. (2000). Prevention of relapse/recurrence in major depression by mindfulness-based cognitive therapy. *Journal of Counseling and Clinical Psychology, 68*(4), 615–623.

Chapter 12
Clinical Applications of *Steven Universe* in Cognitive Behavioral Therapy

Christy Duan, Gian Ramos Monserrate, Elaine Shen, Rishi Chelminski, Diana Mujialli, and Mamatha Challa

Keywords Steven universe · LGBTQ youth · Children's media · Cognitive behavioral therapy

12.1 Introduction

Steven Universe is a Cartoon Network animated series about the coming-of-age of Steven Universe, a half-human, half-alien boy grappling with his mother's legacy while growing up in a small town on Earth. Steven lives with the Crystal Gems, aliens with female humanoid forms who fought alongside his mother to protect

---

All figure images were illustrated by Elaine Shen, MD.

C. Duan (✉)
Private Psychiatric Practice, New York, NY, USA

Mind Body Seven, Brooklyn, NY, USA

G. R. Monserrate
Universidad Central del Caribe School of Medicine, Bayamon, Puerto Rico
e-mail: gian@geektherapy.org

E. Shen
Department of Psychiatry and Behavioral Sciences, Northwestern University Feinberg School of Medicine, Chicago, IL, USA
e-mail: elaine.shen@northwestern.edu

R. Chelminski
Pace University, Dyson College of Arts and Sciences, New York, NY, USA

D. Mujialli
Worcester, MA, USA

M. Challa
Department of Psychiatry, Harvard Medical School, Cambridge Health Alliance, Cambridge, MA, USA

R. D. Friedberg, E. V. Rozmid (eds.), *Creative CBT with Youth*,
https://doi.org/10.1007/978-3-030-99669-7_12

Earth from their own kind. With help from his friends and family, Steven discovers his gem powers and saves the planet.

Critically acclaimed for its diversity of characters and relationship dynamics, LGBTQ+ representation, and nuanced portrayal of mental health challenges, *Steven Universe* garnered a GLAAD Media Award, Peabody Award, and five Emmy Award nominations. The series gathered a huge following of youth and adults alike, which led to a feature-length film and *Steven Universe Future*, an epilogue limited series of Steven as an adolescent struggling with posttraumatic stress symptoms. The show affirms that differences are to be celebrated, everyone faces challenges, and each person is deserving of validation and acceptance.

The following chapter will outline why *Steven Universe* can serve as a uniquely useful adjunct to therapy for children who are fans of the show (particularly for children who are LGBTQ+ or otherwise minoritized). Several sample exercises will be provided, making use of themes from the show to facilitate the development of introspective, prosocial, and regulatory repertoires using techniques common to various modalities of child therapy.

12.1.1   LGBTQ+ Representation

Steven Universe pushed the boundaries of LGBTQ+ representation in the media and made history as one of the first children's shows to feature a same-gender marriage proposal. It is also the first major animated series created by a female-identified person, Rebecca Sugar, who has more recently come out as a bisexual and non-binary woman (Zane, 2018). According to Insider's database of LGBTQ+ characters, *Steven Universe* has more than 40 queer-coded characters, including several gender non-conforming and non-binary characters who make essential contributions to the storyline (White & Chik, 2021). This comes at a time when the depiction of queerness in children's media—particularly queer-coded pre-teen or young-teen characters—is extremely rare (Kelso, 2015). As Sugar said in an interview: "We absolutely must tell LGBTQ+ children that they belong in this world and they deserve to be loved" (Romano, 2018). *Steven Universe*'s broad appeal and critical acclaim is an indication of an appetite for more positive LGBTQ+ representation in popular media for children.

12.1.2   Mental Health Representation

Steven Universe depicts mental health challenges, including those clustered around PTSD and complex trauma, in a way that is both positive and conceptually sound. This is unusual in popular media, which commonly portrays characters suffering from generic, sometimes inaccurate, mental health symptoms that are not reasonably contextualized. These characters are labeled as "deviant" or "undesirable," until they receive hospitalization or medication, often in absence of cognitive/behavioral interventions (Henderson, 2018). A 2003 review of mental health representation in children's media found similarly problematic themes as those in the media at large (Wahl, 2003). By contrast, *Steven Universe's* characters face these struggles using solutions that are cognitive/behavioral in nature, such as developing their introspective repertoires, and practicing skills for emotional regulation and cognitive restructuring. During their respective journeys, they are provided social support that includes normalization and acceptance of their struggles. For the past two decades, children's shows with more responsible depictions of both mental health and LGBTQ+ issues have emerged alongside *Steven Universe*, such as *Adventure Time, Legend of Korra, She-Ra and the Princesses of Power,* and *Muppet Babies.*

Popular media is the layperson's primary source of information regarding mental health issues. Because of this, content creators increasingly report a sense of responsibility to provide useful and accurate mental health education for the common good (Henderson, 2018). In a video statement for the National Alliance on Mental Illness, Sugar said, "My team and I framed a story about mental illness and posttraumatic stress in a way that would be accessible for a young audience...I felt hopeful that this could spark conversations within families, and give kids an understanding that they could carry with them if they were ever to be in a traumatic event, or if they had experienced one already" (NAMI, 2021).

In the United States, 61.8% of youth have been exposed to at least one trauma by age 17 and there is a 4.7% lifetime prevalence of posttraumatic stress disorder (PTSD) in adolescents, with many who suffer from comorbid depression, anxiety, and substance abuse (McLaughlin, 2013). Almost two-thirds of adults report experiencing at least one adverse childhood experience (ACE), such as abuse or neglect of an emotional, physical, or sexual nature; substance abuse, mental illness, and intimate partner violence in the household (Merrick, 2018). The more ACEs a person experiences, the more they are at risk of injury, infectious disease, chronic disease, mental illness, substance abuse, and poor outcomes within maternal-fetal health, education, and occupation. For this population, access to useful and accurate mental health education can serve as a vital adjunct to clinical interventions, providing salient modeling and reinforcement of behavioral skills (Merrick, 2018).

To this end, *Steven Universe* uses a variety of stories and metaphors to demonstrate how Steven and his friends process difficult emotions and experiences. Character development arcs and musical-style songs are used to thoughtfully explore grief, anxiety, PTSD, and interpersonal relationships in a way relatable to both children and adults. Fans of the show have expressed how the realistic complexity of characters has given them insight into their own struggles with depression, trauma, and gender identity (Mellon, 2017). As the series progresses, characters fight in an intergalactic war, have multiple near-death experiences, and witness the deaths of loved ones. There is a recurring theme of Steven feeling pressure to live up to the legacy of his mother, who defended Earth as a rebel army leader, while figuring out his own identity and sense of self-worth. In *Steven Universe Future*, an older teenage Steven manages posttraumatic stress symptoms that originated from his adverse childhood experiences. Across both series, characters demonstrate use of both adaptive and maladaptive coping mechanisms, which the show contextualizes using their individual life experiences and personalities.

In the following section, clinical applications of *Steven Universe* for mindfulness and cognitive behavioral therapy are presented. For young fans of the series, these applications may be especially useful as references to the show may have greater salience than more generic therapeutic content.

12.2   A Mindfulness Education

Mindfulness can be a first step in creating a safe space for children to explore their thoughts and feelings. Mindfulness-based interventions are increasingly common in a variety of therapeutic modalities (Simkin & Black, 2014), and have demonstrated clinical utility for a variety of mental illnesses (Goldberg et al., 2018). Fans of *Steven Universe* are primed to explore mindfulness, as it is depicted throughout the show.

12.2.1   The Mindful Self

In *Steven Universe*, gems are superpowered aliens who appear with a gemstone—such as a garnet, amethyst, or pearl—embedded in their body. The small gem (a type of advanced computer) contains their consciousness, and is the only truly immutable part of their body; the rest of their physical form is a type of hard light projection from the gem, the appearance of which reflects various aspects of their conscious and unconscious, and personality traits and states. This parallels Jungian concepts: the gemstone is a Gem's *true self* while their projected humanoid form is the *persona* presented to the public (Wilde, 2011). As a mindful exploration of self, a therapist can ask the child about their gem—or their key attributes and strengths—and ask them to draw it. Refer to Table 12.1 for questions and guiding comments that can facilitate this process. Figures 12.1, 12.2, 12.3, and 12.4 include examples that you can use.

12.2.2   Mind-Body Awareness

By establishing a connection with his gem, Steven is able to unlock his powers and weapon. As this mind-body awareness strengthens, he is able to control his healing powers and rose-colored shield with greater proficiency. Just like Steven, developing mind-body awareness can unlock a child's strengths (Perry-Parrish et al., 2016). Exercises that can facilitate this include:

- Body scan
  - Have the child settle into a comfortable position. Consider leading the child in a deep breathing, relaxation, or other grounding exercise first. Ask the child to share their current feelings and body sensations. Then, start a "body scan" by systematically asking the child to describe how each part of the body feels—head, fingers, chest, belly, legs, etc. Ask the child where they feel their stated emotion and ask what it feels like. Explain that feelings are connected to the body, and describe how awareness of this connection can strengthen the child's understanding of how they experience their feelings so they can use this valuable information to make good choices.
- Coloring your gem and feelings in the body
  - See Fig. 12.5 on the next page. Have the child draw their gem on a human analog like the one depicted and use the discussion of their gem as a starting point for localizing feelings on their body. Expand the conversation by having them talk about emotions they commonly feel, and choose colors and shapes to represent those emotions on parts of the body where they localize these feelings. Remind them that the localization of their feelings is unique to them, and therefore something they must explore on their own.

12.3   Here Comes a Thought, Feeling, and Behavior

Once the foundation of mindful self and mind-body awareness has been established, the therapeutic work shifts to the cognitive-behavioral triangle by exploring the relationship between thoughts, feelings, and behaviors (Cohen et al., 2012). In Season 4, Episode 4 "Mindful Education," Steven's best friend Connie Maheswaran is struggling with shame after accidentally harming another student (Cartoon Network, 2021). In a musical number "Here Comes a Thought," Garnet educates Connie on the importance of mindfulness and reflection, and shows Steven how to support his friend in processing this difficult event (Cartoon Network, 2021):

Take a moment to think of just
Flexibility, love, and trust...
Take a moment, remind yourself
Take a moment to find yourself...
(Cartoon Network, 2021)

Garnet identifies initial thought problems, recognizes how thoughts caused alarm and harm, and finally suggests how to let them go. The musical segment uses butterflies as a visual metaphor to demonstrate how thoughts can be beautiful, overwhelming, natural, and capable of being freed (Cartoon Network, 2021).

Aaron T. Beck's Cognitive Behavioral Triangle (Cohen et al., 2012) can be adapted to *Steven Universe* by centering the gem—or the child's *true self* and values—in their pattern of thoughts, feelings, and behaviors as in Fig. 12.6. The

Table 12.1 Questions about a child's gem and other resources

Questions	Comments
What kind of gem would you have (ruby, sapphire, diamond, etc.)? What shape and color is your gem? Why?	While the child's gem can be a purely artistic choice, it's important to ask them why they chose those features and understand how it relates to the child's self. See Fig. 12.1
Where can others see your gem?	Gem location can indicate important character traits. For example, Pearl acts very logically and uses rationalization as a coping mechanism. Her gem— a pearl— – is located on her head. Steven is very empathic and bases his decisions on gut feelings. His rose-colored gem is located on his navel. Asking a child where their gem is located can help them consider where their thoughts, feelings, and actions come from. See Fig. 12.2
What kind of body would your gem make?	A child may choose to draw or describe a body similar to theirs, or a body that is very different. Be sure to ask why the gem projects this body and how these aspects relate to the child's self. See Fig. 12.2
How do you shapeshift? Does it depend on the situation? What makes it easier to shapeshift? What makes it more difficult to shapeshift? What does it feel like to shapeshift for fun, vs shapeshifting because others want you to? How do you imagine that makes others feel?	All gems have the power to temporarily shapeshift, and will eventually return to their default form—the true self— because it takes a lot of energy to shapeshift, or project a persona. Some gems are not as capable of shapeshifting and can only "stretch" a little. Other gems, like Amethyst, are skilled shapeshifters who can morph into other gems, humans, animals, cars, helicopters, and much more. The exertion required to shapeshift is potentially a useful metaphor of explaining the difficulty of being forced to alter one's persona to pass in different social circles
What other powers and weapons does your gem give you?	Gems have special powers and weapons that can be summoned from their gem. For example, Garnet has a literal third eye with the power of future vision. She can see many future outcomes and the probability that each will occur. Her weapon is a pair of gauntlets, or armored gloves, used to punch in battle. Asking a child about their powers or weapons is an invitation to understand their abilities and values. See Fig. 12.3
What other coping tools would you pack into your cheeseburger backpack?	In Season 1, Episode 3 "Cheeseburger Backpack," Steven gets a new backpack in the mail and overpacks for a dangerous mission to the Lunar Sea Spire with the Crystal Gems. Though not all of Steven's ideas worked, the Crystal Gems were impressed by his creative solutions involving sweaters and bagels. See Fig. 12.4

therapist explains how the cognitive behavioral triangle works by providing examples of how thoughts, feelings, and behaviors can impact each other and lead to both desired and undesired outcomes. These exercises orient the child to external outcomes of their thoughts/feelings/behaviors. The therapist may then supplement this by using mindfulness exercises to orient the child to internal outcomes within their own body. The therapist should also encourage the child to come up with their own examples by applying this model to their own life with the exercise in Table 12.2.

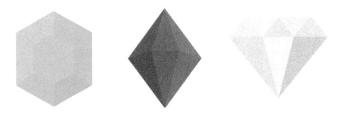

Fig. 12.1 Examples of gems

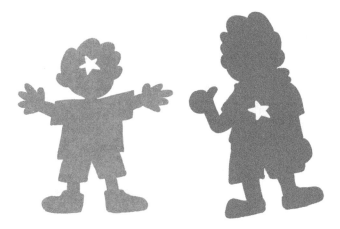

Fig. 12.2 Examples of gem location on a child's body

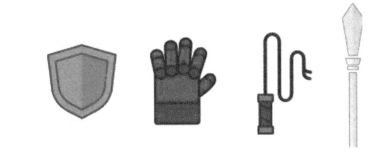

CHARACTER	Steven	Garnet	Amethyst	Pearl
WEAPON	Shield	Gauntlets	Whip	Spear
REPRESENTATION	Safety, protection	Strength, power	Confidence, flexibility	Precision, skill

Fig. 12.3 Examples of gem weapons and their representations

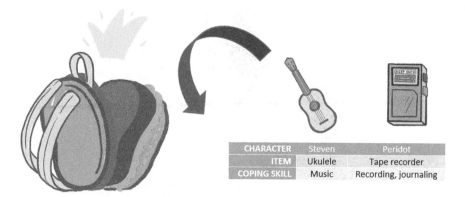

CHARACTER	Steven	Peridot
ITEM	Ukulele	Tape recorder
COPING SKILL	Music	Recording, journaling

Fig. 12.4 Examples of items and coping tools for a child's cheeseburger backpack

12.3.1 Cognitive Distortion Cactus

Throughout *Steven Universe Future*, Steven has difficulty expressing his thoughts for fear of burdening his family and friends. In Episode 10, "Prickly Pair," Steven accidentally creates a sentient cactus. At first, Steven finds relief by venting his insecurities to the cactus, including a fear that his friends do not need him anymore and are leaving him behind. As Steven continues to vent, the cactus grows more humanoid and learns how to speak. The cactus begins to resemble Steven in appearance and speech. Cactus Steven quickly becomes an external, physical representation of Steven's inner "prickly" thoughts. Before running away from home, Steven puts a box over Cactus Steven with the hope that no one will hear it repeating his innermost thoughts. As Steven continues to hide his feelings, Cactus Steven grows bigger and starts attacking the gems. Steven realizes that he is at fault for Cactus Steven's actions and that his cactus just needs love. In an act of self-love, Steven hugs the cactus. Though the hug is prickly and painful for Steven, Cactus Steven grows pink flowers and stops attacking everybody. While it's painful to face difficult emotions, doing so will bring peace and new growth. Therapists can use the story of Cactus Steven to identify cognitive distortions and corrections.

In Fig. 12.7, cactus names and thought bubble labels are related to psychological concepts that therapists commonly teach children. There are three different cacti which represent different types of self-awareness that one may experience when confronted with difficult emotions:

Automatic Cactus refers to one's automatic thoughts or "initial thoughts."

Curious Cactus signifies the child's "mindful thoughts." The Curious Cactus gazes at the initial thoughts of Automatic Cactus with an expression of detached curiosity that can be interpreted as appreciative and loving—as opposed to concerned, confused, or frustrated. The purpose of this facial expression is to model being a non-judgmental observer of oneself.

Wise Cactus refers to "wise mind," which expands on Mindful Cactus' observations by contextualizing them within other facts about the child's life. The "expanded

COLORING YOUR GEM & FEELINGS IN THE BODY

Draw and color your gem in the body below. Remember that gems are like feelings – they are both connected to your body! Feelings can be felt in the body. Feelings come and go, and don't last forever. Sometimes you can even have more than one feeling at the same time!

List as many feelings as you can on the lines below. Find a color that describes each feeling. Color in the squares next to the feelings you came up with.

Choose a feeling that you'd like to focus on. Imagine having that feeling right now. Find out where that feeling is in your body. Color in the places on the body where you have these feelings. Now, try the same thing with a few more different feelings.

Finally, draw and color your gem weapon and powers.

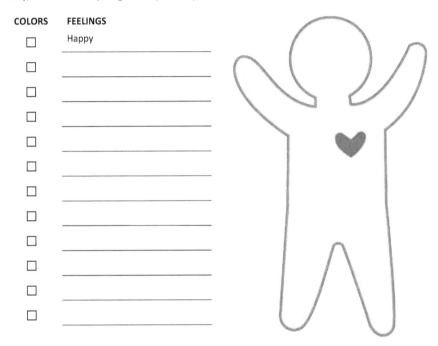

COLORS   FEELINGS

☐   Happy

☐   _____

☐   _____

☐   _____

☐   _____

☐   _____

☐   _____

☐   _____

☐   _____

☐   _____

☐   _____

☐   _____

Fig. 12.5 Worksheet for coloring your gem and feelings in the body

thoughts" label is also important to remove a sense of judgment or rejection of the automatic "initial thoughts" and reference an "expanded state" of enlightened thought.

It is important to convey that all three states self-awareness are equally valid and important (including the automatic thoughts), and that they are part of an interconnected system that helps the child respond to the world. The "expanded state" of Wise Cactus should be presented as useful, but not inherently superior to one's initial reactions or mindful observations. For this reason, it is important to avoid using

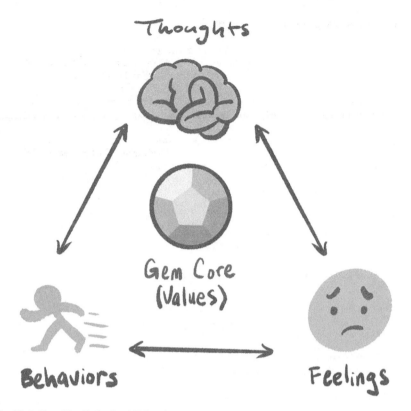

Fig. 12.6 Cognitive Behavioral Triangle

Table 12.2 Here comes a thought, feeling, and behavior exercise

CBT concept	Relevant song lyric	Questions and suggestions
Thought	"Here comes a thought"	• What initial thoughts came up in your mind? • Were there any thinking errors or cognitive distortions in those automatic thoughts? • Can you expand those thoughts and reframe the situation in a more helpful way?
Feeling	"How did it alarm you? How did it harm you?"	• How did those thoughts make you feel? • Validate your feelings—it's okay to feel what you're feeling
Behavior	"Is this how we fall apart?"	• How did you react to those thoughts and feelings? • What would acting differently have done?
Mindfulness	"Take a moment to find yourself"	• Take a step back from the situation • Try a deep breathing, relaxation, or grounding exercise • Re-center around your gem—your true self, values, and strengths

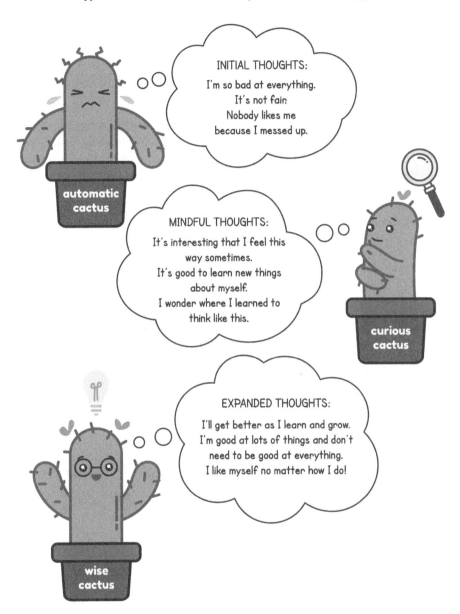

Fig. 12.7 Example of cognitive distortion cactus exercise

labels like "negative" or "maladaptive" for the more difficult parts of the child's experience.

Figure 12.7 provides examples of thoughts that would be appropriate to put in the thought bubble of each cactus, which may be useful to reference while children fill out their own blank thought bubbles in Fig. 12.8. The language chosen for this exercise overlaps with language used across multiple modalities of child therapy, including Dialectical Behavioral Therapy (Perepletchikova, 2018), Acceptance and Commitment Therapy (Turrell et al., 2016), Mentalization-Based Therapy (Midgley et al., 2017), and Mindfulness-Based Stress Reduction (Purcell & Murphy, 2014).

Finally, the child can choose how they would like to acknowledge their cactus in Fig. 12.8. They can choose to hug their cactus like Steven, give the cactus a high-five or a thumbs up, or something totally different! It is important to present neutral models of saying "hi" to their cactus and to avoid suggesting that a particular reaction—like hugging or being emotionally or physically intimate—is a necessary progression of the child's experience. The child can pick their own version of a healthy outcome.

The exercise of filling out Fig. 12.8 can be expanded upon using Fig. 12.9. Using this worksheet, the therapist teaches the child how to identify how initial thoughts, feelings, and behaviors arise from situations, and how they may use a "cactus reframe" (referencing cognitive reframing) to adapt to those situations in a healthier way (Cohen et al., 2012).

12.4   Beach City—Identifying Networks of Safety and Support

Throughout *Steven Universe*, a common theme is empowerment through family, friends, and the Beach City community. Steven learns that he cannot take on the burden of saving Earth by himself and needs support in order to thrive. It can be helpful to have the child identify their network of safety and support in Fig. 12.10. Questions that can facilitate the activity include:

- What kinds of people do you find in different parts of the city (the boardwalk, the home/beach, in town)?
- If you were fighting an intergalactic war, which *Steven Universe* characters would you want on your team?
- Are these characters like anyone in your real life? How so?
- Where in your own community can you find the people you need to support you? Who are they?
- In what ways can these people support you? What are their strengths and limitations?

12.5   Determining Your Path

In *Steven Universe*, gems are manufactured for a specific purpose and face severe punishment if they diverge from that path. For example, Jaspers are created to be elite soldiers, Peridots are created to be engineers, and Lapis Lazulis are created to

MY CACTUSES

Cactuses can be prickly, just like some of our thoughts! What would your cactus say? What would your cactus do? Draw thorns on your cactus and label them with what your cactus would say or do.

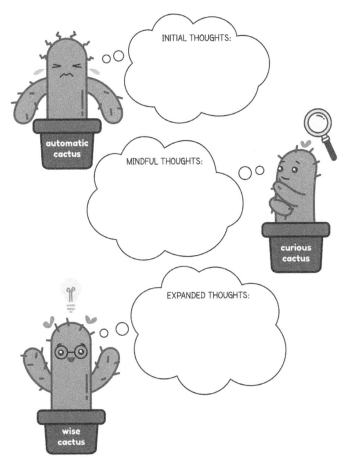

How can you say "hi" to your cactus? Steven gave his cactus a hug, but you can do something totally different – like give your cactus a high-five or a thumbs up! The cool thing is that YOU get to decide!

Fig. 12.8 Worksheet for cognitive distortion cactus exercise

be terraformers. Steven's mother rebelled against that concept. For instance, she encouraged her Pearl to become a warrior, even though Pearls were created to be servants.

Individual differences among gems are also suppressed as much as possible. For example, Amethyst was created to be an elite soldier similar to the Jaspers, but an error in her creation led to her being smaller and weaker than others in her caste. She

MY CACTUS JOURNAL

Situation	Initial Thoughts	Feelings	Behaviors	Cactus Reframe
Bad grade on a test	"I'm terrible." "Everything is ruined."	Anger Sadness Anxiety Fear	Give up on the class Avoid studying for the class	"If every pork chop were perfect, there would be no hot dogs!" - Greg Universe, Steven's Dad

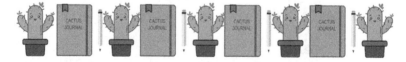

Fig. 12.9 Thought record using cognitive distortion cactus

is seen within Gem Society as defective and fundamentally useless. Gem Society doesn't view her as being worthy of her intended path, doesn't allow her to choose a different path in life, and doesn't recognize that she can contribute as a warrior or as another role.

When Steven's mother insisted that gems be empowered to choose their own destiny and that individual differences be celebrated, an intergalactic war broke out. The concept of self-determination and celebration of diversity is a theme that LGBTQ+ youth commonly struggle with. A therapist may start discussion around these themes by asking:

MY BEACH CITY

Draw and describe who you'd want supporting you in your very own Beach City.

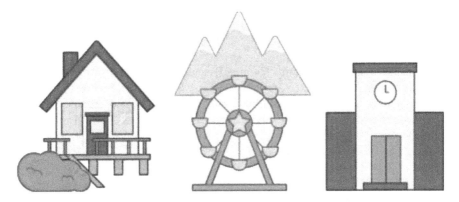

	HOME	FUNLAND	SCHOOL
Who can I find here?			
Why are they here?			
How do they support me?			

Fig. 12.10 Worksheet for identifying networks of safety and support

- What do other people around you see you being the best at? The worst?
- What do you see yourself being the best at? The worst?
- In what ways do you see yourself the same way others see you? In what ways do you see yourself differently?
- How do people's expectations affect you? How do you imagine your expectations affect other children?
- Which people around you are best at seeing "the real you?" How do you identify these people? How can you also become good at seeing "the real" part of other children?

- How can you help other people understand "the real you" better? How can you take care of "the real you" and make sure it isn't pushed aside by the expectations of others? How can you support other children in this way?

12.6   Wrapping Up Therapy with a "Poof"

At the conclusion of therapy, the "Poofing" Exercise can create a space for children to reflect on their progress. In *Steven Universe*, when gems suffer great injuries in battle, they "poof." Their physical form disappears into their gem, and they undergo a recovery process in which they must reflect on their mistakes and growth. This process may take minutes or days, until the gem has reflected and is ready to reform themselves to show their new self. For this exercise, the child is encouraged to reflect on how they looked before and after the therapeutic intervention. At present, the challenges discussed in therapy as the cause of the child's "poofing," Have them imagine how they would look after they've reflected on these challenges in a therapeutic setting. Questions to ask include:

- What did you look like before "poofing" into therapy?
- How have you changed after "poofing" and reflecting during our therapy sessions?

    – Are there changes to the physical appearance of your gem?
    – Do you have any new powers?

By answering these questions, the child can reflect on how they and their perspectives have changed over the course of therapy.

12.7   Conclusion

The acclaimed series *Steven Universe* is a thoughtful and inclusive children's television show that highlights important themes of identity and mental health. Many episodes include direct and age-appropriate introductions to therapeutic concepts like mindfulness, understanding emotions, identity formation, and self-acceptance. In this chapter, we have outlined specific ways that therapists can use ideas from Steven Universe as a lens for exploring key CBT principles with clients. In particular, these strategies can be used to help children practice mindfulness exercises, reflect on their strengths, understand how their thoughts influence their mood and behavior, and learn cognitive restructuring skills to reduce their negative thought patterns. In turn, the fun and LGBTQ-affirming nature of this series may help increase children's comfort and level of engagement in CBT work with their therapists.

References

Cartoon Network. (2021, September 17). "Here comes a thought" | Steven Universe | Cartoon Network [Video]. YouTube. Retrieved from https://www.youtube.com/watch?v=dHg50mdODFM

Cohen, J. A., Mannarino, A. P., & Deblinger, E. (2012). *Trauma-focused CBT for children and adolescents: Treatment applications.* Guilford Press.

Goldberg, S. B., Tucker, R. P., Greene, P. A., Davidson, R. J., Wampold, B. E., Kearney, D. J., & Simpson, T. L. (2018). Mindfulness-based interventions for psychiatric disorders: A systematic review and meta-analysis. *Clinical Psychology Review, 59,* 52–60. https://doi.org/10.1016/j.cpr.2017.10.011

Henderson, L. (2018). Popular television and public mental health: Creating media entertainment from mental distress. *Critical Public Health, 28*(1), 106–117. https://doi.org/10.1080/0958159 6.2017.1309007

Kelso, T. (2015). Still trapped in the U.S. Media's closet: Representations of gender-variant, pre-adolescent children. *Journal of Homosexuality, 62*(8), 1058–1097. https://doi.org/10.108 0/00918369.2015.1021634

McLaughlin, K. (2013). Trauma exposure and posttraumatic stress disorder in a national sample of adolescents. *Journal of the American Academy of Child and Adolescent Psychiatry, 52*(8), 815–830.e14. https://doi.org/10.1016/j.jaac.2013.05.011

Mellon, A. (2017). *4 ways Steven universe saved my mental health.* The Odyssey Online. Retrieved from https://www.theodysseyonline.com/5-ways-steven-universe-saved-mental-health

Merrick, M. (2018). Prevalence of adverse childhood experiences from the 2011-2014 behavioral risk factor surveillance system in 23 states. *JAMA Pediatrics, 172*(11), 1038–1044. https://doi.org/10.1001/jamapediatrics.2018.2537

Midgley, N. J., Ensink, K., Lindqvist, K., Malberg, N., & Muller, N. (2017). *Mentalization-based treatment for children: A time-limited approach (illustrated edition).* American Psychological Association.

NAMI. (2021, September 16). Rebecca sugar NAMI statement [video]. YouTube. Retrieved from https://www.youtube.com/watch?v=1XNRX%2D%2Dwsgo

Perepletchikova, F. (2018, November 1). Dialectical behaviour therapy for pre-adolescent children. The Oxford Handbook of Dialectical Behaviour Therapy. https://doi.org/10.1093/oxfordhb/9780198758723.013.25.

Perry-Parrish, C., Copeland-Linder, N., Webb, L., & Sibinga, E. M. S. (2016). Mindfulness-based approaches for children and youth. *Current Problems in Pediatric and Adolescent Health Care, 46*(6), 172–178. https://doi.org/10.1016/j.cppeds.2015.12.006

Purcell, M. C., & Murphy, J. R. (2014). *Mindfulness for teen anger: A workbook to overcome anger and aggression using MBSR and DBT skills* (1st ed.). Instant Help.

Romano, N. (2018). Steven universe shows a groundbreaking same-sex marriage proposal. Entertainment Weekly. Retrieved from https://ew.com/tv/2018/07/05/steven-universe-same-sex-marriage-proposal-the-question/

Simkin, D. R., & Black, N. B. (2014). Meditation and mindfulness in clinical practice. *Child and Adolescent Psychiatric Clinics of North America, 23*(3), 487–534. https://doi.org/10.1016/j.chc.2014.03.002

Turrell, S. L., Bell, M., & Wilson, K. G. (2016). *ACT for adolescents: Treating teens and adolescents in individual and group therapy (illustrated edition).* Context Press.

Wahl, O. (2003). Depictions of mental illnesses in children's media. *Journal of Mental Health, 12*(3), 249–258. https://doi.org/10.1080/0963823031000118230

White, A. & Chik, K. (2021). 259 LGBTQ characters in cartoons that bust the myth that kids can't handle inclusion. Insider. Retrieved from https://www.insider.com/lgbtq-cartoon-characters-kids-database-2021-06?page=explore-database

Wilde, D. J. (2011). *Jung's personality theory quantified.* Springer Science & Business Media.

Zane, Z. (2018). Steven universe creator Rebecca sugar comes out as 'non-binary woman'. Out Magazine. Retrieved from https://www.out.com/popnography/2018/7/17/steven-universe-creator-rebecca-sugar-comes-out-non-binary-woman

Chapter 13
Integrating Psychodrama [Experiential] and CBT with Adolescents in Groups

Thomas W. Treadwell and Debora J. Dartnell

Keywords Experiential · Action · Psychodrama · Automatic thought record · Cognitive distortion · Negative automatic thoughts

13.1 Introduction

Making CBT user friendly to adolescents involves the integration of existing cognitive behavioral techniques with innovative approaches. In this chapter, a discussion of teenagers' hierarchy of needs is addressed along with reviewing negative self-thoughts and common thinking distortions. As teenagers experience grief, obstacles, or worry, thoughts can easily become negative. Frequently, negative self-thoughts (NSTs) can take over and dominate feelings about one's self worth and life in general. Cognitive Behavioral Experiential Group Therapy (CBEGT) is an effective model for working with teen groups. The model incorporates cognitive behavioral and psychodrama interventions, allowing group members to identify and modify negative thinking, behavior, and interpersonal patterns while increasing engagement in positive and success-based experiences. The environment creates a safe and supportive climate where clients can practice new thinking and behaviors and share their concerns freely with group members (Treadwell et al., 2004).

T. W. Treadwell (✉)
Center for Cognitive Therapy, University of Pennsylvania and West Chester University, Philadelphia, PA, USA
e-mail: ttreadwe@pennmedicine.upenn.edu

D. J. Dartnell
West Chester University, Morgantown, PA, USA
e-mail: DDartnell@wcupa.edu

R. D. Friedberg, E. V. Rozmid (eds.), *Creative CBT with Youth*, https://doi.org/10.1007/978-3-030-99669-7_13

13.1.1 Research Support

Cognitive Behavioral Therapy (CBT) is an evidence-based therapy which has been used extensively in the treatment of depression, anxiety, and personality disorders. With the increasing popularity of CBT techniques, especially those developed by Beck and his colleagues (Beck et al., 1979), the treatment has been applied to a wide range of disorders from anxiety and depression to schizophrenia in both individual psychotherapy and group therapy settings. Psychodrama, an interactive method of roleplaying past situations in the present, is often used within group therapeutic settings to facilitate insight and problem-solving. Although traditional psychodrama is conceptualized in terms of three main techniques—warm-up, action, and sharing—there is no dearth of techniques that may be applied in those three phases (Treadwell et al., 2004). The versatility of psychodrama stems from the variety of techniques that have been borrowed or adapted from various individual and group psychotherapy modalities (Wilson, 2009; Hamamci, 2002, 2006; Baim, 2007).

13.1.2 Clinical Application

Cognitive Behavioral (Psychodrama) Experiential Group Therapy (CBEGT) is an effective model for working with teen groups. The model incorporates cognitive behavioral and psychodrama interventions, allowing group members to identify and modify negative thinking, behavior, and interpersonal patterns while increasing engagement in positive and success-based experiences (Shay, 2017; Treadwell et al., 2016). The environment creates a safe and supportive climate where clients can practice new thinking and behaviors and share their concerns freely with group members (Treadwell et al., 2004).

Initially, all members are assessed using various instruments to establish the nature and severity of presenting issues and to uncover other relevant information. The first one or two sessions are devoted to establishing group norms, providing psychoeducation about Cognitive Behavior Therapy (CBT) and schemas, as well as describing the session format. These initial didactic sessions are intended to explain the group format as a problem-solving approach for working through various interpersonal, educational, psychological, and health-related conflicts. The sessions include information about the nature of the structured activities so participants have realistic expectations about how the group will run. Each group member signs informed consent and audiovisual recording consent forms as every session is recorded. The audiovisual recordings create an ongoing record of group activities and serve as a source for feedback for the individuals when requested.

Here's how the model looks with a group of ten teenagers, ranging in age from 13 to 17. In session one, the facilitator introduces the Beck Depression Inventory-II (BDI), Beck Anxiety Inventory (BAI), and Beck Hopelessness Scale (BHS; Beck,

1988; Beck & Steer, 1993; Beck et al., 1996), explaining the importance of completing each scale on a weekly basis. These instruments are administered before the start of each session and are stored in personal folders to serve as an ongoing gauge of participants' growth in action group therapy (Treadwell et al., 2008). In addition, the GRIT Survey for teenagers is administered, pre and post, to assess group members desire and determination to stick with and carry out a desired goal (Baruch-Feldman, 2017).

In the second or third session, additional data on early maladaptive and dysfunctional schemas and core beliefs are obtained when group members complete Young's schema questionnaire (Young et al., 2003; Young & Klosko, 1994; Young, 1999). A list and the definitions of dysfunctional schemas and core beliefs are given to participants during the initial session (Treadwell et al., 2008).

Each group session in CBEGT is divided into three sections typically found in psychodramatic interventions: *warm-up*; *action*; and *sharing* (Moreno, 1934). During the **warm-up** phase, individuals engage with one another utilizing cognitive and behavioral techniques including identifying upsetting situations, automatic negative thoughts and triggered moods; writing balanced thoughts to counter negative automatic thoughts; and recognizing distortions in thinking and imprecise interpretations of difficult episodes. The second portion, **action**, employs psychodramatic techniques such as role-playing, role reversal, and mirroring, which facilitate the examination of various conflicting situations individuals experience within the group context. This segment enables group members to better understand the nature of negative thoughts triggered by situations and their effects on moods. The last stage, *sharing*, involves the protagonist (i.e., the client) listening to and working with the auxiliaries (i.e., group members assisting the protagonist) as they share their experiences with the protagonist. At this stage, the facilitator may provide additional guidance to the protagonist regarding ways to begin resolving the actual situation in real life. Normally, the protagonist will be asked to complete a homework assignment that will be reviewed at the next session.

13.1.3   Multi-cultural Considerations

In my experience, multi-cultural issues can be addressed in the model utilizing specific psychodrama techniques, including role interview and surplus reality (e.g., where one imagines or creates significant others to avoid reproaching relationships) present another's point of view. Additionally, during the warm-up, the protagonist has the opportunity to discuss and expand on what is important in his/her culture, utilizing the genogram, Maze worksheet, and teen automatic thought record. The genogram, (i.e., Family Tree) is useful in capturing a picture of family and cultural relationships, while the Maze Worksheet allows the group member to record their thoughts and emotions to situations as they identify automatic thoughts, also known as "hot thoughts." These materials assist in educating the group members gain insight into the protagonist's values and beliefs. The psychodrama takes place within the cultural context that the protagonist defines. For example, when acting out a scene, the protagonist has control over which group members serve as auxiliaries and provides, through role interview and role reversal, insights into the auxiliaries' reality. The protagonist can continue providing direction to the auxiliaries as the psychodrama unfolds. This ensures that the psychodrama accurately depicts his/her environment and cultural realities.

The following case study presents Angelica[1], a teenager struggling to fit in at her new school and neighborhood. In this case study, Angelica emerges as the protagonist, the main client for the session, and other members of the group serve as auxiliaries, members assisting Angelica, and the audience, those listening and watching the session unfold. The main group[1] members include Riley, 15, who was recently cut from the soccer team; Kia, 13, whose grandmother just passed away and Angelica, 16, whose parents recently got divorced, causing her to move towns and change schools. Jan, 17, who worries about being able to afford to go away to college; both Lauren, 15, and Dak, 13, have no close friends; Bobby, 16, and Jenny, 14, are failing classes due to problems at home; Tyler, 17, and Marta, 13, both have social anxiety. Tyler is afraid of graduating from high school and moving on to an unfamiliar environment; Marta is new to the school and doesn't know how to navigate new social relationships.

13.2   One Teen's Story

A case conceptualization based on Beck's rubric (2011) is presented below and applied as an ongoing therapeutic tool. After three or four sessions, the therapist explains and teaches the main ideas behind the technique and asks group members to complete the case conceptualization form on an ongoing basis as the group progresses. A member discusses his or her completed form with the group on an assigned day. Case conceptualization may help group members reflect on their various rules, conditional assumptions, beliefs, and means of coping. Please see Fig. 13.1 for Angelica's conceptualization.

The conceptualization leads to the more specific cognitive triad of negative thoughts explaining how Angelica's thoughts reflect themes of loss, emptiness, and failure creating a depressive/failure mindset. Typically, this characterization is distorted, making case formulation useful in challenging the teen's view of self, the world, and the future. Presenting it in the group during warm-up can be helpful for the action phase and provides structure for the group, ensuring all members feel heard. The cognitive triad is best conveyed to group members using this visual representation (*see* Fig. 13.2).

Angelica is a 16-year-old girl who recently moved to a new school. She was eager to make friends, she was feeling very down that she had not made any interpersonal connections yet. Angelica joined a therapy group for teens dealing with depression and anxiety and began the work by telling the group a story about an uncomfortable situation that had recently come up.

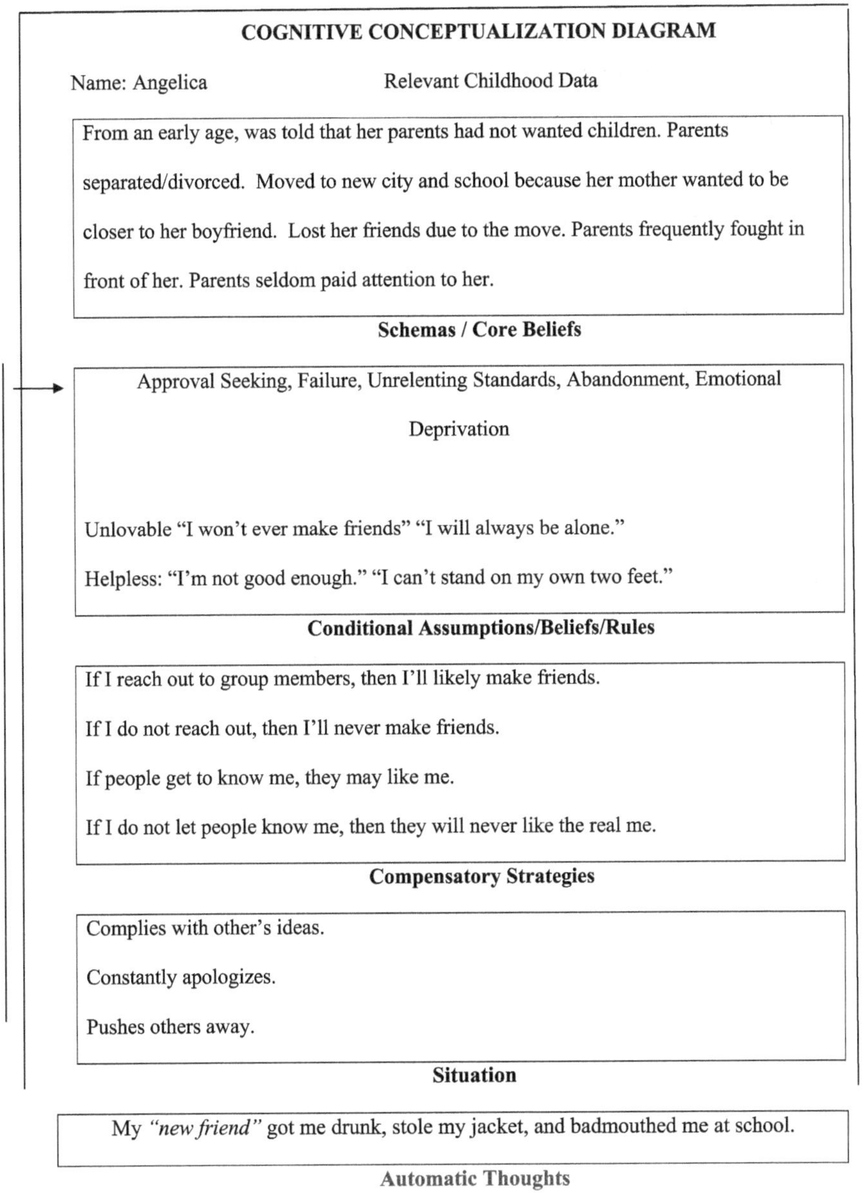

COGNITIVE CONCEPTUALIZATION DIAGRAM

Name: Angelica   Relevant Childhood Data

From an early age, was told that her parents had not wanted children. Parents separated/divorced. Moved to new city and school because her mother wanted to be closer to her boyfriend. Lost her friends due to the move. Parents frequently fought in front of her. Parents seldom paid attention to her.

Schemas / Core Beliefs

Approval Seeking, Failure, Unrelenting Standards, Abandonment, Emotional Deprivation

Unlovable "I won't ever make friends" "I will always be alone."

Helpless: "I'm not good enough." "I can't stand on my own two feet."

Conditional Assumptions/Beliefs/Rules

If I reach out to group members, then I'll likely make friends.

If I do not reach out, then I'll never make friends.

If people get to know me, they may like me.

If I do not let people know me, then they will never like the real me.

Compensatory Strategies

Complies with other's ideas.

Constantly apologizes.

Pushes others away.

Situation

My *"new friend"* got me drunk, stole my jacket, and badmouthed me at school.

Automatic Thoughts

Fig. 13.1 Cognitive Conceptualization Diagram

13.2.1 Warm-Up

During the warm-up and while completing the Maze Worksheet, a type of thought record, Angelica described a situation where she had been invited to a party by a

I am such a jerk

How could I let this happen?

I never drink

I just wanted to fit in

I only want someone to like me

My parents fought so much that they didn't even know I was around

I'm not important to anyone

I'll never have any friends

I'm a loser

I'm not good enough for anybody

Meaning of Automatic Thought(s)

I am never a priority to others.

I am scared that I am going to be alone; I fear that I will never fit in and have friends

Emotion

Betrayed

Stupid

Sad

Angry

Ashamed

Lonely

Afraid

Behaviors

Avoids reaching out to form new friendships.

Ignores her own feelings in favor of others.

Takes chancy risks in order to fit in.

Fig. 13.1 (continued)

popular girl in her class. Although that she does not over consume alcohol, Angelica became intoxicated at the party and the popular girl offered to take her home. When

Fig. 13.2 Cognitive Triad

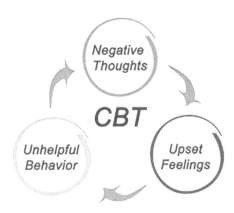

Angelica arrived home, her mom was awake and her *"new friend"* said she would stay with Angelica to make sure she was alright. She passed out and when she woke up, her "friend" was gone and so was her leather jacket. The next day at school, her "new friend" ignored her, and Angelica heard the friend telling everyone what a loser Angelica is.

After identifying Angelica's moods, the facilitator of the group began to lead her through testing her automatic thoughts. Using the downward arrow technique by repeatedly asking her questions to evoke the automatic thoughts, the facilitator helped Angelica to consider which underlying thoughts or beliefs caused her feelings to arise in this situation. Angelica eventually identified her negative self-thought. Her schemas of abandonment and approval seeking and core beliefs that she was unlovable and helpless emerged as she completed the Maze worksheet. A portion of Angelica's Maze worksheet can be seen in Fig. 13.3.

The protagonist, Angelica, selected Riley, another group member, to be her double. The role of the double is to communicate thoughts and feelings the protagonist is having but cannot express. Angelica was very distressed and had trouble moving forward to articulate her defeated attitude. The facilitator used the soliloquy technique, encouraging Angelica to walk around the room with her double, freely associating her thoughts and feelings. Ultimately, this led her to calm down and express her feelings of rejection. The monologue permitted her inner feelings and thoughts to emerge and gave the facilitator, the group therapist, direction to set the stage allowing Angelica to move gradually into the action phase. Angelica paced around the room, with her shoulders slumped, thinking/talking aloud, expressing her concerns, discomfort, and hopes. Angelica's double, Riley, walked with her, articulating the thoughts he imagined Angelica was thinking but not outwardly expressing. Angelica echoed the beliefs that she agreed with and dismissed those that were not on target. The technique enabled her to relax, focus, and prepare for the action stage. Additionally, this method allowed other group members to engage and focus on the upcoming action.

As Angelica walked around the room with her double, she realized how her parents' tumultuous marriage and recent divorce, along with the move from her house

1. Explain a recent situation that caused you to feel upset.

> My *"new friend"* got me drunk, stole my jacket, and made fun of me at school.

2. List the emotions you felt immediately following the situation. Rate them on a scale from 0 to 10.

    (0 = Not at All, 10 = Very Strong)

> Betrayed 10
> Stupid 10
> Sad 10
> Angry 10
> Ashamed 10
> Lonely 10
> Afraid 8

3. What were your immediate thoughts about yourself following the situation? Circle the thought

    that makes you feel the worst. This is your **"Negative Self-Thought"**.

> I am such a jerk
> How could I let this happen?
> I never drink
> I just wanted to fit in
> I only want someone to like me
> My parents fought so much that they didn't even know I was around
> I'm not important to anyone
> I'll never have any friends
> I'm a loser
> **I'm not good enough for anybody** ➡ **Negative self-thought**

4. List experiences throughout your life that support your **"Negative Self-Thought"**.

> My parents never wanted kids.
> Even though I cried when they fought, they didn't stop.
> I was always the last kid picked for teams.
> I wanted to stay in the area where we used to live but my mom wanted to be closer to her boyfriend.
> I don't have any friends at my new school.
> People make fun of me.
> My boyfriend from home hasn't called me since I moved.
> Most of my old friends don't check in with me to see how I'm doing.

Fig. 13.3 The Maze

to a small apartment with her mom had affected her. She understood that she was consistently looking for acceptance from others and latched on to anyone who seemed to like her. When the facilitator asked Angelica what she needed to do to

5. List experiences throughout your life that **do not** support your **"Negative Self-thought"**.

> I was good enough to be picked to travel with my old school's band.
> My dad came to all of my concerts.
> I have two friends that I've had since 1st grade and we talk or text every week.
> My dad calls once a week and I see him once a month.
> My mom and I have a girl's night once a month.

6. Is there anything helpful about your **"Negative Self-Thought"**? (optional)

7. Use an experience from #4, and #5 to create a "balanced thought" and rate how much you believe this thought on a scale of [0 not at all – 10 very strong].

   Balanced thought may look something like this: *Even though I'm struggling to fit in at my new school, I met some people at soccer tryouts, and they asked me to hang out.(7)*

> Even though I don't have any friends at my new school yet, I do have 2 friends from 1st grade that I talk to or text every week.   6
> Even though my parents didn't notice me or my feelings when they were fighting, they each spend special one on one time with me every month. 7
> Even though I was always the last one picked for teams, I was picked to travel with my old school's band. 8
> Even though my parents never wanted kids, my dad came to all of my concerts.   9

8. Re-rate the emotions listed in #2. Add and rate any new emotions.

> Betrayed 10
> Stupid 9
> Sad 10
> Angry 8
> Ashamed 6
> Lonely 10
> Afraid 5

Fig. 13.3 (continued)

address the way she felt, she recognized that she had "no self-confidence and was desperate for social acceptance."

The facilitator asked Angelica to select a new group member to play one of her long-term friends from her previous home. She chose Kia to play her friend long-term friend, Nicole. The facilitator used the interview in role reversal to help Kia understand and play the role of Nicole. Using this technique, Angelica got into the character and mindset of Nicole, giving Kia information about the role. Once the interview in role reversal completed, Kia was prepared to play the role of Nicole, setting the stage for Angelica and "Nicole" to start a conversation. Angelica told "Nicole" how sad she was about not having anything to offer and felt she would never make new friends. She and "Nicole" reversed roles many times, attempting to get Angelica to recognize her strengths and good qualities but, even with the assistance of Riley, her double, she could not see herself as anything but a flawed person who would never have friends again. The facilitator asked Angelica if it might be helpful to explore a role opposite to her perceived "flawed" roles. Angelica was interested and receptive to the idea. When the facilitator asked her to identify the roles she currently plays, Angelica quickly responded: ugly duckling, nerd, lost girl, peacemaker, and perfect student. She admitted that the "lost girl" is the dominant role she inhabits and that she slips into the perfect student role when she feels like the lost girl is swallowing her up. She also realized that the ugly duckling and nerd roles feed her lost girl and sometimes prevent her from trying to form new friendships. As the peacemaker, she realized that she is always thinking about how others feel, while ignoring herself. She said she is always walking on eggshells no matter who she is with. Thinking about her current roles, Angelica recognized that she needed to develop a confident role to help her see clearly what she has to offer others.

To address the confident role struggle role training involves a person delineating a specific aspect of functioning they wish to improve or develop to foster a new role. Usually begin with a specific situation where the person wishes to acquire, role training involves the dramatic setting up of an enactment of a situation. To further explore Angelica's roles, chairs were placed in the middle of the room and Angelica played each role: ugly duckling, nerd, lost girl, peacemaker, and perfect student, as she expressed her thoughts and emotions about each role. Her double, Riley, sat with her in each role, expressing thoughts and feelings he imagined she was having but not expressing. Another member of the group, Bobby, was chosen, as an auxiliary, to play the "lost girl" and Jenny and Marta acted as the "ugly duckling" and "nerd," respectively. Lauren took the auxiliary role of "peacemaker." After several attempts, Angelica, in her confident role, was unable to shut down these powerful roles. Simultaneously, the facilitator learns information from the roles and understand which role to focus on to bring about change. This takes minimal time in session. Another member of the group, Dak, was chosen to play the confident role. After seeing him model this role, Angelica, with the help of her double, was finally able to shut the negative roles down. The final step in the action phase was to have Angelica, using the empty chair technique, address her *"new friend"* about what she did to her at the party and, afterward, at her house and at school. This technique fosters interpersonal development by asking Angelica to imagine that person sitting in the empty chair and confronting her *"new friend."* She was able, with help from her double, Riley, to confidently express her anger about the situation. Furthermore, she told her *"new friend"* that she was worth more and deserved healthy relationships. As Angelica moved further into her confident role, her body language shifted from a lump shouldered little girl to a more powerful young woman. Use of the "Empty Chair" gives the protagonist freedom or flexibility to express thoughts without having the fear of retaliation. This information lets the facilitator prepare the person for future face-to-face interactions.

Doubling, modeling, and role training are crucial in learning how to get unstuck from repeated negative behavioral interactions. Many protagonists are anxious when learning a new role; it is therefore important to support them as they practice it in the group session.

Before the final stages of sharing and assigning homework to the protagonist, the double, all auxiliaries, and Angelica were de-roled. This de-roling technique is an important procedure which allows members of the action group to transition from the role they were assigned to and return to their own identity. Thus, from each role assigned to auxiliaries, they share their sense of being in character, and let go of any negative emotions that may have arisen from their participation as an auxiliary. De-roling is key in returning group members back to their original role.

13.2.2 Sharing

Following the action phase, group members shared and discussed what occurred, commenting on how the situation affected them. As a rule, no advice is to be offered by group members, only sharing their thoughts from their perspective. Angelica took a huge risk, exposing her feelings and inner struggles; hearing group members share similar painful feelings and experiences led to feelings of acceptance, support, and understanding. Sharing is essential for both the protagonist and for each of the group members as they process the experience, reflect, and learn from each other. Sharing is a key component in developing and enhancing group cohesion. The sharing phase provides time for group members to discuss the events that took place in the action phase.

13.2.3 Alternative Behavior Plan (Homework)

At the end of the session, the protagonist is assigned homework to it encourages the continue the new role development explored in the session. Role development requires practice for habituation to take place and to move the protagonist to feel safe in the new role. Thus, the facilitator addresses the protagonist's core beliefs and schemas with a behavioral strategy. Homework is a critical factor in encouraging members to practice learned strategies in their own environment (Beck, 2011).

In Angelica's case, practicing the new confident role was crucial. Angelica, the group, and the facilitator collaboratively designed situations where she could rehearse this new role in her everyday life and practice for developing healthy relationships. In her case, situations were designed to focus on developing a schedule to reach out to group members to develop healthy relationships. The goal was established to create mutual respect between her and a peer and an opportunity to develop lasting friendships. To promote Angelica in this new endeavor, she was asked to choose two people in the group to spend time with before the next session. Although initially reluctant to ask anyone, she asked Riley, her double, and Jenny, who enthusiastically agreed.

Clients like Angelica find CBT components of the psychodrama helpful in becoming aware of their habitual dysfunctional thought patterns and belief systems that play an important role in mood regulation; the action component allows them to see and feel the dysfunction. The schema-focused techniques present an opportunity for a deeper level of insight and merge well with the psychodramatic framework. The schemas and core beliefs provide a deeper understanding into the etiology of clients' presenting problems and form the basis for treatment planning.

13.2.4 Drawbacks

Teens with severe social anxiety may initially find CBEGT too demanding and may opt to seek individual therapy prior to joining a group. While their experience may be trying, they will likely benefit from the group interaction and support and will, ultimately, choose to participate as a protagonist.

It is important that the facilitator? be cognizant of participants' BDI, BAI, and BHS scores to ensure a client is ready to act as the protagonist. Additionally, the director must be prepared to address any spin-off dramas that occur as a result of the protagonist's psychodrama.

The following exclusions are recommended:

(a) Individuals with self-centered personality traits and conduct disorders who display strong resistance to group work. They tend to lack spontaneity and are rigid in their portrayals of significant others; that is, they either insulate or attempt to dominate others in the group;
(b) Individuals with narcissistic, obsessive compulsive (severe), and antisocial personality disorders for whom individual therapy is more suitable; and
(c) Individuals with cluster A personality disorders and impulse control disorders have difficulty functioning in a group.

13.3 Conclusions

CBT and action techniques can be used effectively within the context of psychodrama. In our experience, teenagers, adults, college students, and clinical populations respond well to this approach and, as a result, are able to develop an awareness of their dysfunctional thought patterns and beliefs that play an important role in mood regulation. Other CBT techniques, not discussed in this chapter, such as coping cards and the advantages/disadvantages matrix, are easily integrated into CBEGT during role play or as homework. Although some resistance from group members can be expected, particularly around the Maze Worksheet being completed on time or disclosed in the group, this diminishes as trust and cohesion grow (Yalom & Leszcz, 2005). As group members recognize the usefulness of the structured CBT and action techniques, intimacy and spontaneity tend to increase, creating and supporting a safe space for sharing.

One of the most important elements of CBEGT is that it is data-based. Group members keep track of their dysfunctional thoughts and depression, anxiety, and hopelessness scores from week to week along with reviewing their GRIT scores from pre-to post testing. They can easily see changes resulting from group therapy that make the therapeutic process worthwhile. The use of CBT techniques aligned with psychodrama provides a balance between an exploration of emotionally laden situations and a more concrete, data-based, problem-solving process. CBEGT adds a new dimension to both the fields of cognitive behavior and group therapy and is built on a proven efficacious model. The integration of these methods may be beneficial for clients who have not responded to more traditional approaches.

References

Baim, C. (2007). Are you a cognitive psychodramatist? *British Journal of Psychodrama and Sociodrama, 22*(2), 23–31.

Baruch-Feldman, C. (2017). *The grit guide for teens; A workbook to help you build perseverance, self-control & a growth mindset.* Instant Help Books; New Harbinger Publications.

Beck, A. T., Rush, A. J., Shaw, B. F., & Emery, G. (1979). *Cognitive therapy of depression.* New York: The Guilford Press.

Beck, A. T. (1988). *Beck hopelessness scale.* The Psychological Corporation.

Beck, J. S. (2011). *Cognitive behavioral therapy: Basics and beyond* (2nd ed.). The Guilford Press.

Beck, A. T., & Steer, R. A. (1993). *BAI: Beck anxiety inventory manual.* The Psychological Corporation.

Beck, A. T., Steer, R. A., & Brown, G. K. (1996). *Beck depression inventory—II manual.* The Psychological Corporation.

Boury, M., Treadwell, T., & Kumar, V. K. (2001). Integrating psychodrama and cognitive therapy: An exploratory study. *International Journal of Action Methods, 54*(1), 13–25.

Fisher, J. (2007). Congenial alliance: Synergies in cognitive and psychodramatic therapies. *Psychology of Aesthetics, Creativity, and the Arts, 1*(4), 237–242.

Hamamci, Z. (2002). The effect of integrating psychodrama and cognitive behaviour therapy on reducing cognitive distortions in interpersonal relationships. *Journal of Group Psychotherapy, Psychodrama & Sociometry, 55,* 3–14.

Hamamci, Z. (2006). Integrating psychodrama and cognitive behavioural therapy to treat moderate depression. *The Arts in Psychotherapy, 33,* 199–207.

Moreno, J. L. (1934). *Who shall survive? A new approach to the problem of human interrelations.* Nervous & Mental Disease.

Shay, J. J. (2017). Contemporary models of group therapy: Where are we today? *International Journal of Group Psychotherapy, 67,* 7–12.

Treadwell, T., Dartnell, D., Travaglini, L., Staats, M., & Devinney, K. (2016). *Group therapy workbook: Integrating cognitive behavioral therapy with psychodramatic theory and practice.* Outskirts Publishing.

Treadwell, T., Kumar, V. K., & Wright, J. (2004). Enriching psychodrama via the use of cognitive behavioral therapy techniques. *Journal of Group Psychotherapy, Psychodrama, & Sociometry, 55,* 55–65.

Treadwell, T., Kumar, V. K., & Wright, J. (2008). Group cognitive behavioral model: Integrating cognitive behavioral with psychodramatic theory and techniques. In Scott Simon Fehr (Ed.) 101 Interventions In Group Therapy. New York: The Hayworth Press.

Treadwell, T., Travaglini, L., Reisch, E., & Kumar, V. K. (2011). The effectiveness of collaborative story building and telling in facilitating group cohesion in a college classroom setting. *International Journal of Group Psychotherapy, 61*(4), 502–517.

Wilson, J. (2009). An introduction to psychodrama for CBT practitioners. *Journal of the New Zealand College of Clinical Psychologists, 19*, 4–7.

Yalom, I. D., & Leszcz, M. (2005). *The theory and practice of group psychotherapy* (5th ed.). Basic Books.

Young, J. E., & Klosko, J. S. (1994). Reinventing your life. New York, NY: Plume.

Young, J. E. (1999). Cognitive therapy for personality disorders: A schema-focused approach. Sarasota, FL: Professional Resources Press.

Young, J. E., Klosko, J. S., & Weishaar, M. (2003). *Schema therapy: A practitioner's guide.* Guilford Publications.

Chapter 14
Integrating Popular Culture, Movie Clips, and Improvisation Theater Techniques in Clinical Supervision; Add a Dash of Spice to CBT Supervision

Robert D. Friedberg and Erica V. Rozmid

Keywords CBT supervision · Superhero therapy · Improv supervision · Youth CBT · Cinemedicine

14.1 Introduction

> Why do we fall? So we can learn to pick ourselves back up.
> —Batman

The process of becoming a therapist is no easy feat. During graduate school, students learn how to sit (or play!) in the room with a patient, assess their symptoms, formulate a case conceptualization and treatment plan as well as work to improve the patient's quality of life. Figuring out this process can leave clinicians feeling plagued with anxiety about making mistakes and not doing a "good enough" job. At the same time, supervisors are tasked with encouraging clinicians to remain engaged in this learning process while teaching supervisees to become effective therapists. When trainees stumble, supervisors teach them how to pick themselves up!

CBT is the gold standard treatment for various psychiatric disorders in youth (Beidas et al., 2012; Friedberg et al., 2014) yet barriers exist in implementing this treatment in clinical practice; either the treatment is not delivered with fidelity or is not delivered flexibly enough to meet the individual needs of patients (Kendall & Frank, 2018). CBT

R. D. Friedberg (✉)
Palo Alto University, Palo Alto, CA, USA
e-mail: rfriedberg@paloaltou.edu

E. V. Rozmid
Clarity CBT and DBT Center, Los Angeles, CA, USA
e-mail: hello@claritycbt.com

R. D. Friedberg, E. V. Rozmid (eds.), *Creative CBT with Youth*,
https://doi.org/10.1007/978-3-030-99669-7_14

241

supervisors teach the techniques and process of CBT while also training student clinicians the fundamental basics of conducting therapy sessions (i.e., how to validate and provide empathy, best practices to assess for risk, etc.). In traditional graduate training programs, supervisees typically work under the same supervisor for approximately a year which can be rather overwhelming, and quite impossible, for a supervisor to impart all their CBT wisdom to trainees. Integrating popular culture, humor, and improv in the therapeutic process emphasizes the flexibility and idiographic approach to CBT. Similarly, the use of videos, popular culture, and improvisational theater propels clinicians to learn fundamental therapeutic techniques that can be generalized and implemented with their own patients. In this chapter, we introduce the role of supervision and then discuss how movie clips, popular culture, superheroes, and improvisational theater are vehicles to deliver CBT supervision for children and adolescents.

14.2 CBT Supervision

Evidence-based supervision is just as critical as evidence-based treatment. If we want our patients to receive the highest quality of treatment, then supervisors should prioritize educating the next generation of clinicians to utilize evidence-based treatment. Supervision is a process of education, mentorship, monitoring progress, and consistent feedback in order to teach trainees how to become independent clinicians (Friedberg et al., 2009). Supervisors utilize powerful techniques to teach trainees how to absorb and process information as well as execute treatment interventions successfully. Just as we want our patients to be involved and engaged from the first moment they meet their therapist, we want supervisees to have a similar experience with their CBT supervisor.

14.2.1 Teaching and Training with Movie Clips and Popular Culture

During the COVID-19 pandemic, most supervisors adapted their pedagogical tools to be delivered and taught through online platforms. Virtual or hybrid models of supervision are likely to remain. Additionally, making supervision a fun and engaging process is a key to teach the next generation of clinicians who are "digital natives" since many were born into a world where fluency in technology was an imperative (Prensky, 2001). Training with movies and television/movie clips is a great augmentation to CBT supervision. Movies elucidate poignancies and illustrate the complexity of relationships; they are cost-effective, easily accessible, and you can easily find clips that highlight different cultures and diagnoses (Schulenberg, 2003). For example, in DBT groups, trainees teach 6 months of skills to adolescents and their families. While some skills are easy for trainees to read and then subsequently teach on their own, other skills require a more in-depth explanation.

Conducting a chain analysis in DBT is complex as patients gain an understanding of their emotions that lead them to engage in specific, ineffective behaviors (i.e., when Micky* felt very sad, he thought no one cared about him, withdrew to his room, and self-harmed). Working with youth who have suicidal thoughts and self-harming behaviors can feel very daunting for student clinicians. Clinicians-in-training may feel frozen as they sit in a therapy room with Micky, attempting to uphold the ethical principle of non-maleficence and personally help Micky through reducing his self-harming behaviors. Therefore, teaching the skills, like a chain analysis, is easier when trainees feel calm and more self-regulated.

Supervisors can show movie clips to demonstrate a scene of a character engaging in an ineffective behavior while the trainees practice completing the chain analysis worksheet to describe the situation, thoughts, and feelings that led to the behavior. A few examples include Hulk (Lee, 2003) when Bruce is on the floor and expresses to Talbot "you're making me angry" as he transforms into Hulk; the scene from Frozen when Elsa and Anna get into a fight and Elsa refuses to give Anna the blessing to marry; or the scene from the TV show Parenthood when Crosby throws beer onto Adam's back after denouncing him as the Best Man for his wedding. Using a popular culture figure or fictional character as the identified patient enables trainees to practice skills in real time, allowing for in vivo feedback. This approach is not only feasible and acceptable to graduate students but can also improve the learning experiences of trainees as training materials are delivered through engaging methods (Gary & Grady, 2015).

Trainees can also watch a movie and construct a case conceptualization on an identified character. For example, when viewing *Wonder (Chbosky,* 2017), a movie about a boy named Auggie with facial differences who never attended mainstream school until the fifth grade and has a difficult time making friends, students develop a cognitive behavioral case conceptualization and present the formulation in a group discussion. This process drives a richer discussion and is potentially more generalizable and engaging compared to a one-page case conceptualization. In group therapy supervision settings, videos are an adjunctive teaching method to increase learning retention outside of session, facilitate learning of an initial concept, and vary the teaching methods to increase attention and engagement.

In this digital era, supervisors and trainers are well-advised to leverage technology and alternative platforms that students find easily accessible. The days are likely over when students flock to a library and check out hard-copy books. The new generation of graduate students and clinicians connects through social media, the internet, and technology. Accordingly, educational teaching methods that actively involve students in these learning processes are necessary.

14.2.2 Integrating Superheroes and Therapy

Superheroes are not only reminiscent of favorite childhood movies, but they also demonstrate vital psychological concepts, including how they overcome fears (i.e., Batman with his fear of bats), cope with loss (i.e., when Miles Marker told

Spiderman, "No matter how many hits I take, I always find a way to come back"), and deal with grief (i.e., when Doctor Strange said "death is what gives life meaning"). Patients who identify with a superhero's struggles may feel validated and motivated to overcome these obstacles (Dantzler, 2015). Integrating the use of superheroes as a metaphor in therapy is not new (Dantzler, 2015). Primarily, current literature focuses on clinicians' anecdotes. These reports largely showcase the use of superheroes as a play therapy component in eclectic therapy or psychodynamic therapy but not cognitive behavioral therapy. However, in this chapter, we integrate superheroes in CBT training.

14.2.3 Implications for Training, Teaching, and Supervision

Supervision typically involves scaffolding and modeling using more traditional techniques. Using popular culture, superheroes, and humor in supervision provides supervisees with an environment that welcomes fun and embracing making mistakes as a learning tool. Supervision in the early process focuses on skill development and case content (Schwitzer et al., 2005). Barriers to effective case conceptualization include gathering enough critical information during the intake process. When trainees are tasked with forming diagnostic treatment plans, they may forget to ask important questions that would be useful in generating an accurate case conceptualization. However, utilizing popular culture mitigates these barriers and allows the supervisees to focus on the main task of improving their case conceptualization skills. Because superheroes and fictional characters are available throughout mainstream media, trainees can easily relate to the character development; superheroes embody superhuman traits, fight for the good of humanity, and usually have a pretty good sidekick. Trainees are empowered to freely explore their own experiences, attitudes, and beliefs about conceptualizing a character's story rather than placing undue focus on gathering pertinent information. Below is a case example that can propel students' learning of these foundational therapeutic skills:

Shawna* is a graduate-level clinician who is learning DBT and starting to conduct sessions with older children and younger adolescents. Shawna read through the DBT manuals developed by Marsha Linehan and wanted to improve her own case conceptualization of her patients who engage in impulsive behaviors. She was assigned homework to watch Frozen and utilize the biosocial theory to develop a conceptualization of Elsa and search for themes of extreme emotional states. Shawna presented her findings from the movie and suggested that biologically, Elsa had a higher sensitivity to emotions (i.e., feeling emotions more strongly than her sister, Anna) and a higher biological reactivity (i.e., as evidenced by the way her body responds to emotions where she freezes the world around her). She then formulated that Elsa had a history of invalidation as seen when Elsa accidentally hurt Anna and was subsequently told by her parents that her powers were harmful. The transaction between Elsa's biological emotional tendencies and social invalidation led her to feel more emotionally dysregulated. For example, the more Elsa *experienced intense emotions, the more she froze the world around her, which led to others rejecting her. According to Shawna, Elsa either felt strongly and was rejected or she attempted to hide her own emotions which further pushed people away. Shawna then describes how the song lyrics in the movie clearly highlighted Elsa's emotional extremes (i.e., Let it Go vs. Conceal Don't Feel). These emotional extremes reflect the emotional "states of mind" in DBT as emotion mind (feeling very strong emotions) vs. reasonable mind (only logic, no emotions)* (see Fig. 14.1).

Utilizing film as a training tool is documented in the literature. Presenting the biopsychosocial model to medical residents was studied under the context of "cinemeducation" or "cinemedicine," a tool to integrate teaching medicine with film (Alexander, 2002; Kadivar et al., 2018). In one study, medical residents were tasked with watching films that highlighted psychosocial factors among common medical challenges (Kadivar et al., 2018). They ranked their level of agreement on items relating to cinemedicine on a Likert scale of 1–4 (*strongly agree to strongly disagree*). Results indicated that 84% of the students preferred the movie over the traditional lecture, while 89% of the residents agreed or strongly agreed that watching these medical and mental health related films were useful (Kadivar et al., 2018). Instructors and supervisors can integrate the films into the course material. After watching a film for educational purposes, the instructors should debrief and assess whether the trainees understood the key learning concepts (Schulenberg, 2003; Berk and Trieber 2009; Baños & Bosch, 2015).

Analyzing characters from popular fiction and entertainment media assists trainees in the development of assessment, diagnosis, conceptualization, and treatment planning (Schwitzer et al., 2005). Baños and Bosch (2015) noted that Mary Shelley's (1818) **Frankenstein** is an appropriate film to highlight the ethical principles of

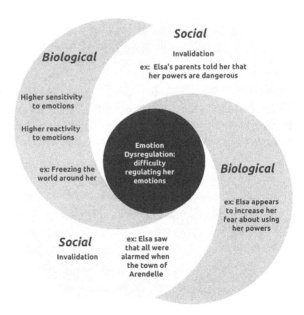

Fig. 14.1 Biosocial Theory of Elsa from the movie Frozen

biomedical research, while Marguerite Johnson, a character from Maya Angelou's (1979) *I Know Why the Caged Birds Sing* was used to highlight depression (Schwitzer et al., 2005). Supervisors and clinical instructors can curate films to highlight characters from different cultural backgrounds. Films that highlight characters from specific cultural backgrounds and diagnoses lends itself well to culturally enhanced CBT supervision. For example, the Disney movie *Moana* (Musker & Clements 2016) tells the story about a girl from Polynesia who sets out on a daring adventure to save her community by restoring the islands' vegetation and fish resources. This movie made cultural references to the beliefs of Polynesians (i.e., Demigods as heroes, explanation of Polynesian mythology) and included Polynesian music throughout. The emphasis on family and generational bonds highlighted the uniqueness of Moana's culture. As trainees watch Moana, they can consider the various life lessons taught within the movie's cultural context (i.e., emphasis on family and generational bonds, overcoming fears, and embracing differences). Throughout this process, trainees will learn to flexibly conceptualize youth patients from different backgrounds within a CBT framework.

Cinemedicine also encourages enhanced feedback from colleagues to improve peer consultation skills when used in a group setting. For example, if a trainee is responsible for relaying the patient's information, factual information is inherently lost like in the game of telephone. Instead, identifying the central patient within a film or book, peers have access to the same information and can offer each other feedback (Schwitzer et al., 2005). There are a variety of ways to include popular culture and film in the trainee process. Groups work together to generate a group case conceptualization which can be conducted during grand rounds or other clinical meetings. It is recommended to practice group consultations with a wide array of practitioners at varying levels of experience to help students refine their own critical thinking skills. Specifically, case conceptualization should focus on fictional characters to diminish concerns of over pathologizing a celebrity which can lead to uncomfortable feelings about diagnosing and treating a person who is not in treatment. Additionally, it is important to note that American mainstream media often lacks appropriate cultural metaphors and perpetuates "popular" characters that maintain negative and inaccurate perceptions for different subgroups. Consequently, an appreciation of the value of diversity is frequently attenuated (Cerny et al., 2014). Box 14.1 contains a list of recommendations for CBT supervisors to consider when incorporating multimedia and popular culture into supervision.

Box 14.1 Recommendations for CBT Supervisors to Consider when Incorporating Multimedia and Popular Culture into Supervision
Assign media clips and films as a way for students to practice skills and formulating case conceptualizations
- If media clips are assigned as independent homework or shown during class, debrief as a group to ensure students learned the key concepts.
- Supervisors should review all content prior to assigning. It's important to demonstrate culturally appropriate examples and diverse characters.

14.3 Improvisational Theater and Supervising Trainees in CBT with Youth

You know how sports teach kids teamwork and how to be strong and brave and confident? Improv was my sport. I learned how to not waffle and how to hold a conversation, how to take risks and actually be excited to fail.—Emma Stone

As supervisors, our goal is to train clinicians who are proficient, confident in their abilities, tolerant of discomfort, accepting of uncertainty, ethical, willing to take reasonable risks, embracing of their imperfections, interpersonally graceful, and engaging in their work with patients. Incorporating improvisational (improv) theater exercises into conventional CBT supervision may foster these qualities in supervisees. In this section, we define improv theater training, illustrate its application to clinical training, demonstrate the potential fit with CBT supervision, and offer some handy guidelines for CBT supervisors willing to add a dash of improv to spice up their supervision recipes.

14.3.1 Improvisational Theater Training

Improv theater is an art form that dates to the Italian Renaissance period and derives from *commedia dell arte* (Bedore, 2004; Sheesley et al., 2016; Strohbehn et al., 2020). The development of modern improv in the United States is credited to Viola Spolin (1939) who used the methods to enhance immigrant children's creativity and self-expression (Felsman et al., 2020; Sheesely et al., 2016). In general, improv theater performances are unscripted, spontaneous narratives (Gao et al., 2019). While fun and laughter often occur during improv exercises, comedy is not the goal. Rather, honesty, flexibility, empathy, tolerance of uncertainty, divergent thinking, and spontaneity are emphasized (Watson, 2011). Finally, training in this form of theater is done experientially (Bayne & Jangha, 2016)

There are several key elements in improv training (Huffaker & West, 2005; Strohbehn et al., 2020). The first fundamental practice is referred to as accepting offers from others. This is often referred to as adopting a *"Yes and…"* perspective. *Yes and* involves incorporating others' ideas and adding to them. This stance serves to maintain interpersonal flow between individuals, attenuate biases, and promote collaboration. Remaining present or embracing a here and now focus is another crucial imperative. Staying present allows greater tolerance of uncertainty and enables risk-taking. Active authentic listening is an obvious essential precept. Finally, openness and willingness to change are required. Consequently, teaching improv to health care providers seems a natural fit.

Training health care providers in improv is an emerging form of education, training, and supervision (Fessell et al., 2020; Gao et al., 2019; Harendza, 2020). Eminent medical institutions such as Northwestern University, Boston University, University of Washington, Johns Hopkins University, Indiana University, and University of

Michigan are including improv classes in their curriculum (Gao et al., 2019; Rossing & Hoffman-Longtin, 2018). Many counseling programs also integrate improv exercises in their coursework (Bayne & Jangha, 2016 Bermant, 2013; Harendza, 2020; Hoffman et al., 2008; Lawrence & Coaston, 2017, Romanelli et al., 2017; Romanelli & Berger, 2018). Although few clinical psychology training programs are experimenting with improv, we nonetheless endorse incorporating improv in psychotherapy classes and supervision for reasons articulated below. Therefore, the following sections delineate the relevance of improv to clinical work and offer several practical guidelines for use in supervision/training.

14.3.1.1 Application to Clinical Work

Improv is readily applied to clinical work. Various authors contend improv fosters elemental psychotherapeutic skills ranging from proficiencies in basic micro-counseling skills to more advanced techniques and processes. Improv training promotes rudimentary competencies such as listening and empathic responding (Bayne & Jangha, 2016; Gao et al., 2019; Lawrence & Coaston, 2017; Misch, 2016; Watson, 2011). Many diversity trainers also employ improv techniques with their trainees (Boal, 1979, 2002). Moreover, this work could lay the foundation for better cultural alertness and responsiveness by increasing attention to stereotyping, attenuating implicit biases, and managing micro-aggressions (Hobson et al., 2019). In sum, skills developed via improv training may add to the "secret sauce" that seems to characterize successful treatment relationships.

The level of empathy produced by this theatrical training facilitates better interviewing and case conceptualization (Bayne & Jangha, 2016; Schochet et al., 2013). For example, Schochet and colleagues explained, "The medical interview has notoriously been extremely difficult for students to learn and to move beyond competency toward excellence. It requires managing multiple cognitive skills such as question asking, retaining detailed information and integrating the patient's story with medical knowledge and clinical reasoning. When building a patient's history, medical students need to be able to improvise (p. 123)". In this way, a rich understanding of patients' stories is potentially achieved.

CBT is a phenomenological approach and works to accelerate change in "here and now" moments during treatment sessions. Therefore, the use of immediacy in session is demanded. Training in improv advances skills in optimizing powerful psychotherapeutic moments (Farley, 2017; Gao et al., 2019; Romanelli & Berger, 2018). In short, improv enables supervisees to be "fully present in the face of uncertainty and anxiety (Fessell et al., 2020, p. 87)."

Doing psychotherapy is hard work and frequently occurs in a high stress environment. Periodically feeling uncertain and doubting one's abilities is common to both beginning and experienced clinicians. Nonetheless, in highly stressful and ambiguous situations, good clinical reasoning, adaptive problem solving, and flexible thinking are especially important. Fortunately, improv training catalyzes these skills (Bermant, 2013; Farley, 2017: Fessell et al., 2020; Gladwell, 2005; Lawrence &

Coaston, 2017; Misch, 2016; Schochet et al., 2013 Watson, 2011). Gladwell (2005) argued, "how good people's decisions are under the fast moving high stress conditions of rapid cognitions is a function of training and rehearsal (p. 114)." An optimistic outlook, tolerance for uncertainty, creative problem solving, and divergent thinking skills are spurred by improv (Felsman et al., 2020; Hoffman-Longtin et al., 2017; Huffaker & West, 2005; Lewis & Lovatt, 2013). Improv training helps students accept uncertainty as well as catalyze reasoned risk-taking, creativity, and poise under pressure (Misch, 2016).

The route to clinical wisdom and competence is filled with potholes. Supervision then involves giving and receiving feedback. As Strohbehn et al. (2020) stated supervisors and trainees alike are well-advised to accept that every learning path is bumpy and marked by mistakes, poor application of skills, and misunderstanding. Many supervisees try to hide their mistakes due to their perfectionistic tendencies and fear of negative evaluation. However, improv increases acceptance of one's imperfections (Misch, 2016; Watson, 2011).

Good supervision facilitates improving competence via experiential learning and directed feedback. Watson (2011) noted that improv training helps learners accept and incorporate corrective feedback. Tolerating uncertainty, doubt, and making mistakes build professional development, competence, and clinical wisdom. Lewis (2016) argued that the "use of moments of uncertainty to teach the students that the process of finding out the correct answer (diagnosis, medication, formulation) is the most important task in psychiatry (p. 954)." It turns out Emma Stone was exactly right!

Due to improv training's powerful pedagogical characteristics, it is recommended in a number of medical, psychological, and counseling training settings (Bayne & Jangha, 2016 Bermant, 2013; Harendza, 2020; Hoffman et al., 2008; Lawrence & Coaston, 2017; Misch, 2016; Romanelli et al., 2017; Romanelli & Berger, 2018; Watson, 2011; Watson & Fu, 2016). Improv training improved medical students' listening, communication skills, and confidence (Hoffman et al., 2008). Schochet et al. (2013) studied the effectiveness of using improv to train medical students in clinical interviewing. Their course content included improv games that focused on mindfulness, active listening, comprehension, agreement, acceptance, thoughtful responding, and clear articulation. They found that 81% of the students considered this experience to be "tremendous." Eighty-five percent of the class noted that improv was very relevant to their clinical practice. Schochet et al. concluded, "This creative experiential process allowed students to both practice and gain confidence in their interpersonal skills thereby giving them insight to draw upon when facing unique iterative moments in clinical encounters (p. 122)."

Fesell and collaborators evaluated the impact of improv workshops on medical students' clinical competencies. Their results showed that 90% of the attendees reported the workshops improved their insight and team work skills. Overall, 90% of the medical students gave training favorable ratings. Misch (2016) concluded, "So for physicians, improv training is an opportunity to enhance typically underdeveloped right brain emotional life to feel, read, interpret, and express emotions (p. 346)."

Kaplan-Liss et al. (2018) reported on their efforts regarding teaching an elective communication skills class for medical students. Working in collaboration with the Alda Center for Communicating Science at Stony Brook University, they designed a course employing innovative methods. In particular, the Alda Method emphasizes training in *Improvisation for Scientists* and *Distilling Your Message*. The *Improvisation for Scientists* module focuses on explaining medical/scientific concepts in an understandable, accessible, and jargon-free manner, tolerating uncertainty, and building empathic listening skills. The *Distilling Your Message* pod teaches students to communicate their ideas through engaging analogies and storytelling. The course received very favorable evaluations with 96% of students endorsing the very highest ratings for the class. Students reported improving their understanding of patients' lived experiences, enhancing their listening skills, and increasing their comprehension of medical knowledge.

Integrating improv theater courses into psychotherapy training curricula appears promising (Romanelli et al., 2017; Romanelli & Berger, 2018). Romanelli and colleagues (2018) claimed "psychotherapy can be seen as a kind of improvisational theater where therapists and clients co-create the reality of every moment (p.26)." This "here and now" focus is quite congenial with contemporary views of CBT with youth (Friedberg & McClure, 2015; Gosch et al., 2006). More specifically, when discussing therapeutic process issues in CBT with children and adolescents, Friedberg and Gorman (2007) argued "psychotherapeutic moments are charged with the urgency and genuineness of emotional experience in present tense and real time (p.189)." The use of improv theater games in treatment seems to enliven the clinical encounter, general excitement in sessions, facilitate the exploration of heretofore neglected possibilities, and model appropriate social risk-taking (Romanelli et al., 2017; Romanelli & Berger, 2018). Consequently, incorporating these methods in CBT supervision and training is well-advised.

Romanelli et al. (2017) designed and studied a semester long course combining training in improv methods with more psychodynamically oriented psychotherapy. Students' comments revealed very favorable course evaluations. In particular, they reported their clinical intuition, spontaneity, flexibility, playfulness, presence, use of immediacy, and confidence increased as a result of the seminar. Romanelli and his co-authors concluded the course propelled students' skills in being "mindfully aware," "present in the moment," and "openly animated." It is noteworthy that many of these processes are also explicitly rated on the Cognitive Therapy Rating Scale for Children and Adolescents (CTRS-CA; Friedberg, 2014) which is used to evaluate clinicians' competencies in conducting CBT with youth (Friedberg, 2019; Gudino, 2020; Johnson & Phythian, 2020).

Several authors have also integrated improv training into a traditional counseling courses (Bayne & Jangha, 2016; Farley, 2017; Lawrence & Coaston, 2017). Their course content included common improv exercises that were selected due to their focus on emotional awareness, tolerating uncertainty, and embracing spontaneity. Lawrence and Coaston (2017) concluded that training in improv may propel counselors' collaborative abilities and capacity to engage patients.

In sum, improv theater exercises foster multiple clinical skills ranging from basic micro-competencies to more advanced proficiencies. Empathy, critical reasoning, cultural alertness, use of immediacy in session, and enhanced therapeutic presence are some of the practices fueled by this training. Good decision-making while under pressure, tolerance of uncertainty, and increased emotional awareness are also strengthened. Thus, incorporating improvisational theater games into supervision of CBT with youth is a meritorious notion.

14.3.2   CBT Supervision and Improv: Arranged Marriage or Perfect Union?

Fusing CBT principles and practices with improv methods represents a perfect union. The two paradigms share many features. The common focus on collaboration, authenticity, presence, and experiential learning empower integration. CBT supervision with youth is facilitated by supervisors who are authentic, supportive, collaborative, and foster robust learning environments (Corrie & Lane, 2015; Friedberg, 2018; Gordon, 2012; Newman & Kaplan, 2016). Collaboration and guided discovery are central aspects of CBT supervision (Friedberg, 2018; Newman & Kaplan, 2016). Improv training aligns precisely with these conventions. Improvisation techniques change the communication landscape between supervisors and supervisees. Rossing and Hoffman-Longtin (2018) claimed that improv disables the power imbalance between teacher and learner. More specifically, improv shifts the pedagogical focus from delivering information "to" trainees to constructing an educational partnership with them.

Friedberg (2015) argued CBT with youth is not the same as treating mini-adults. Playfulness, transparency, and fun are essential when working with young patients. In our experience, beginning child clinicians are disinclined to appear whimsical or even somewhat goofy in session. By using improv in training, trainees can liberate themselves from the chains of unnecessary orthodoxy. Boal (2002) aptly remarked, "If everyone is ridiculous, then no one is (p. 92)."

Improv exercises and practices can be seamlessly assimilated into traditional supervisory methods. CBT supervisors routinely ask trainees to summarize supervisory sessions and elicit feedback from them. Improv training offers a unique and compelling take on this practice. Rossing and Hoffman-Longtin (2018) recommended asking three basic summary questions to help students acquire and apply skills learned in improv (e.g., What? So What? and Now What?). The "what" questions prompts recall of the session. "So what" calls on students to discern the skill's relevance. Finally, "Now What" encourages learners to act their new found knowledge and skills.

Socratic dialogue is a staple in both CBT supervision and training in improvisation. Strohbehn et al. (2020) asserted that "Socratic or open-ended questioning is especially useful in promoting critical reasoning and represents one manifestation of improv pedagogy (p. 390)." Socratic dialogues enable learners to interrogate their own belief systems and create new perspectives. The ability to see clinical phenomena from multiple angles is essential for professional development.

Both CBT with young patients and improv foster presence a here and now focus and experiential learning. Experiential learning nourishes increased self-efficacy, approach behavior, and believable cognitive reappraisals (Kendall et al., 2006) Like the Elvis Pressley (1968) classic song, youth prefer "a little more action, a little less conversation" in CBT (Friedberg, 2015). Incorporating improvisational methods in supervision teaches supervisees to maximize pivotal moments in therapy and emphasize action.

14.3.3   Tips for CBT Supervisors

Using improvisational theater exercises to train clinical students calls for numerous supervisory skills (Bayne & Jangha, 2016; Hoffman-Longtin et al., 2017; Misch, 2016). Supervisors are encouraged to be enthusiastic and energetic when leading games (Bayne & Jangha, 2016). Further, providing a rationale to trainees for experimenting with exercises during supervision is recommended. Supervisees need to know how improv is relevant to their clinical work and professional development. Hoffman-Longtin and colleagues urged supervisors to explicitly communicate to their mentees that improv games are designed to facilitate a specific mindset or perspective which embraces ambiguity and spontaneity.

Remembering the importance of "here and now" moments in supervision and training is crucial. When supervising psychiatric residents, Lewis (2016) disclosed, "I try to remind myself that each moment on clinical service may be the important moment that changes a student's perspective (p. 953)." Potentiating the power of here and now moments breathes life into clinical supervision. Trainees are far more likely to apply their acquired skills and knowledge when they see them as relevant and memorable. Further, if supervisees have played the game themselves in supervision, they are more likely to use the exercise with their patients.

Hoffman-Longtin et al. (2017) alerted supervisors to expect trainee avoidance. Practicum students, interns, and post-docs may be reluctant to take risks posed in improv exercises due to pressure to prove their worth and desire to belong (Rossing & Hoffman-Longtin, 2018). Rossing and Hoffman-Longtin believed that professional staff who are overly invested in prestige will approach improv timorously.

Graduated tasks will enable most trainees to scaffold their skills and may mitigate their apprehensiveness. Indeed, graduating these tasks is similar to delivering exposure. The key is to coach supervisees to lean into discomfort with unfamiliar exercises. Additionally, just as Newman (1994) urged therapists to gently persist (p. 94) when patients avoid so too are supervisors to do the same with avoidant trainees. For instance, a supervisor could invite the trainee to explore their reluctance by saying, "Yes this game makes you feel a bit uneasy and how *willing on scale of 1–10* are you to give it a try?" Then the supervisor may continue by saying,

"What makes you a __, right now?" and "What do you expect to happen?" This type of Socratic dialogue allows the trainer to set up the game as an experiment.

Like exposure, debriefing improvisational theater exercises is crucial. It is recommended that supervisors help their mentees make sense of their experiences. Debriefing catalyzes the learning by molding conceptual anchors. Questions such as "What is the take-away message from this game?" "What was useful/not useful about this exercise?" "Based on your experiences in the game, what things can you use in your work with young patients?" and "When you got stuck during the game, what did it teach you about doing CBT?" Box 14.2 contains some additional helpful Socratic debriefing questions culled from the literature.

Box 14.2 Useful Debriefing Questions
Lawrence and Coaston (2017)
    What was this experience like for you?
    What did you notice in the pattern of your responses
    How difficult was this? How easy?
    What risks did you take? Avoid?
    What did this teach you about ____?
Bayne and Jangha
    What was it like for you to be in the here and now?
    What is the value of this game?

Finally, fostering spontaneity, flexibility, tolerance of imperfection, a sense of universality, and FUN are the goals when integrating improvisational theater games into supervision for CBT with youth. Supervisors should welcome trainees' discomfort and errors. Everyone gets stuck when doing both CBT and improv. Creating an atmosphere where stuck points are abided, reasoned risk-taking is championed, and sharing imperfections are applauded is vital. Remaining mindful of these tips can avoid improv becoming "um-prov" where supervisees are hesitant and halting participants who pause and say "Um" (Box 14.3).

Box 14.3 Recommendations for Supervisors
Be enthusiastic and energetic
    Specifically link improv procedures to clinical skill development
    Explain that improv is designed to train tolerance for ambiguity and appreciation of spontaneity
    Emphasize the importance of the here and now
    Expect and process avoidance
    Employ graduated tasks

14.3.4   Improv in CBT: Specific Examples

CBT supervisors may need a stockpile of improv exercises. There are a number of excellent texts which contain many improv exercises (Bedore, 2004; Boal, 2002; Rooyackers, 1998) Additionally, various internet sources list valuable improv exercises (www.medicalimprov.org). Finally, Table 14.1 presents a selection of games culled from several scholarly articles and texts.

I (RDF) began to integrate improv in supervision while training child psychiatry fellows and post-doctoral psychologists in the Cognitive Behavioral Therapy Clinic for Children and Adolescents at Penn State Milton Hershey Medical Center. Initially, the fellows and post-docs were initially reluctant and skeptical. Their many work demands and time constraints made them wary of "wasting" any time on irrelevant activities. However, by giving them a clear rationale, setting up a comfortable environment, and providing some coaxing, their willingness increased. Subsequently with greater exposure, practice, and laughter, they increasingly embraced the games. In the paragraphs below, I describe a few games we played in supervision.

One word story (Bedore, 2004) is a group game where players work as a team to construct a story one word at a time. The group creates a story by members adding one word each when it is their turn. This game teaches supervisees the value of listening, cooperation, reciprocity, and cognitive flexibility.

Famous Movie Lines is a game that involves a player reciting familiar lines from popular movies (e.g. "Say hello to my little friend," "You had me at hello," "Mama, what's my destiny?"). However, the player must express an emotion not readily associated with the particular line. The lines are written on slips and placed in a box. Various emotion cards (e.g., mad, sad, ashamed, excited, fearful, etc.) are put in another box. Students then pick one line and an accompanying emotion. For instance, a student may have to say "You had me at hello" in an angry agitated tone. Often, this exercise is a nice ice-breaker and introduction to silliness.

Many beginning and even advanced behavioral health clinicians struggle to explain diagnoses, case conceptualizations, assessment findings, and the course of

Table 14.1 Improvisational exercises and their foci

Game	Focus
Sound Ball (Farley, 2017)	Warm-up
Bippity-Boppity Bop (Farley, 2017)	Warm-up
Hoy (Farley, 2017)	Warm-up
What are you doing (Farley, 2017)	Spontaneity
One word proverb (Farley, 2017)	Spontaneity
Group Think (Lawrence & Coaston, 2017; McCloud, 2010)	Spontaneity
Two Minute Drill (Farley, 2017)	Risk-taking
Gibberish (Farley, 2017)	Embracing change and uncertainty
Sound and Motion Circle (Boal, 2002; Bodenhorn & Starkey, 2005	Empathy

treatment to patients and their families in understandable ways. Often, their stilted language is flooded with jargon. Consequently, treatment engagement and adherence suffers. Learning to talk to patients so they understand is a pivotal skill.

Time traveler (Fessell et al., 2020) is an improvisational game that promotes clear and cogent communication. In this exercise, players take turn explaining a new invention (cell phones, the internet, vaccines, cable TV, self-driving cars, etc.) to a time traveler from the fourteenth century. Trainees need to bring down these technological and scientific advances into simple, jargon free explanations so the traveler from the distant past understands. Supervisors give the players corrective feedback when the players fall back on professional patter or arcane shop talk.

The Blind Car (Boal, 2002) is a favorite game I (RDF) used in supervision as well as in family treatment (Friedberg, 2006). The exercise involves one blindfolded trainee being "driven" in a room by a second team member. The car is steered by the driver applying gentle pressure to the shoulders of the member playing the car (e.g., pressure to right shoulder turns right, press on both shoulders go forward, etc.). Obstacles can be set up in the room so the car has to turn, go in reverse, and so on. Not surprisingly, this game enhances trainees' capacity to trust, give up control, and tolerate uncertainty.

Improv exercises are welcome additions to training large groups of practicing professionals. They facilitate more active participation and fun in long training sessions. Additionally, some of the games are also used in CBT with youth so students get the opportunity to experience the exercise for themselves. A favorite group training game is *Group Photo* (Rooyackers, 1998) and it is also applicable to treating socially anxious young patients (Friedberg & McClure, 2015). *Group Photo* involves several group members working together to pose for a picture doing a common activity (e.g., going to an amusement park, attending a surprise birthday party, standing in a long line waiting the bathroom, etc.). Players not involved in the photo try to guess the scene.

14.4 Conclusion

I have one super power. I never give up.—Batman

Like Batman, supervisors want their trainees to never give up learning and developing. Supervisors are challenged to come up with new ways to instruct and inspire their mentees. Getting stuck in the same sometimes tired routines is a common problem. In this chapter, we presented the idea of integrating movies, popular culture, and improvisational theater techniques into supervision for conducting CBT for youth. Ideally, these strategies may foster supervisors and trainees achieving their superpowers.

*All case examples have been sanitized.

References

Alexander, M. (2002). The doctor: A seminal video for cinemeducation. *Family Medicine, 34*(2), 92–94.

Angelou, M. (1979). I know why the caged bird sings. New York: Random House.

Baños, J. E., & Bosch, F. (2015). Using feature films as a teaching tool in medical schools. *Medical Education, 16*(4), 206–211.

Bayne, H. B., & Jangha, A. (2016). Utilizing improvisation to teach empathy skills in counselor education. *Counselor Education and Supervision, 55*, 250–262.

Bedore, B. (2004). *101 Improv games for children and adolescents*. Hunter House.

Beidas, R. S., Mychailyszyn, M. P., Edmunds, J. M., Khanna, M. S., Downey, M.M., & Kendall, P.C. (2012). Training school mental health providers to deliver cognitive-behavior cognitive-behavioral therapy. *School Mental Health, 4*, 197–206.

Berk, R. A., & Trieber, R. H. (2009). Whose classroom is it anyway? Improvisation as a teaching tool. *Journal of Excellence in College Teaching, 20*, 29–60.

Bermant, G. (2013). Working with (out) a net: Improvisation theatre and enhanced well-being. *Frontiers in Psychology, 4*, 929. https://doi.org/10.3389/fpsyg.2013.00929/

Boal, A. (1979). *Theatre of the oppressed*. Theatre Communication Group.

Boal, A. (2002). *Games for actors and non-actors* (2nd ed.). Routledge.

Bodenhorn, N., & Starkey, D. (2005). Beyond role-playing: Increasing counselor empathy through theatre exercises. *Journal of Creativity in Mental Health, 1*, 17–27.

Cerny, C., Friedman, S., & Smith, D. (2014). Television's "Crazy Lady" trope: Female psychopathic traits, teaching, and influence of popular culture. *Academic Psychiatry, 38*(2), 233–241.

Corrie, S., & Lane, D. A. (2015). *CBT supervision*. Sage.

Chbosky, S. [Director]. (2017). Wonder [motion picture]. United States: Lionsgate.

Dantzler, J. Z. (2015). How the marvel cinematic universe represents our quality world: An integration of reality therapy/choice theory and cinema therapy. *Journal of Creativity in Mental Health, 10*(4), 471–487.

Farley, N. (2017). Improvisation as a meta-counseling skill. *Journal of Creativity in Mental Health, 1*, 115–128.

Felsman, P., Gunawardena, S., & Seifert, C. M. (2020). Improv experience promotes divergent thinking, uncertainty tolerance, and affective well-being. *Thinking Skills and Creativity, 35*, 100632.

Fessell, D., McKean, E., Wagenschutz, H., Cole, M., Santen, S. A., Cermak, R., ... Alda, A. (2020). Medical improvisation for all medical students:3 year experience. *Medical Science Educator, 30*, 87–90.

Friedberg, R. D. (2006). A cognitive-behavioral approach to family therapy. *Journal of Contemporary Psychotherapy, 36*, 159–165.

Friedberg, R. D. (2014). *Cognitive therapy rating scale for children and adolescents (CTRS-CA) manual*. Center for the Study and Treatment of Anxious Youth.

Friedberg, R. D. (2015). Where's the beef: Concrete elements in supervision with CBT with youth. *Journal of the American Academy of Child and Adolescent Psychiatry, 54*, 527–553.

Friedberg, R. D. (2018). Best practices in supervising cognitive behavioral therapy with youth. *World Journal of Clinical Pediatrics, 7*, 1–8.

Friedberg, R. D. (2019, October). *Measuring up: First-session competency ratings in the cognitive therapy rating scale for children and adolescents (CTRS-CA) for eight practicing clinicians*. Poster presentation delivered at the annual meeting of the American Academy of Child and Adolescent Psychiatry, Chicago, Ill.

Friedberg, R. D., & Gorman, A. A. (2007). Integrating psychotherapeutic processes with cognitive behavioral procedures. *Journal of Contemporary Psychotherapy, 37*, 185–193.

Friedberg, R. D., Gorman, A. A., & Beidel, D. C. (2009). Training psychologists for cognitive-behavioral therapy in the raw world: A rubric for supervisors. *Behavior Modification, 33*(1), 104–123.

Friedberg, R. D., Hoyman, L. C., Behar, S., Tabbarah, S., Pacholec, N. M., Keller, M., & Thordarson, M. A. (2014). We've come a long way, baby!: Evolution and revolution in CBT with youth. *Journal of Rational-Emotive & Cognitive-Behavior Therapy, 32*(1), 4–14.

Friedberg, R. D., & McClure, J. M. (2015). Clinical practice of cognitive therapy with children and adolescents: The nuts and bolts (2nd. Edition). New York: Guilford.

Gao, L., Peranson, J., Nyhof-Young, J., Kapoor, E., & Rezmovitz, J. (2019). The role of "improve" in health professional learning: A scoping review. *Medical Teacher.* https://doi.org/10.108 0/0142159x.2018.1505033

Gary, J. M., & Grady, J. P. (2015). Integrating television media into group counseling course work. *The Journal of Counselor Preparation and Supervision, 7*(2), 3.

Gladwell, M. (2005). Blink: The power of thinking without thinking. New York; Back Bay Books.

Gordon, P. K. (2012). Ten steps to cognitive behavioural supervision. *The Cognitive Behaviour Therapist, 5*(4), 71–82.

Gudino, O. G. (2020, October) *Improving child and adolescent CBT competence using competency-based supervision.* Clinical panel presentation delivered as a part of R.D. Friedberg (Chair), Training others to deliver a proper dose of CBT to youth, 2020 presented at the annual meeting of the American Academy of Child and Adolescent Psychiatry, San Francisco, CA.

Gosch, E. A., Flannery-Schroeder, E., Mauro, C. F., & Compton, S. N. (2006). Principles of cognitive behavioral therapy for anxiety disorders in children. *Journal of Cognitive Psychotherapy, 20*, 247–262.

Harendza, S. (2020). Improvisation—a new strategy in medical education. *Journal for Medical Education, 37*(4), Doc44. https://doi.org/10.3205/zma001337

Hobson, W. L., Hoffman-Longtin, K., Loue, S., Love, L., Liu, H., Power, C. M., & Pollart, S. M. (2019). Active learning on center stage: Theater as a tool for medical education. *MedEdPORTAL, 15*, 10801. https://doi.org/10.15766/medp_2374-8265/10801

Hoffman, A., Utley, B., & Ciccarone, D. (2008). Improving medical student communication skills through improv theatre. *Medical Education, 42*, 513–543.

Hoffman-Longtin, K., Rossing, J., & Weinstein, E. (2017). Twelve tips for using applied improvisation in medical education. *Medical Teacher, 40*, 351–356.

Huffaker, J. S., & West, E. (2005). Enhancing learning in the business classroom: An adventure with improv theater techniques. *Journal of Management Education, 29*, 852–869.

Johnson, L., & Phythian, K. (2020, October). *Implementation of a competency-based supervision model using a standardized measure (CTRS-CA) of clinician practice.* Clinical panel presentation delivered as a part of R.D. Friedberg (Chair), Training others to deliver a proper dose of CBT to youth, 2020 presented at the annual meeting of the American Academy of Child and Adolescent Psychiatry, San Francisco, CA.

Kadivar, M., Mafinejad, M. K., Bazzaz, J. T., Mirzazadeh, A., & Jannat, Z. (2018). Cinemedicine: Using movies to improve students' understanding of psychosocial aspects of medicine. *Annals of Medicine and Surgery, 28*, 23–27.

Kaplan-Liss, E., Lantz-Gefroh, V., Bass, E., Killebrew, D., Ponzio, N., Savi, C., & O'Connell, C. (2018). Teaching medical students to communicate with empathy and clarity using improvisation. *Academic Medicine, 93*, 440–443.

Kendall, P. C., & Frank, H. E. (2018). Implementing evidence-based treatment protocols: Flexibility within fidelity. *Clinical Psychology: Science and Practice, 25*(4), e12271.

Kendall, P. C., Robin, J. A., Hedtke, K. A., Suveg, C., Flannery-Schroeder, E., & Gosch, E. (2006). Considering CBT with anxious youth? Think exposures. *Cognitive and Behavioral Practice, 12*, 136–148.

Lawrence, C., & Coaston, S. C. (2017). Whose line is it anyway? Using improvisational exercises to spark counselor development. *Journal of Creativity in Mental Health, 12*, 513–528.

Lewis, A. (2016). How the principles of improvisational theater can set our educational potential free. *Academic Psychiatry, 40*, 953–955.

Lewis, C., & Lovatt, P. J. (2013). Breaking away from set patterns of thinking: Improvisation and divergent thinking. *Thinking Skills and Creativity, 9*, 46–58.

Lee, A. [Director] (2003). Hulk [motion picture] United States: Universal Pictures and Marvel Studios.

McCloud, H. (2010). Free association. Retrieved from http://learnimprov.com/?p=132

Misch, D. A. (2016). I feel witty oh so witty. *JAMA, 315*, 345–346.

Musker, J., & Clements, R. [Directors]. (2016). Moana [motion picture]. United States: Walt Disney Pictures.

Newman, C. (1994). Understanding client resistance: Methods of enhancing resistance to change. *Cognitive and Behavioral Practice, 1*, 47–70.

Newman, C., & Kaplan, D. A. (2016). *Supervision essentials for cognitive-behavioral therapy.* American Psychological Association.

Prensky, M. (2001). Digital natives, digital immigrants part 2: Do they really think differently? *On the Horizon, 9*(6), 1–6.

Romanelli, A., & Berger, A. (2018). The ninja therapist: Theater improvisation tools for the (daring) clinician. *The Arts in Psychotherapy, 60*, 26–31.

Romanelli, A., Tishby, O., & Moran, G. S. (2017). Coming home to myself: A qualitative analysis of therapists' experience and interventions following training in the theater improvisation skills. *The Arts in Psychotherapy, 53*, 12–22.

Rooyackers, P. (1998). *Drama games for children.* Hunter House.

Rossing, J. P., & Hoffman-Longtin, K. (2018). Making sense of science: Applied improvisation for public communication of science, technology, and health. In T. R. Dudeck & C. McClure (Eds.), *Applied improvisation: Leading, collaborating, and creating beyond the theatre* (pp. 245–266). Methuen Drama.

Schochet, R., King, J., Levine, R., Clever, S., & Wright, S. (2013). "Thinking on my feet": An improvisation course to enhance students' confidence and responsiveness in medical interviewing. *Education for Primary Care, 24*, 119–124.

Schulenberg, S. E. (2003). Psychotherapy and movies: On using films in clinical practice. *Journal of Contemporary Psychotherapy, 33*(1), 35–48.

Schwitzer, A. M., Boyce, D., Cody, P., Holman, A., & Stein, J. (2005). Clinical supervision and professional development using clients from literature, popular fiction, and entertainment media. *Journal of Creativity in Mental Health, 1*(1), 57–80.

Shelley, M. (1818). Frankstein. United Kingdom: Lankington, Hughes, Harding, Mavor, & Jones.

Sheesley, A. P., Pfeffer, M., & Barish, B. (2016). Comedic improv therapy for the treatment of social anxiety disorder. *Journal of Creativity in Mental Health, 11*, 157–169.

Strohbehn, G. W., Haffe, T., & Houchens, N. (2020). Sketching an approach to clinical education; What we can learn from improvisation. *Journal of Graduate Medical Education, 12*(4), 388–391.

Watson, K. (2011). Serious play. Teaching medical skills with improvisational theater techniques. *Academic Medicine, 86*, 1260–1265.

Watson, K., & Fu, B. (2016). Medical improv: A novel approach to teaching communication and professionalism skills. *Annals of Internal Medicine, 165*, 591–592.

Chapter 15
The Last Stanza: Creativity, Ingenuity, and Wisdom

Erica V. Rozmid and Robert D. Friedberg

Keywords CBT · Youth · Evidence-based therapy · Superheroes · Improvisational theatre · Play therapy

15.1 The Last Stanza?

> Creativity is intelligence having fun.—Albert Einstein

We titled this final chapter, "The Last Stanza" because we wanted to highlight the recurring themes that pervaded the preceding chapters. Of course, we know we are taking some liberties with the strict literary definition of stanzas, but this book is all about stretching traditions, practices, and principles without breaking their theoretical boundaries. In this chapter, we add our final thoughts to the inventive chapters that formed the core of the book. Einstein's opening quote succinctly captures the material in this book–intelligent clinician scholars having fun while doing CBT with youth.

No matter how much we love our work as cognitive behavioral therapists, our job remains challenging. We make progress with one young patient or family and the next one takes a step or two backward. So we surf the sinusoidal curve riding the cresting and falling waves of emotional growth and recession with each case. We

E. V. Rozmid
Clarity CBT and DBT Center, Los Angeles, CA, USA
e-mail: erozmid@claritycbt.com

R. D. Friedberg (✉)
Palo Alto University, Palo Alto, CA, USA
e-mail: rfriedberg@paloaltou.edu

R. D. Friedberg, E. V. Rozmid (eds.), *Creative CBT with Youth*,
https://doi.org/10.1007/978-3-030-99669-7_15

look for new and improved ways to care for our patients. Ideally, this text helps clinicians in this journey.

Creativity and fun in CBT with youth are encouraged by contemporary scholars and clinicians alike (Friedberg & McClure, 2015; Friedberg et al., 2011; Kendall & Beidas, 2008; Kendall et al., 1992, 1998, 2008; Knell, 1993; Stallard, 2005). Indeed, "children feel freer to express themselves in a creative and fun environment (Friedberg et al., 2011, p. 59)." Anecdotally, clinicians also appreciate the flexibility and liberty to work with their patients in a fun and creative manner. What's better than teaching youth to challenge their negative thoughts while simultaneously incorporating their favorite movie characters in the process? The chapters in this book focused on boosting young patients' engagement in CBT.

Ingenuity is another central theme. After reading this book, it is apparent that we see CBT as a hero. Similar to the superheroes mentioned in several chapters, CBT is also flawed. Despite the voluminous data base, CBT does not help everyone. Reaching non-responders is a crucial task, and mobilizing our ingenuity is essential. Atul Gawande (2007) in his compelling book noted that ingenuity is an indispensable ingredient for success in medicine. However, ingenuity requires a bit of courage. As Gawande explained ingenuity "demands more than anything a willingness to recognize failure, to not paper over the cracks, and to change. It arises from deliberate, even obsessive reflection on failure and a constant searching for new solutions (p. 9)." Like many of you, I (RDF) was traditionally trained in various clinical psychology orthodoxies. Deviating from established doctrine comes with some anxieties. Nonetheless, we have to manage our fears of change and uncertainty to find new ways to care for young patients.

Pablo Picasso famously remarked, "Learn the rules like a pro, so you can break them like an artist." All the chapter authors are genuine "pros" who have metabolized the rules of CBT spectrum approaches with youth. We urge readers to do the same and learn the CBT orthodoxies. Then, like the chapter authors *and* Picasso you can become CBT artists making faithful adaptations and modifications to the traditional procedures.

15.2   Humor

Humor and laughter in therapy are explicitly addressed in Chaps. 2–4. This is a welcomed and perhaps overdue discussion. Clinical work undoubtedly is serious business, but it does not preclude light moments and laughter. Langer (1962) eloquently concluded "as speech is the culmination of a mental activity, laughter is the culmination of feeling-the crest of a wave of felt vitality (p. 248)." Moreover, humor and laughter are important ways children and adolescents can gain a sense of self-efficacy over stressors and negative emotional states (Martin, 2007). Laughter is also a way people connect with others (Bergson, 1962; Martin, 2007). Borcherdt (2002) claimed that humor enhanced transparency, emotional tolerance, and treatment engagement while also reducing guardedness as well as defensiveness. Finally, the competent use of humor in therapy communicates clinicians' humanness (Franzini, 2001).

As Chaps. 2–4 demonstrated, the artful application of humor in CBT requires considerable skillfulness. We agree with Meredith (1962) who noted, "...to touch and kindle the mind through laughter demands more than sprightliness, a more subtle delivery (p. 206)." A subtle and nuanced approach is imperative in treatment sessions. Castro-Blanco, Buerger and Miller as well as Stephanou, and colleagues exemplified this sophisticated clinical manner.

15.3 Play

And this I believe, that the free, exploring mind of the individual human is the most valuable thing in the world.—John Steinbeck, East of Eden

Play is often a neglected part of CBT with youth. Chapters 5–8 rectify this oversight and illustrate the free exploring minds Steinbeck valued in his writing. Integrating stories, games, costumes, drawing, music, and theatre exercises into the psychotherapeutic process is congenial with fundamental CBT (Friedberg & McClure, 2015; Knell, 1993; Peterman et al., 2014). "Play is the medium by which inaccurate internal dialogues are elicited and more adaptive coping methods are taught (Friedberg & McClure, 2015, p. 175)." Davis et al. (2019) cogently concluded that play in CBT serves three important functions. First, it enhances the relationship between young patients and their providers. Second, play facilitates identification of children's thoughts and images. Finally, play enables more productive problem-solving, perspective-taking, and constructive cognitions.

Learning about CBT play therapy from the master, Dr. Susan Knell, provided a deep dive into her innovative clinical methods. Specific applications of play with evidence-based CBT practices (Park and Kim) and directed to aggressive youth (Feindler and Schira) as well as to patients diagnosed with OCD (Herren and colleagues) demonstrated wide suitability. Ingenuity, creativity, and clinical savvy abounded in these chapters.

15.4 Superheroes and Popular Culture Characters

Loverd et al. (2018) wrote

> Walk into any large scale research laboratory and take a stroll through the offices. If you are a betting person, you can comfortably put your retirement portfolio down on the wager that there will be in among half marathon ribbons, coffee cups with pithy statements about Mondays and photos of loved ones, you will find an action figure of Spock, Yoda, Neo, Wonder Woman, Marvin the Martian, or a Cylon. These are the characters that influenced and inspired our current generation of scientists (p. 1310).

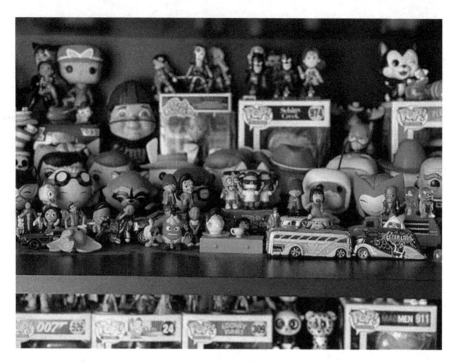

Fig. 15.1 Character shelf

I (RDF) confess I display my figures in my office (Please see Fig. 15.1). They remain a source of inspiration for me and a conversation topic for my young patients. For instance, while I was working at Penn State University Milton Hershey Medical Center, a 10 year old came into my office, surveyed my character shelf, and asked, "So are you a collector too?" Almost 30 years ago, Kendall et al. (1992) endorsed integrating superheroes in CBT with youth. Presently, Chaps. 9–11 teach proper contemporary practices for using superheroes in therapy with youth These contributions made us think, "What is it about superheroes that speak to children, adolescents, and adults?"

Loeb and Morris (2005) explained, "But it's very reasonable to suggest that the superheroes have been around for so long and have continued to be so popular, in part, because they speak to our nature, as well as to both our aspirations and fears (p. 16)." Nearly all superheroes own a tragic origin story. Life comes hard for them. Resilience in the face of adversity makes these characters relatable and suitable coping models for youth.

Persistence is another common characteristic. Despite hardships and barriers, they do not give up! Loeb and Morris (2005) remarked, "the superhero shows us nothing worth doing is easy (p. 17)." And isn't this a lesson for everyone? In particular, we work to help our patients persist when they become stuck, inert, or even immobilized by their stressors.

Superheroes are also flawed beings. Superman has his kryptonite, Batman has a dark side, and Wonder Woman is mortal. In short, these characters are like us, they have limitations. The late Chadwick Boseman who played King T'Challa in *Black Panther* said in an interview, "The thing I love about Marvel in general is that they deal with people. They deal with the human being first. Who is inside the suit? Who is the person that obtained this power or ability?"

So in response to the question about what's so special about superheroes? The answer is they are essentially human. Like all of us, they aspire, worry, strive, fail, and persevere. In short, they make for excellent coping models. Superheroes seem to communicate that whether you wear a cape or not, individuals are faced with confronting stressors. The chapters written by Pimental and DeLapp (Chap. 9), Nabors and Sanyaolu (Chap. 10), Letamendi (Chap. 11), and Duan and colleagues (Chap. 12) all told this story about coping. Their inventive and resourceful use of characters ideally catalyzed your desire to use these characters in your own work with children and adolescents.

15.5 Improv in CBT Practice and Training

You can't use up creativity, the more you use, the more you have.—Maya Angelou

Any fan of Robin Williams, *Who's line is it anyway?* and *Saturday Night Live* has heard about improv. But what place does improv theatre exercises have in CBT? Chapters 13 (Treadwel and Dartnell) and 14 (Friedberg and Rozmid) aimed to answer this question.

Ryan Stiles, improviser extraordinaire, said, "I'm convinced that all you have to do is listen to what people are saying to you and then just add more information to what they have just said. That's all there is to improv but it's the hardest thing to do." Isn't this what we try to do in CBT and when we train others in the model? Absorbing young patients' subjective experiences and then adding new perspectives through Socratic dialogues and behavioral experiments represent our role in the therapeutic partnership. Mindfully attending to supervisees' accounts of their work and supplementing their practice with our constructive ideas characterizes training. Improv exercises help us *really l*isten.

Improv and good CBT take place in the NOW. They are both phenomenological approaches. Perhaps, this is what makes improv, psychodrama, and CBT so congenial with each other. Writing about improv in training medical students, Mehta and colleagues (2021) concluded, "Listening, observing, and responding in the moment deepen the human capacity to be present (p. 265)." Therapeutic presence is essential to good CBT.

Finally, as mentioned in the chapters, improv theatre exercises build cognitive flexibility. Learning to think quickly in multiple directions is critical in our work with young patients. Being cognitively nimble when managing difficult risk situations, stuck points in therapy, and other challenging circumstances enables us to maintain therapeutic momentum.

15.6 Just Do It

If you want to learn to swim you have to throw yourself in the water.—Bruce Lee

What do the Nike Slogan and Bruce Lee have in common? A willingness for change. The expert authors in this book have demonstrated a keen curiosity for utilizing the therapeutic interventions that are the most effective and enhancing them even further. Throwing ourselves into the work with our young patients require us to "just do it."

I (EVR) remember practicing to be irreverent with my teenager patient who was suicidal. I kept contemplating how I could utilize this strategy for change from DBT without coming across like a rude therapist. It was scary. I would have rather remained comfortable by addressing their suicidality with seriousness. And then I did it! I made the irreverent comment "you seem so certain about what death entails and that it will solve your problems. But there's no research your problems die with you." And my patient laughed. A laugh that caught them off course, instantly bonded us, and they decided to engage with me further.

It's not just those who are beginning to learn a new mode of therapy that will be forced with throwing ourselves into the moment. With each patient, we are challenged in a novel and different way. For example, I (EVR) had a TikTok loving 8-year-old who had social anxiety. While the treatment for social anxiety with her was straightforward, TikTok was not! Throwing myself into therapy meant learning TikTok dances so that I could join my patient during her in-session exposures. And if you can remember the famous lines of Dr. Seuss "you'll never be bored when you try something new. There's really no limit to what you can do!"

We hope that after reading this book that you are motivated and excited to "just do it"-to incorporate fun, humor, superheroes, and improv into your youth psychotherapy sessions.

15.7 Conclusion

By three methods, we may learn wisdom. First, by reflection, which is noblest; Second, by imitation which is the easiest, and third, by experience, which is the bitterest.
Confucius

Just as the wise Confucius proposed over 2000 years ago, reflection-based learning is the noblest. Beginning clinicians and late-career clinicians, alike, engage in the humbling act of contemplation. Psychological science improves, and new behavioral theories emerge over time. We must always be open to change, reflect when our patients are not improving and continue to improve the methods with which we utilize to improve the lives of the young patients we serve. As I (EVR) was trained by Dr. Robert Friedberg, I clearly remember him telling our lab group "when you don't know where to go in session, do not go rogue!" We can continue to rely on the behavioral principles and theories that exist today, flexibly apply our interventions, and be open to new science and information.

Each chapter of this book is done by wise authors. They are well-trained, reflective, and clinically experienced. These insightful works are clear-headed, clever, and learned. We hope you have mined some golden nuggets for your work with young patients that add to your clinical wisdom. A.A. Milne from Winnie the Pooh wrote, "It is more fun to talk with someone who doesn't use long, difficult words but rather short, easy words like, 'What about lunch?'." The musings of Pooh Bear is quite sound. Adapting clinical expertise from years of graduate school, training, research, and clinical work poses a challenge when working with youth who rely on concrete metaphors. Children and adolescents are naturally playful, do not always want to be in therapy, and are struggling immensely. Children may come to session without ever hearing the word "clinician" or "therapist" before. What a fun task to translate the science and our expertise into something that anyone, of any age or developmental level understands.

We conclude with fitting wisdom from *Alice in Wonderland* by Lewis Carroll who wrote, "Begin at the beginning, the King said very gravely, and go on till you come to the end, and then stop!"

References

Bergson, H. (1962). Laughter. In M. Felheim (Ed.), *Comedy: plays, theory, and criticism* (pp. 205–214). Harcourt, Brace, & World.

Borcherdt, B. (2002). Humor and its contributions to mental health. *Journal of Rational-Emotive and Cognitive Behavioral Therapy, 20,* 247–257.

Davis, J. P., Palitz, S. A., Knepley, M. J., & Kendall, P. C. (2019). Cognitive behavioral therapy with youth. In K. S. Dobson & D. J. A. Dozois (Eds.), *Handbook of cognitive-behavioral therapies* (4th ed., pp. 349–382). Springer.

Franzini, L. R. (2001). Humor in therapy: The case for training therapist and its uses and risks. *Journal of General Psychology, 128,* 170–193.

Friedberg, R. D., Gorman, A. A., Hollar-Wilt, L., Buickians, A., & Murray, M. (2011). *Cognitive behavioral therapy for the busy child psychiatrist and other mental health professionals.* Routledge.

Friedberg, R. D., & McClure, J. M. (2015). *Clinical practice with children and adolescents: The nuts and bolts* (2nd ed.) Guilford.

Gawande, A. (2007). Better. Henry Holt.

Kendall, P. C., & Beidas, R. S. (2008). Smoothing the trail for dissemination of evidence-based practices for youth: Flexibility within fidelity. *Professional Psychology: Research and Practice, 38,* 13–20.

Kendall, P. C., Chansky, T. E., Kane, M. T., Kim, R. S., Kortlander, E., & Ronan, K. R. (1992). *Anxiety disorders in youth: Cognitive-behavioral interventions.* Allyn & Bacon.

Kendall, P. C., Chu, B., Gifford, A., Hayes, C., & Nauta, M. (1998). Breathing life into a manual. *Cognitive and Behavioral Practice, 5*, 177–198.

Kendall, P. C., Gosch, E., Furr, J., & Sood, E. (2008). Flexibility within fidelity. *Journal of the American Academy of Child and Adolescent Psychiatry, 47*, 987–993.

Knell, S. M. (1993). *Cognitive behavior play therapy*. Jason Aronson.

Langer, S. (1962). The great dramatic forms. In M. Felheim (Ed.), *Comedy: Plays, theory, and criticism* (pp. 241–253). Harcourt, Brace, & World.

Loeb, J., & Morris, T. (2005). Heroes and superheroes. In T. V. Morris & M. Morris (Eds.), *Superheroes and philosophy: Truth, justice, and the socratic way* (pp. 11–20). Open Court.

Loverd, R., ElShafie, S. J., Merchant, A., & Sachi Gerbin, C. (2018). The story of science and entertainment exchange, a program of the National Academy of Sciences. *Integrative and Comparative Biology, 58*, 1304–1311.

Martin, R. A. (2007). *The psychology of humor: An integrative approach*. Academic.

Meredith, G. (1962). Comedy and uses of the comic spirit. In M. Felheim (Ed.), *Comedy: Plays, theory, and criticism* (pp. 205–214). Harcourt, Brace, & World.

Peterman, J. S., Settipani, C. A., & Kendall, P. C. (2014). Effectively engaging and collaborating with children and adolescents in cognitive behavioral therapy sessions. In E. S. Sburlati, H. J. Lyneham, C. A. Schniering, & R. M. Rapee (Eds.), *Evidence-based CBT for anxiety and depression in children and adolescents* (pp. 128–140). Wiley-Blackwell.

Stallard, P. (2005). Cognitive behavior therapy for pre-pubertal children. In P. Graham (Ed.), *Cognitive behaviour therapy for children and families* (2nd ed., pp. 121–135). Cambridge University Press.

Index

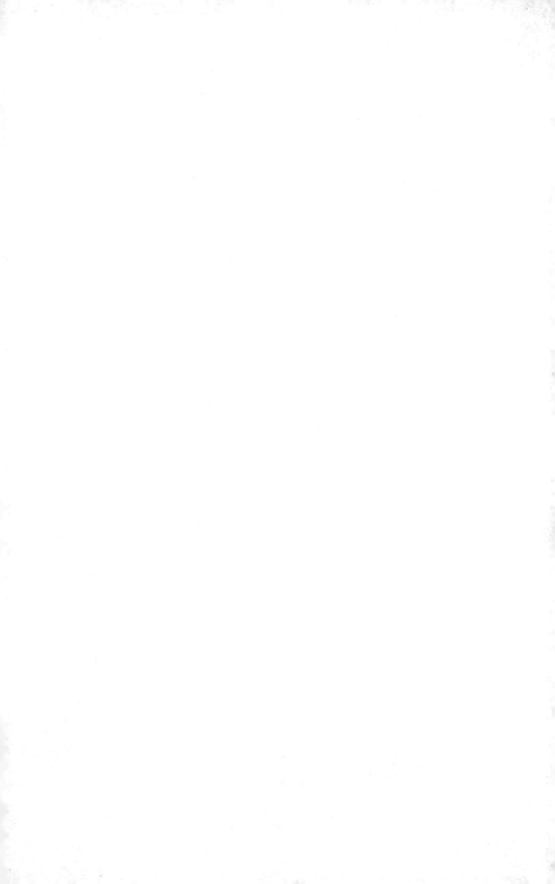

9 783030 996680